Handbook of Obstetrics
and Gynaecology

Handbook of Obstetrics and Gynaecology

Fourth edition

Edited by

Leo R. Leader
Senior Lecturer

Michael J. Bennett
Professor and Head

and

Felix Wong
Professor

School of Obstetrics and Gynaecology
UNSW, Sydney

CHAPMAN & HALL MEDICAL

London · Glasgow · Weinheim · New York · Tokyo · Melbourne · Madras

Published by Chapman & Hall, 2-6 Boundary Row, London SE1 8HN, UK

Chapman & Hall, 2-6 Boundary Row, London SE1 8HN, UK

Blackie Academic & Professional, Wester Cleddens Road, Bishopbriggs, Glasgow G64 2NZ, UK

Chapman & Hall GmbH, Pappelallee 3, 69469 Weinheim, Germany

Chapman & Hall USA., 115 Fifth Avenue, New York, NY 10003, USA

Chapman & Hall Japan, ITP-Japan, Kyowa Building, 3F, 2-2-1 Hirakawacho, Chiyoda-ku, Tokyo 102, Japan

Chapman & Hall Australia, 102 Dodds Street, South Melbourne, Victoria 3205, Australia

Chapman & Hall India, R. Seshadri, 32 Second Main Road, CIT East, Madras 600 035, India

First edition 1979
Second edition 1985
Third edition 1989
Reprinted 1990
Fourth edition 1996

Typeset in 10/12 Palatino by Acorn Bookwork, Salisbury, Wilts
Printed in Great Britain by St Edmundsbury Press, Bury St Edmunds, Suffolk

ISBN 0 412 58530 8

A Catalogue record for this book is available from the British Library

Library of Congress Catalog Card Number. 95-74635

∞ Printed on permanent acid-free text paper, manufactured in accordance with ANSI/NISO Z39.48-1992 and ANSI/NISO Z39.48-1984 (Permanence of Paper).

Contents

Contributors

Michael J. Bennett, MB, ChB MD (UCT), FCOG(SA), FRCOG, FRACOG, DDU
Professor and Head, School of Obstetrics and Gynaecology UNSW, Sydney, Australia

John A. Eden, MD, FRACOG, MRCOG, CREI
Senior Lecturer, School of Obstetrics and Gynaecology UNSW, Sydney, Australia

Stephen P. Gatt, LRCP, MRCS, MD, DCH, FFARCS, FFA Int Cr, FANZCA, FFICANZCA
Senior Lecturer, Discipline of Anaesthesia UNSW, Sydney, Australia

Jagdish Gupta, MB BS MD, DCH, MRCP, MRACP
Associate Professor, School of Paediatrics UNSW, Sydney, Australia

Graeme J. Hughes, MB BS, MRCOG, FRACOG
Senior Lecturer, School of Obstetrics and Gynaecology UNSW, Sydney, Australia

Leo P. Lacy, MB, BS, Dip Obst, DA, FAZCA
Staff Anaesthetist, Royal Hospital for Women, Sydney, Australia

Leo R. Leader, MD, FRACOG, FRCOG, FCOG (SA), DA (RCS London)
Senior Lecturer, School of Obstetrics and Gynaecology UNSW, Sydney, Australia

Rosie McInnes, MB BS, RACGP
Lecturer, School of Obstetrics and Gynaecology UNSW, Sydney, Australia

Kate H. Moore, MB BS, MRCOG, FRACOG, CU
Senior Lecturer, School of Obstetrics and Gynaecology UNSW, Sydney, Australia

Felix Wong, MB BS, M Med (Sing) MD, FRCS (Edin), FHKCOG (HK), FRCS (Glas), FRACOG

Professor, School of Obstetrics and Gynaecology UNSW, Sydney, Australia

Barry G. Wren, MD, MB BS, MHPed, FRACOG, FRCOG
Director, Centre for the Management of the Menopause, Royal Hospital for Women, Sydney, Australia

Preface

The *Handbook of Obstetrics and Gynaecology* was initially written in 1974 to assist local students to understand the core of knowledge required for the curriculum at the University of New South Wales in Sydney, Australia. The *Handbook* was designed to contain only information which was thought to be essential for the undergraduate course and it was published with a specific size in mind – that it would slip easily into a ward coat pocket.

Since then there have been three further publications of this book and it is widely used by students in many parts of the English-speaking world. The original concepts have been maintained but new ideas and advancing technology have required a continual need for updating.

In this, the fourth edition of the *Handbook* the original editorial team of Dr Barry Wren, who has edited all previous versions, and Dr Rogerio Lobo have retired, and a new team at the University of New South Wales has taken over.

Some new chapters have been added, while the rest have either been revised, or completely rewritten. Many of the diagrams have been replaced and improved. The editors acknowledge the contributions made by all the previous authors in previous editions.

We hope that this new edition of the *Handbook of Obstetrics and Gynaecology* will remain as popular as the earlier versions. In spite of the extensive revisions made, it should still be regarded as a guide for undergraduates and not as a major reference manual. The text remains logical, easy to understand and has simple diagrams covering all common obstetric and gynaecological conditions, making it highly suitable for medical and nursing students, as well as interns. We hope that those who use this book will find it of practical value both before and after graduation.

Leo R. Leader
Michael J. Bennett
Felix Wong
1995

1

History-taking and physical examination

1.1 GENERAL INSTRUCTIONAL OBJECTIVE

The students are expected to develop competence in taking a history and performing a physical examination so that obstetric or gynaecological abnormalities can be recognized and appropriate management initiated.

1.2 SPECIFIC BEHAVIOURAL OBJECTIVES

1. Elicit a relevant history from a patient with an obstetric or gynaecological problem.
2. Examine the pelvis and abdomen of a patient with an obstetrical or gynaecological problem.
3. Discuss the history, physical findings and possible diagnosis of a patient with obstetric and gynaecological problems.
4. Demonstrate care, consideration, tact and kindness when taking a history, examining or managing a patient who presents with an obstetric or gynaecological problem.

1.3 REASONS FOR LEARNING TO TAKE A RELEVANT HISTORY AND PERFORMING A SPECIFIC OBSTETRIC AND GYNAECOLOGICAL EXAMINATION

Most medical students are taught to take a good general history and to perform an adequate physical examination, but at first they tend to ask too many questions, to ask far too many irrelevant time-and-space-filling questions, or to fail to obtain sufficient information on an important symptom. It is, however, necessary to focus on only the more relevant facts and to ask for some very specific information. Without knowledge regarding the relevance of material or the knowledge of the pathophysiology of the disease, it becomes very difficult for students to sort out the important from the unimportant facts that a patient may offer to a doctor. Specific and leading questions may never be asked unless the student knows that a certain symptom may be the key to opening the diagnosis. Symptoms that the patient may regard as irrelevant may hold the answer to the diagnosis. It is important that the student is aware not only of some of these specialised symptoms, but also how to obtain a history from a female patient.

There is often a reluctance on the part of the patient to state what actually the problem is. Female patients may feel embarrassed to talk to strangers about vaginal discharge, sexual problems or other personal gynaecological symptoms. Students should be aware of the problem and show sympathy. Questions should be open-ended, beginning with such queries as 'How did you feel?', 'What happened then?', 'Tell me about it'. Students should avoid the use of any questions implying a judgment such as 'Why did you do that?'. The justification necessary to answer such questions may make the patient defensive, tense and anxious, so that a correct easily expressed history is not obtained.

If possible, students should avoid writing answers immediately to all questions. It is more natural and comforting to a patient for the doctor to appear to be having a chat or pleasant talk than to be conducting a staccato interview. Facts such as age, parity and marital state should be obtained and recorded early – then the doctor must relax and let the patient tell her story. It is important only to interrupt in order to clarify a certain point. When she has finished, the doctor will have a better idea of what is wrong and can then ask the specific, probing and detailed questions that allow a diagnosis to be made.

Without the ability to take a good history and to perform an adequate examination, no medical practitioner can assist women who attend complaining of obstetric or gynaecological problems.

The specific questions that it may be necessary to ask include the following:

<h2 style="text-align:center">1.4 OBSTETRIC HISTORY</h2>

1. Name and address
2. It is best to obtain the actual date of birth. People age from year to year but the birth date remains the same.
3. Gravidity and parity. Gravidity refers to the number of times a woman has conceived, while parity refers to the number of pregnancies, of more than 20 weeks of amenorrhoea, she has delivered. Parity is noted, for example, as P2 + 3, meaning the woman has delivered two babies and also had three pregnancies that have terminated before 20 weeks of amenorrhoea.
4. Last normal menstrual period (LNMP). This should be recorded from the first day of the last normal period. Ask about its duration, the volume of flow, any associated pain or other symptoms. Did it appear normal or was it merely 'spotting'? If the latter was the case then the second-last menstrual period should also be recorded, and, if that was also abnormal, keep going back until the last normal menstrual period can be ascertained. Abnormalities of 'menstrual flow' are frequently found in such conditions as dysfunctional uterine haemorrhage, fibromyomata, threatened abortion, implantation bleed and ectopic pregnancy.
5. Menstrual cycle. The normal cycle varies from 3 to 5 days every 21–35 days. It may become grossly irregular in a variety of states, particularly dysfunctional uterine haemorrhage and certain infertility problems. A regular pattern generally suggests a normal hypothalamic–pituitary–ovarian function.
6. Period of amenorrhoea should be calculated accurately by counting from the first day of the last normal period. The length of time should *always* be recorded accurately in weeks and days (a month is *not* a scientific measure of time!).
7. Expected date of confinement (EDC). A rough guide for doctor and patient is achieved by the knowledge that most infants will deliver 280 (± 14) days after the first day of the last normal period. An easy ready reckoner is achieved by adding 9 months and 7 days to the date of the LNMP to determine the EDC.

e.g. If LNMP was 8 April 1993,

then add 7 days and 9 months	Days	Months	Year
	8	4	1993
	7	9	
and the EDC is approximately	15	1	1994

8. Nationality may be important, as Mediterranean peoples have a higher incidence of thalassaemia, tuberculosis and other locally acquired diseases.
9. Does the patient smoke, drink or take drugs? All of these may have a deleterious effect on a pregnancy and the medical officer should warn the patient.
10. Obstetric record

Pregnancy No.	Year	Complications of pregnancy	Length of labour	Type of delivery	Weight	Sex	A SB NND

A, alive; SB, still birth; NND, neonatal death.

11. Medical history. Some medical diseases are particularly relevant to pregnancy and care must be taken to enquire about these, such as heart disease, rheumatic fever, hypertension, tuberculosis, asthma, bronchitis, urinary tract infection or 'fits'.
12. Surgical history. Take particular care to record such previous operations as dilatation and curettage, abdominal operations or accidents, as well as blood transfusions.
13. Family history. Enquire about illness in close relatives, such as tuberculosis, diabetes, hypertension, multiple pregnancy or congenital abnormalities.
14. Social history. Enquire about marital status, financial support, smoking and drinking habits, work or occupation, and knowledge regarding social benefits, reproductive education, baby care, contraception, sexual attitudes and community child-care centres.
15. Gynaecological history regarding her menstrual life, contraception and sexual intercourse. Difficulty, pain or ignorance

in any areas would suggest that either counselling or further investigation may be necessary.

1.5 HISTORY OF THE PRESENT PREGNANCY

1. Ask about the common symptoms of pregnancy, such as:
   (a) Nausea or vomiting
   (b) Breast tenderness or swelling
   (c) Frequency of micturition
   (d) Fainting
   (e) Vaginal discharge
2. Determine when fetal movements are first felt. In primigravida women they are usually first detected at about 18–20 weeks of amenorrhoea. In multigravida, because of prior experience, they are usually first detected at about 16–18 weeks. Movements are usually felt as 'bubbles' or like a butterfly.
3. Abnormal symptoms may be pain, vaginal bleeding and an abnormal discharge. Specific questions should be asked, and further inquiries made if the response is affirmative.
4. If there is any response that indicates the presence of an abnormality, it is wise to investigate all the associated factors by careful inquiry or by physical examination.

1.6 OBSTETRIC EXAMINATION

General impression

Note anything obvious such as height, weight, accent, configuration and gait.

General examination

1. Blood pressure, pulse, hands, nails.
2. Feet, varicose veins, oedema.
3. Mouth, tongue and teeth.
4. Neck, thyroid.
5. Thorax and breasts (observe the nipples, areola, Montgomery tubercles, veins and breast secretions).
6. Listen to heart and lungs for abnormal sounds.

Abdominal examination

1. Inspect the abdomen for the presence of striae, scars or bruises.
2. Palpate for the liver, spleen, kidneys and uterus.

Uterine palpation

The uterus grows from a small organ, 8 cm long, in the pelvis to a large mass, 30–35 cm long, which reaches to the subcostal margins by the 36th week of a normal pregnancy. The regular palpation and observation of changes in parameters of the growing uterus allow an attendant to determine normal and abnormal growth patterns, and to modify the antenatal care as necessary. The parameters that should be closely examined as often as necessary and recorded on a chart are as follows:

1. **Fundal height** (Fig. 1.1). Clinically the fundal height is recorded using a tape measure to record the distance between the symphysis pubis and the uterine fundus. This is just palpable above the symphysis pubis by the 12th week of pregnancy, reaches approximately to the umbilicus by the 24th week, and finally ceases to ascend at about the 36th week. When the uterine fundus is about halfway from

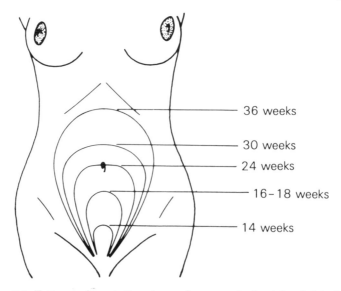

Figure 1.1 Estimated gestational age from equivalent fundal heights.

the symphysis pubis to the umbilicus, the gestational age is about 16 weeks (soon after, the fetal movements may be first felt). From the umbilicus to the subcostal margins, the uterine fundus grows at a rate equivalent to one finger's breadth (2 cm) every 2 weeks. (Note that the umbilicus becomes flattened after 24 weeks due to the intra-abdominal distension.) The fundus of the uterus generally remains at about the level of the xiphisternum (or the subcostal margins) from the 36th week until the time of delivery (38–42 weeks), unless the head actually engages in the pelvis – in which case, as the head and body descend, so will the fundus appear to decrease in height (to the 32 or 34 weeks' fundal height). This phenomenon is known as lightening.

2. **Fetal lie** (Fig. 1.2). The fetal lie is the relationship of the long axis of the fetus to the long axis of the mother. The fetal axis can generally be detected easily by finding the two ends (poles) of the fetus. The head is usually harder and rounder than the large, diffuse, soft bottom of the fetus. A line drawn between these two poles is the fetal axis. To confirm the lie, the fetal back can also be palpated parallel to the axis. An oblique or transverse lie usually indicates some abnormality.

3. **Fetal presentation**. Over 95% of all babies present by the fetal head and less than 5% are found to have a breech,

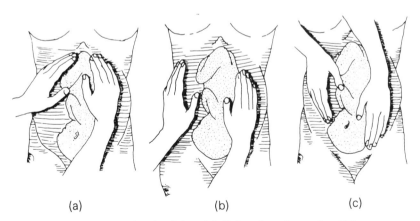

(a)   (b)   (c)

Figure 1.2 Palpating the fetal lie. (a) Palpating the soft, diffuse, upper pole of the fetal breech; (b) Palpating the broad, firm back of the fetus. Note that there is little resistance to the convex front of the fetus; (c) Palpating the firm, round, mobile head of the fetus.

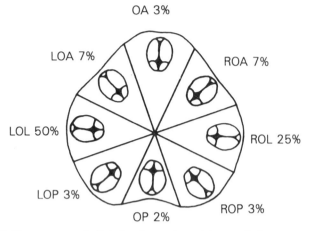

Figure 1.3 Frequency of distribution of positions of the occiput at the onset of labour.

shoulder or other form of presentation. The head is generally easily palpated lying in the lower segment as a firm, round, mobile mass, but if doubt exists an ultrasound examination should be taken after the 34th week to confirm the presence of breech or other abnormal presentation.

4. **Fetal position**. This is the relationship of the denominator of the presenting part of the fetus to the mother's pelvis. When the head is presenting with one of the usual degrees of flexion, then the occiput is the denominator. The position is stated as being occipito-anterior (OA), occipito-lateral (OL) or occipito-posterior (OP) in relationship to the maternal pelvic brim. The common positions before the onset of labour are: left occipito-lateral (LOL), 50%: and right occipito-lateral (ROL), 25% (Fig. 1.3). However, at the end of labour, 60% of positions are found to be left occipito-anterior (LOA) and 30% are right occipito-anterior (ROA), indicating that internal rotation to an anterior position is the most common outcome during labour. Other positions may be related to the mentum (face) and sacrum (breech) presentations.

5. **Fetal attitude**. The fetal head is normally universally flexed so that the fetal head presents the smallest diameters (9.5 cm) to the maternal pelvic brim. However, when the fetus is in the occipito-posterior position, its back is against the maternal back and the maternal lumbar lordosis causes

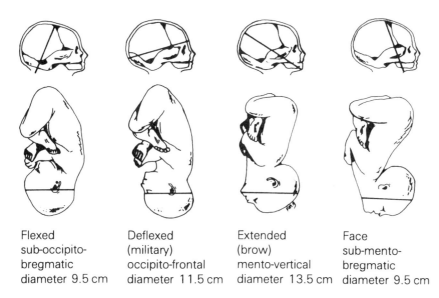

| Flexed
sub-occipito-
bregmatic
diameter 9.5 cm | Deflexed
(military)
occipito-frontal
diameter 11.5 cm | Extended
(brow)
mento-vertical
diameter 13.5 cm | Face
sub-mento-
bregmatic
diameter 9.5 cm |

Figure 1.4 Fetal attitude.

the fetus to present with a degree of extension of the back, neck and head (the 'military' attitude). This extension means that a larger diameter – occipito-frontal (11.5 cm) or mento-vertical (13.5 cm brow presentation) – presents at the maternal pelvic brim (Fig. 1.4).

6. **Fetal engagement** (see Fig. 6.9). This is the term used when the largest diameter of the presenting part has passed through the pelvic brim. With a well-flexed fetal head, the sub-occipito-bregmatic diameter and the biparietal diameter are both about 9.5 cm and will easily pass through a pelvis that has dimensions of average size. However, a fetal head that is extended due to an occipito-lateral or occipito-posterior position may not engage until strong labour contractions cause flexion and then descent of the head. Engagement may be detected either by abdominal palpation or by vaginal examination.

7. **Amniotic fluid volume**. The uterus is balloted to assess the volume of amniotic fluid. Oligohydramnios (decreased volume) is associated with renal agenesis (Potter's syndrome) and may be one of the earliest signs of intrauterine growth retardation (IUGR). Polyhydramnios (increased volume) is associated with diabetes, congenital abnormal-

ities of the central nervous system and gastrointestinal tract.

8. **Uterine irritability**. The uterus is usually relaxed through-out pregnancy until 32 weeks of gestation when the mother starts to experience painless contractions known as Braxton–Hicks contractions. These lead to the formation of the lower uterine segment. Inappropriate uterine activity may indicate the patient is at risk of preterm labour or may be one of the earliest signs of IUGR.

9. **Fetal movements**. Mothers are asked whether their fetuses are moving normally. Asking about maternal perception of fetal activity is an important part of the antenatal examination.

10. **Fetal heart rate**. This is usually between 110 and 160 per minute and is detected over the portion of the fetal chest that lies closest to the uterine wall.

Determining the fetal position

1. First determine the presentation. If the head presents, the denominator will almost always be the occiput.

2. The occiput always lies on the same side of the fetal body as the back, so palpate for the back. Palpate across the abdomen at the level of the umbilicus. The back is detected as a broad band of resistance on one side. Palpate along the back to the breech and then down to the shoulder and the head. The portion of the fetal head that is first palpated after the fetal back is the occiput.

3. Having determined the side on which the occiput lies, it is relatively easy to determine whether the occiput is anterior, lateral or posterior. The fetal head is an oval shape, with the occiput at one end and the synciput at the other. A line drawn through the occiput and synciput passes along the sagittal suture, and a line drawn at right-angles to the sagittal suture will pass through the tips of both fetal shoulders (Fig. 1.5). Knowing this simple geometry allows one to palpate not only the back but the shoulder, occiput and the synciput, and so by spatial imagery to determine the fetal position. Final confirmation can be obtained at a vaginal examination to feel the sagittal suture, the anterior and posterior fontanelles or even the fetal ear if the head is well down in the pelvis.

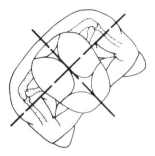

Figure 1.5 Showing that a line drawn through the two shoulders will be at right-angles to a line drawn through the sagittal suture. This piece of geometry is helpful when determining the position of the fetus during labour.

Abdominal palpation to determine fetal lie, presentation, position and engagement

It is essential in obstetrics that from the 30th week of pregnancy, medical practitioners can accurately palpate the lie, presentation, position and engagement of a fetus. It is by mastering these skills that they can diagnose such conditions as breech, transverse lie, twins, disproportion, occipito-posterior position, polyhydramnios and may suspect other conditions such as placenta praevia, hydrocephalus or failure of fetal growth.

Medical practitioners who do not have these skills in palpation will be seriously handicapped in management of normal pregnancy and will fail to diagnose problems that might be present. Students who fail to master the steps and techniques of fetal palpation will be unable to assist in antenatal clinics or in the labour ward.

Steps in palpation of uterus at more than 30 weeks

1. Ensure that the patient is lying comfortably in a bed (or on an examination couch), on her back and with her abdominal muscles completely relaxed.
2. Expose the whole abdomen from the symphysis pubis to the xiphisternum. Make sure that underclothes are pulled below the level of the hips and symphysis.
3. Observe the configuration of the uterus. It is generally oval

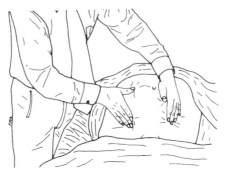

Figure 1.6 Demonstrating that to palpate an abdomen satisfactorily, the position of the body must allow the flat of the hands to press against the fetus.

in shape with the long axis parallel to the long axis of the mother. Abnormal shapes to the uterus may be due to transverse lie, subseptate uterus, multiple pregnancy, poly-hydramnios or disproportion.

4. Palpate the uterine outline. Stand in a position so that you face either the head or the feet of your patient – in this way you can place a hand easily on either side of the uterus without undue effort. Use the flat of the hand and fingers when palpating, as it causes less discomfort than when one or two fingers are pressed into the abdominal wall (Fig. 1.6). Run your hands gently over the uterus to feel its configuration. This gentle palpation helps in two ways. First, you can determine the general outline of the uterus and can confirm that it is indeed of an oval (or an uneven) shape; secondly, by being gentle with your initial palpation you can assist in relaxing the patient for the next steps in palpation.

5. Now determine the lie of the fetus. Using both hands on either side of the uterus and approximately at the same level, palpate the fetus as it lies within the uterus. Usually it will be lying longitudinally; it is then easy to feel the fetal back as a broad, firm and resistant mass on one side. Having found the back, move both hands up and down (on either side of the uterus), following the back to the two ends (poles) of the fetus. Determine very carefully the size and consistency of the two poles. A line drawn between the midpoint of each pole is the axis of the fetus. To obtain

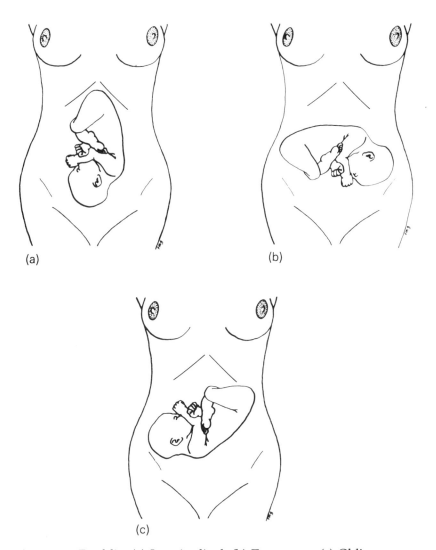

Figure 1.7 Fetal lie. (a) Longitudinal; (b) Transverse; (c) Oblique.

the lie, relate the axis of the fetus to the axis of the uterus. An oblique lie will have the lower pole lying in one iliac fossa, while a transverse lie will have both poles lying in the flanks (Fig. 1.7).

6. The presentation is usually the head, which is felt as a firm, round mass. A breech is usually soft, diffuse and often feels larger than the head. Again, palpation should be with both hands working opposite each other on either side of

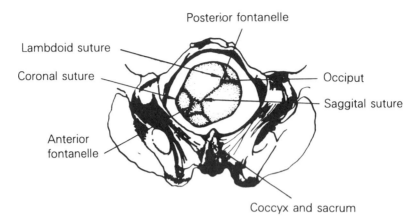

Posterior fontanelle

Lambdoid suture

Coronal suture

Occiput

Saggital suture

Anterior
fontanelle

Coccyx and sacrum

Figure 1.8 Fetal skull within the bony pelvis. The skull sutures can be easily palpated to determine the fetal position. In this case it is left occipito-anterior.

the uterus. Be gentle but firm with all palpation and avoid 'playing the piano' when palpating. Irregular movement in palpation is more likely to produce a uterine contraction or cause pain so that further palpation is difficult.

7. Finding the position can be difficult, but remember that the occiput and the sacrum both lie on the same side as the fetal back. If you can palpate the firm, resistant back at the level of the umbilicus and can follow this down to the lower pole, then the denominator is easily detected. As the head usually presents, the first part of the head that is palpated after moving off the back must be the occiput (Fig. 1.8). Mostly the fetus will be in the occipito-lateral position, and this can be confirmed by pressing down on the fetal occiput and the synciput to ascertain that both lie approximately equidistant from the skin over the anterior abdominal wall.

8. It is sometimes difficult to be sure whether a head is engaged in the pelvis, but it is easy to decide when it is high above the brim. If your fingers can be made to pass around in front of the head about the symphysis pubis, then it is clearly not engaged. When you cannot get your fingers in front of the head then the head is obviously fitting into the brim. The point of decision between engagement and non-engagement in these cases is a fine one, and

probably not important unless you are considering applying forceps prior to delivery. In this case, a vaginal examination must become the final arbiter.

Vaginal examination in labour (see Chapter 5, Section 5.8)

Vulva: This is inspected for the presence of Herpes simplex lesions, vulval warts and vulval varicosities. A digital vaginal examination is usually performed to determine:

1. The cervical dilatation and effacement and application to the presenting part.
2. The descent of the fetal head and its position in the pelvis.
3. The presence of caput succedaneum or of fetal skull moulding.
4. The shape of the maternal bony pelvis.
5. Whether a prolapsed cord is present following rupture of membranes.

Never perform a digital vaginal examination in the presence of an antepartum haemorrhage unless placenta praevia has been excluded by an urgent ultrasound examination or full preparations should be made for an urgent delivery in case of placenta praevia may be present.

Technique

1. Using sterile gloves, swab the labia and vaginal introitus with antiseptic lotion.
2. Use an antiseptic cream to lubricate the index and middle fingers, then under direct observation, separate the labia with one hand while the two fingers are inserted gently into the vagina.
3. Feel for the fetal head. It can usually be easily felt as a bony hard mass filling the pelvis. A breech may feel firm and is occasionally mistaken for the head, unless care and thought are involved during the procedure.
4. The cervix is usually easily detected, unless effacement is almost complete. Pass the fingers inside the cervix and feel for the extent of dilatation. Try to estimate the diameter of the cervical dilatation and express it in centimetres. The cervix may be thick when only slightly dilated, but

becomes thinner (or effaced) as the cervix dilates beyond 5 cm.

5. When performing a vaginal examination in labour, it is important to determine how far down in the pelvis the presenting part has advanced. The leading part of the head is usually the vertex and this point is related to the ischial spines. The distance of the vertex above or below the ischial spines is assessed in centimetres and expressed as –3,–2,–1,0,+1,+2,+3, etc. to indicate the degree of descent.

6. The skull of the fetus is carefully palpated. Early in labour, before caput formation has occurred, the sagittal suture and the fontanelles can be easily felt, and from this position is usually determined. Late in labour, the degree of moulding and skull bone overlap may be extreme; the fontanelles are difficult to feel and when the head has been pressing against the dilating cervix for some hours, oedmatous thickening of the scalp can be felt (caput succedaneum). The more moulding and caput occurring, the more likely it is that a long difficult labour is taking place. When difficulty is experienced in determining the position (because of caput formation), then a hand slipped over the side of the fetal skull will easily feel the fetal ear if the head is well down. When this is moved backwards and forwards, it is easy to determine the direction of the pinna. The pinna of the ear always points backwards towards the occiput.

7. Maternal pelvic findings (Fig. 1.9). Generally it is difficult

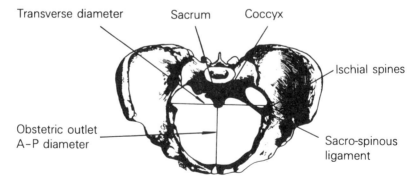

Figure 1.9 Landmarks of bony pelvis showing well-rounded features of a gynaecoid brim shape.

to assess a pelvis from the point of view of obstetric outcome. However, a rough guide can be established:

Pelvic inlet
(a) Feel for the sacral promontory (Fig. 1.10). Generally it cannot be palpated unless the true conjugate diameter is less than 10.5 cm.
(b) Feel along the iliopectineal line. In a normal pelvis, the examining finger can reach no further than one-third of the way round the sidewall of the pelvis.
(c) Feel the retropubic angle. It is usually rounded, but may have straight rami and a narrow angle at the back of the symphysis pubis – this would indicate an android-shape to the brim.

Mid-cavity
(a) Feel for the sacral curve. Generally the sacrum cannot be felt, but in a narrow funnel-shaped pelvis (associated with an android-shaped brim) the first four segments may appear flat.
(b) The sacro-spinous ligament is generally 4 cm or more in length, but a reduction in distance may indicate an increased 'funnelling' of the pelvis.
(c) Feel for the forepart of the pelvic brim. It is usually rounded, but may have straight rami and a narrow angle at the back of the symphysis pubis – this would indicate an android-shape to the brim.
(d) The subpubic angle may be narrow and less than 90° in arc. This would force the fetal head further posteriorly in an attempt to pass out of the pelvis, and is obviously an

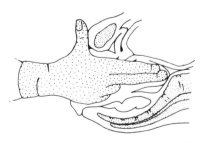

Figure 1.10 Feel for the sacral promontory and then palpate the sacral curve.

additional problem if associated with an android-shaped pelvic brim.

Pelvic outlet

(a) The antero-posterior diameter is the distance from the coccyx to the symphysis pubis.
(b) The transverse diameter is the intertuberous diameter and can be measured clinically.

1.7 VAGINAL EXAMINATION IN GYNAECOLOGY

Speculum examination

Passing a vaginal speculum is an essential skill required by all medical students to enable them to identify and diagnose problems presenting in obstetric and gynaecological patients. Students should be able to display, identify and describe the physical findings of the vagina and cervix without causing hurt or embarrassment to the patients they are examining.

Many females attend a medical practitioner complaining of symptoms that suggest a vaginal or cervical problem. When the patient complains of symptoms referable to the bladder (stress incontinence, dysuria or frequency) or of dyspareunia, a lump in the vagina, then it is important that the speculum used is of single-blade type (Sims' speculum Fig. 1.11). However, when the symptoms are of vaginal discharge, post-coital bleeding or bleeding due to problems in early pregnancy (abortion, ectopic pregnancy, hydatidiform mole), or if a Papanicolaou (PAP) smear is to be obtained, then a bivalve speculum is the more convenient instrument. The better types of bivalve instrument

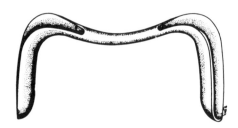

Figure 1.11 Sims' speculum.

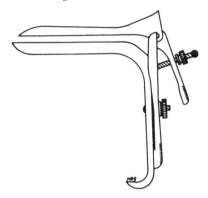

Figure 1.12 Bivalve (Grave's) speculum.

will come apart (Grave's speculum Fig. 1.12), allowing the anterior blade of the speculum to be removed – the posterior blade can then be used as a Sims' speculum.

Whichever speculum is used, several steps should be taken before attempting to pass the speculum.

1. Make sure the speculum is at an acceptable temperature. Warm the speculum in a bowl of water at about 40–45°C.
2. Apply a thin smear of lubricant to the surface of the speculum. Make sure that no lubricant is on the inner (concave) surfaces as it may be mistaken for a discharge, and may also mix with a cervical smear and ruin the cytological examination.
3. Choose all your equipment before the examination and have it ready to hand. You may need Ayre's spatula, sponge-holding forceps, cottonwool swabs, swab-sticks, culture media or transport media.

Passing the speculum (Figs. 1.13–1.22)

Several techniques are employed and all are satisfactory if the condition is displayed adequately without causing hurt or embarrassment to the patient. A common method for passing a Grave's speculum is described:

1. Position the patient on her back so that the buttocks are over the end of the couch or table and the feet are supported on a ledge or in stirrups.

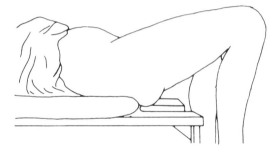

Figure 1.13 Demonstrating that to obtain the best position to examine a patient using a speculum, the buttocks must be over the end of the couch.

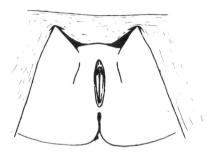

Figure 1.14 Demonstrating that when a patient is draped and lying comfortably on a couch, the labia are apposed and examination is difficult.

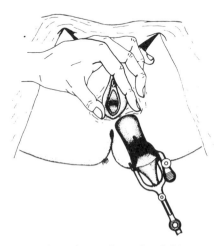

Figure 1.15 Demonstrating that when the labia are widely separated the speculum may be more easily inserted into the vagina.

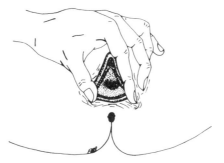

Figure 1.16 Showing that if the index finger and thumb are inserted between the labia and then separated, the vaginal introitus is clearly seen, a speculum can be passed easily and sometimes even the cervix can be visualized.

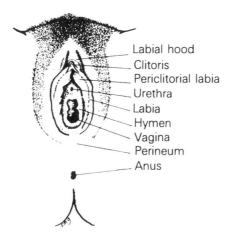

Labial hood
Clitoris
Periclitorial labia
Urethra
Labia
Hymen
Vagina
Perineum
Anus

Figure 1.17 Illustrating the anatomy of the labia and vaginal introitus, which should be carefully inspected when the labia are separated.

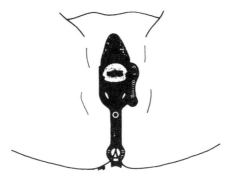

Figure 1.18 Visualization of cervix through the bivalve speculum.

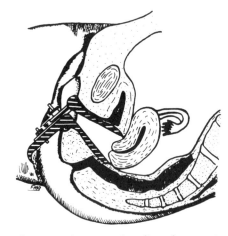

Figure 1.19 Open the speculum to visualize the cervix.

2. Drape the sheet over the lower abdomen and the legs so that the thighs and abdomen are covered but the vulva is easily seen.
3. Explain to the patient that you are about to pass a metal speculum into the vagina.
4. Hold the speculum so that the blades are between the index and middle finger, the handle is held comfortably in the hand and the thumb is resting lightly on the lever of the anterior blade.

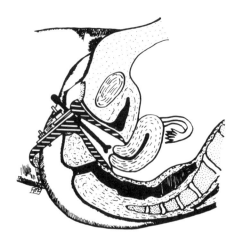

Figure 1.20 To show how a PAP smear is taken using a bivalve speculum.

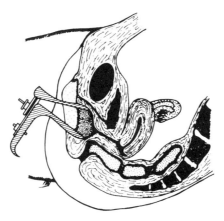

Figure 1.21 Illustrating that if a bivalve speculum is opened before it is fully inserted into the vagina, the walls of the vagina only are seen.

5. Inspect the labia for any signs of masses, inflammation or discharge.
6. Insert the forefinger and the thumb of the other hand between the labia towards the posterior third of the vaginal introitus and then separate the labia as widely as possible. This manoeuvre transforms the introitus from an antero-posterior slit into a triangular shape with the base stretched to a width of about 5 cm between the finger and thumb.

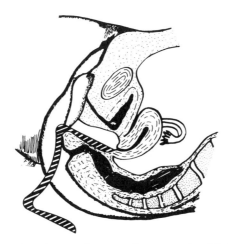

Figure 1.22 Use a Sims' speculum or the posterior blade of a bivalve speculum to visualize the anterior wall of the vagina.

7. Press the speculum against the straight line made by the stretching of the fourchette and then gently insert the speculum so that it enters the vagina in an upward (towards the patient's head) and backward inclination. It should slide easily to the full length of the vagina, but if resistance is felt do not exert a force, just change direction a little until the resistance is overcome.

8. When the speculum is fully inserted into the vagina, open the blades by pressing with the thumb on the lever of the anterior blade. If the speculum has been correctly inserted, the cervix should become clearly visible. (If the speculum is opened when only part way in the vagina, the vaginal walls beyond the speculum will be found to be in position and, to the novice, may appear to be the cervix.)

9. Observe the cervix first, then the os and finally the type of vaginal discharge. When the cervix has been completely inspected, the anterior blade may be removed to disclose the anterior wall of the vagina.

10. Observe the anterior wall of the vagina for any epithelial changes such as neoplasm, atrophic changes or other abnormalities. Note whether the bladder bulges down and if there is a cystocoele, whether it is related to a urethrocoele or if stress incontinence can be elicited.

11. Finally, note the level of the cervix as the speculum is withdrawn. There may be a prolapse of the uterus or bladder. If a prolapse is noted, then it may be graded by degrees depending on its relationship to the vaginal introitus. If the uterus is prolapsed but the cervix is still within the vaginal introitus, it is termed a first-degree prolapse. A second-degree prolapse is found when the cervix passes through the introitus but the body of the uterus is still within the vagina. A third-degree prolapse (or procidentia) occurs when the cervix and the uterus are completely outside the vaginal introitus.

Description of the cervix

When describing the cervix it is best to develop a routine observational check-list which can be used in all written histories and which acts as a base for future reference.

The significant features that should be noted on all cervices are:

1. The condition of the epithelium. Normally the cervix is covered by flat squamous epithelium which meets the endo-cervical columnar epithelium at the margin of the external cervical os. However, under the influence of excessive oestrogen (at menarche, in pregnancy, certain contraceptive pills, postmenopausal oestrogen), the columnar epithelium of the endocervix proliferates and grows out over the endo-cervix. This ectopic columnar epithelium (ECE) is identified as an orange or red (erythroplakia) velvety, irregular-looking epithelium. (It was formerly called an 'erosion' but because there is no loss of epithelium this term is a mis-nomer.) It produces a clear mucous discharge, and if trau-matized may bleed easily. Following stabilization of oestrogen levels, the ectopic columnar epithelium will undergo metaplasia to squamous epithelium. This process often leads to blockage of mucous crypts, so producing retention cysts (Nabothian follicles). It is in this metaplastic area, that neoplasia may occur, so the squamo-columnar junction must be sampled when taking a smear for cytologi-cal analysis.

2. The colour of the epithelium. Normal non-pregnant squa-mous epithelium in a young woman is of a mid-pink colour, but may range from a pale-pink to bright-pink shade. The darker colour is associated with an increase in blood supply to the cervix (such as in pregnancy, neopla-sia, infection) – and if the blood flow is very much increased, the epithelium may even be mauve or plum coloured. In fact a dark-plum colour is regarded as a diag-nostic sign of pregnancy.

    In postmenopausal women the epithelium is often very pale, or may be mottled orange or red. The mottled colour is due to the extremely thin atrophic epithelium allowing the blood vessels below the epithelium to be easily seen. Sometimes, the vaginal epithelium is so thin and fragile that any trauma such as intercourse or passage of a spec-ulum will cause loss of, or a tear of the epithelium, produ-cing minute haematomas or haemorrhages.

    In women who have vaginal infection due to trichomo-nas, the epithelium may show a diffuse red discoloration or may present with punctate red spots ('strawberry' cervix). Monilia results in a bright-pink or red discoloration, with typical white plaques covering patches of the epithelium.

3. Cervical os. The cervical os is usually round or oval shape in a nulliparous woman and the squamo-columnar junction is seen at the ectocervical opening. In multiparas, the cervix often discloses evidence of tears and lacerations so that the os has a distorted appearance. Tears usually take place at the lateral (3 o'clock and 9 o'clock) positions, so that the os has a transverse appearance. The cervix will appear to gape open like two lips pouting, and a large area of columnar epithelium is then seen. This is not ectopic epithelium, for once the speculum is allowed to close, the cervical 'lips' close and normal cervical epithelium is seen. The condition where mucous epithelium is seen in association with cervical tears is called an ectropion.

4. Vaginal discharges. Physiological vaginal discharge may be clear and thin due to transudation across the vaginal epithelium, of a mucousy nature from columnar epithelium, or milky in colour due to the normal desquamation of cells and admixture with other cellular debris.

   Pathological discharges may be difficult to differentiate, but three in particular are relatively easy to identify. Infection with *Trichomonas vaginalis* results in a thin, yellowish discharge (sometimes grey, and at other times greenish in colour), which has a few frothy bubbles present (due to the low surface tension) and has a distinct odour. *Gardnerella vaginalis* has a similar appearance but most times the patient is asymptomatic. Monilial infection results in a white, flaky discharge (like thin cottage cheese), which is intensely itchy. If a secondary bacterial infection occurs in the vagina, the discharge may have a yellowish appearance and appear to be the result of trichomonal infection. Bacterial invasion of columnar epithelium produces a pus-like mucous discharge from the cervix.

5. Neoplastic conditions of the cervix. These may include polyps of endocervical or endometrial aetiology and appear as tear-shaped lesions protruding through the external os. They are covered by mucous epithelium in most cases, are usually a bright-red colour, and vary from several millimetres to a few centimetres in size.

Carcinoma may present as ulcers or a sessile or polypoid lesions. It is usually identified by the presence of haemorrhage, increase in blood vessels, abnormal epithelium (leukoplakia, dysplasia), loss of epithelium and distortion of the normal features of the cervix.

6. Papanicolaou smears. These are now obtained using an Ayre's spatula which should be applied to the cervix so that the spatula, when rotated through 360° around the squamo-columnar junction, scrapes off the superficial cells from this region. Additional endocervical cells are obtained by a cytobrush as a part of the procedure. Smears obtained in this manner are usually classified as:
   (a) Negative – no malignant cells seen
   (b) Doubtful – abnormal cells of doubtful significance – repeat
   (c) Suspicious – suspicion of malignancy
   (d) Positive – cancer cells seen.

A comment of 'absence of endocervical cells' might indicate an inadequate sample as it has failed to sample the squamo-columnar junction. Any abnormal PAP smear must have a colposcopy and biopsy performed to obtain a histological diagnosis before any definite therapy can be initiated. Colposcopy examination is used to define the nature and extent of the lesion producing the abnormal smears. A negative or unsatisfactory colposcopy examination may require a cone biopsy or a curettage to exclude the possibility that the abnormal smear is arising from the endocervix or the endometrial cavity.

Summary of vaginal examination

When passing a vaginal speculum to examine a patient, take the following steps.

1. Choose an appropriate speculum.
2. Position the patient correctly.
3. Lubricate the speculum and make sure it is warmed.
4. Inspect the labia.
5. Separate the labia and inspect the introitus.
6. Pass the speculum in an upward, backward direction for the full length of the vagina.
7. Open the speculum to disclose the cervix.

8. Describe the cervix (epithelium, colour, cervical os, vaginal discharges, any neoplastic lesions).

Digital vaginal examination

Performing a digital vaginal examination is also an important part of a gynaecological examination, but often is difficult to perform, or the findings are incorrectly interpreted. Unless a medical practitioner knows what to feel and how to examine a pelvis, then many pathological conditions may be missed. A suitable technique is described:

1. Wear a glove of suitable size and lightly lubricate the middle and index fingers.
2. Separate the labia and under direct vision insert the two fingers gently into the vagina.
3. Pass the fingers in an upward, backward direction to the full length of the vagina. Normally the thumb will be found to rest firmly on the symphysis pubis and further pressure becomes difficult.
4. Feel for the cervix. It is usually easily felt as a firm rounded mass about 3 cm in diameter. The os is felt as a dimple or pit in the surface of the cervix, and an imaginary rod passing out of the cervical canal through the os would normally point in a downward and backward direction if the uterus was anteverted. When the cervix is felt to point directly downward or in a downward and forward direction, then the uterus is usually in a retroverted position.
5. Determine the consistency of the cervix. Non-pregnant women will have a firm, well-defined cervix, whereas pregnancy usually produces a softening and enlargement of the tissue.
6. When a patient is pregnant it is important that extreme gentleness be employed when feeling for the cervical os. It may be dilated or patulous and the finger can then be accidentally inserted into the canal, introducing infection or precipitating a rupture of membranes (such as in cervical incompetence or late pregnancy). When the cervix is dilated in early pregnancy, it usually indicates cervical incompetence (when no uterine contractions have occurred pre-

viously), or inevitable or incomplete abortion (when uterine contractions have been present).

7. Determine the mobility of the cervix. It will normally move up or laterally by 1–2 cm when pushed by the examining fingers. There may be complete or partial immobility, indicating induration (due to infection or neoplasia) in the surrounding tissue.

8. Pain on moving the cervix is usually minimal, but conditions producing blood, pus or chemical irritation of the pelvic peritoneum will be accompanied by extreme discomfort when the cervix is moved (excitation tenderness). This occurs because the cervix is like one end of a lever that has the uterine fundus (and its covering peritoneum) at the other end, and both can then move around the fulcrum of the lateral cervical ligaments. Lateral movement of the cervix produces a marked movement of the uterine fundus and consequently extreme peritonism in association with ectopic pregnancy, salpingitis and pelvic peritonitis.

9. The uterus. A bimanual examination of the uterus is now performed. The uterus is normally about 8–9 cm long from the cervix to the fundus, and is normally found in an anteverted position with the cervix pointing downwards and backwards (Figs. 1.23–1.25). Determine the size of the

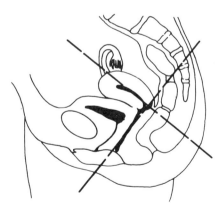

Figure 1.23 Illustrating the axis of various anatomical organs in the pelvis, using the cervix as a fulcrum and a point of reference. The uterus is normally upwards and forwards while the cervix points downwards and backwards. The vagina passes into the pelvis in an upward and backward direction.

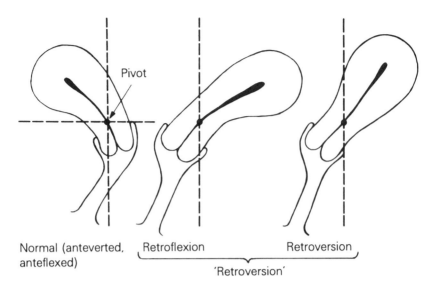

Figure 1.24 When the cervix points downwards and backwards, the uterine fundus is upwards and forwards (anteverted).

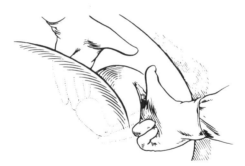

Figure 1.25 Showing vaginal examination using the bimanual digital technique.

    uterus. Try to develop the skill of spatial imagery when
    performing bimanual examinations. Skill and accuracy
    come after many examinations, but may be difficult for the
    beginner to achieve.
10. Determine the size of the uterus, its consistency (normally
    it is firm, but in pregnancy it becomes softer), its outline or
    shape (normally a regular pyriform shape, but pathological
    states produce irregularity), its mobility and any tenderness
    that may be present.

11. Feel for the adnexa. This consists of the parametria, the ovaries and the tubes. Normally the anatomical detail cannot be palpated. However, if a mass is present, it can be felt by passing the examining vaginal fingers into the lateral fornices and then pressing upwards, backwards and laterally towards the abdominal fingers which press down from the pelvic brim towards the vaginal fingers. Determine the size, mobility consistency (solid or cystic, soft or hard) and tenderness of the mass.

SUMMARY

Obstetric and gynaecological history-taking and examination are relatively easy, but do require thought and expertise to be conducted adequately. To learn the techniques it is important that some logical and simple steps be taken. This chapter attempts to clarify the basic concepts in these procedures and explain what can be seen and felt and how to describe the findings.

2

Adverse factors affecting embryo or fetus

2.1 GENERAL INSTRUCTIONAL OBJECTIVE

The students should appreciate the pre-conceptual, antenatal and intrapartum factors that may adversely affect an embryo or fetus so that they can initiate the management of related problems.

2.2 SPECIFIC BEHAVIOURAL OBJECTIVES

1. Take a relevant history to reveal congenital or hereditary factors that may affect the fetus.
2. Discuss the maternal factors that may be associated with inadequate fetal nutrition.
3. Discuss oxygen transfer to the fetus, those factors that may impair or interrupt it, and the effects of hypoxia on the fetus.
4. Discuss the examination, relevant investigations and findings, and their significance in relation to detecting abnormalities of fetal growth.
5. Discuss the initial management when either hypoxia or intrauterine growth retardation is identified by symptoms, signs or by investigations.
6. Explain how induction of labour, vaginal delivery or Caesarean section may adversely affect the fetus.
7. Discuss those factors that contribute to cerebral damage and birth trauma.
8. Discuss those signs during pregnancy that may indicate fetal malformation.
9. Discuss perinatal mortality and identify the major factors contributing to perinatal mortality and morbidity.

10. Describe how a fetus may become infected *in utero*.
11. Discuss the effect of maternal trauma on the fetus.
12. Discuss the formation, constitution and significance of amniotic fluid.

2.3 REASONS FOR LEARNING TO APPRECIATE THE PRE-CONCEPTUAL, ANTENATAL AND INTRAPARTUM FACTORS THAT MAY ADVERSELY AFFECT AN EMBRYO OR FETUS *IN UTERO*

This chapter discusses the major reasons why the medical and paramedical professions should be involved in the care of couples who are either planning or expecting a further addition to their family unit.

A fetus may succumb to noxious influences *in utero*, resulting in miscarriage or stillbirth, or a potentially healthy infant may die in labour or suffer significant morbidity which may affect the whole of his or her often shortened life.

Fortunately many of the causes of antenatal and postnatal morbidity and mortality can be predicted, or at least identified early, so that detrimental effects on the future child can be eliminated or alleviated by appropriate antenatal management. However, medical care itself is not without hazard; iatrogenic damage to the embryo, fetus or newborn must be guarded against, as many of the procedures commonly used with the aim of improving the outcome of pregnancy may lead to increased perinatal mortality and morbidity if used inappropriately or on the basis of misleading information.

As most parents enter a pregnancy in good health, obstetrics is one medical speciality where prophylaxis should be the main aim. This, of course, is not possible unless the medical practitioner appreciates those factors that may adversely affect the fetus, knows how to investigate and identify those problems when they occur, and how to initiate the appropriate management of any such problem.

Perinatal deaths are regrettable, but perinatal morbidity may in many ways disrupt a family unit to a greater extent and produce untold suffering for the child. There is also great cost to the community in the form of special educational facilities or the establishment of total care institutions for the more severely handicapped.

Adverse factors can begin their influence before conception, during the antenatal course, or during labour and delivery. The problems can be broadly divided into two groups: genetic and environmental. Environmental factors include the mother's external environment, the mother's general health and also intrauterine factors. The fetus can be likened to a goldfish in a fish tank, in that it is dependent for survival on the purity of the environment outside the tank (poisons in the air entering the water), as well as the addition of appropriate nutrients and oxygen and competition from other inhabitants of the tank for nutrients.

Only about 2% of ongoing pregnancies after the first trimester result in a child with a significant congenital abnormality. Minor malformations are recognized in a further 5%. The proportion of these abnormalities resulting from drug usage is probably less than 1 in 20. This factor albeit small, is largely avoidable.

2.4 GENETIC AND SOCIAL FACTORS

These are best detected by a careful history and examination when the patient attends for her first visit. Socioeconomic and environmental factors should be noted and modified, if possible, to achieve the optimum results. The history should include:

- Age and parity
- Height and weight
- Occupation and domestic circumstances
- Smoking habits
- Drug and alcohol intake
- Previous obstetric history
- Previous medical history
- Family history of inherited disorders
- Immunity or otherwise to rubella, exposure to animals.

The importance of these individual factors varies. All the factors should be weighted together in an attempt to determine whether the present or planned pregnancy is one with a high risk of morbidity or mortality. Approximately 10–20% of women fall into the high-risk category and account for greater than 50% of the fetal and neonatal deaths. Some of the important characteristics that are associated with the high-risk group include the following:

1. Maternal age and parity. The risk is least between 20 and 29 years of age and between the second and fourth pregnancies. Thus a woman older than 35 years who has more than four children falls into the high-risk category. The nulliparous teenager is also at increased risk.
2. Maternal height. Height has a negative linear correlation to perinatal mortality. Women under 152cm (5 ft) have smaller babies. This may be due to familial trends; however, it may also be due to a poor environment which limited the mother's growth potential. Perinatal mortality is increased for mothers of shorter height and lower socioeconomic class. There is also a greater incidence of pre-eclampsia and Caesarean section in this group of women.
3. Socioeconomic class. The socioeconomic class of the father has a less direct relationship with perinatal mortality than that of the mother, but the lower the class the higher the risk. Where the mother is unsupported and the pregnancy unplanned, the incidence of small-for-gestational-age infants and of perinatal mortality is double that found for married women between 25 and 30 years of age. This group of patients also commonly have several other high-risk social factors, the effects of which are cumulative.
4. Social habits. Smoking more than ten cigarettes a day, significant alcohol intake and/or drug addiction increases the risk of perinatal mortality.
5. Nutrition. Weight gain during pregnancy and pre-pregnancy weight are relevant to the outcome of the pregnancy. Specific associations include the following:
   (a) Iron or vitamin deficiencies are associated with anaemias and infection.
   (b) Poor nutrition is associated with small-for-gestational-age babies.
   (c) Severe nutritional lack in pregnancy can cause impairment of the development of the fetal central nervous system.
   (d) Women with a pre-pregnant weight of less than 50 kg and a pregnancy weight gain of less than 5 kg tend to have low birthweight babies.

6. Trauma. Mothers who are exposed to trauma, especially severe mental trauma, have an increased incidence of pre-term labour and as a result a higher perinatal mortality. Abdominal trauma may rarely cause premature separation of the placenta (accidental haemorrhage) or rupture of the uterus. Massive blood loss leading to shock and decreased placental blood flow can cause an acute hypoxic insult to the fetus. Mothers who are exposed to repeated violence in the home are frequently without emotional or sufficient financial support, all of which may adversely affect the pregnancy and all of which may be aggravated further by the anticipated addition to the family unit.

7. Obstetric history. The patient's previous obstetric history can give a good indication of possible problems in the present pregnancy, and provides a good summary of any high-risk factors that remained or have become worse since the previous pregnancy. Those previous obstetric complications that may indicate a problem in the present pregnancy include:
    (a) Previous stillbirth or neonatal death
    (b) Small-for-gestational-age baby
    (c) Pre-term labour
    (d) Cervical incompetence and/or uterine abnormality
    (e) Previous fetal abnormality
    (f) Antepartum haemorrhage
    (g) Rhesus disease
    (h) Diabetes
    (i) Cardiovascular problems, including congenital heart conditions and hypertension
    (j) Anaemia
    (k) Prolonged labour or difficult delivery
    (l) Caesarean section
    (m) Significant postpartum haemorrhage
    (n) Postpartum depression

    A woman who delivered a pre-term infant in a previous pregnancy has at least a two-fold increased risk of deliver-ing another pre-term infant. A previous perinatal loss is associated with a three-fold increased risk of another such outcome, particularly if the first loss was associated with a low birthweight infant. It has been found that patients who have previously delivered a low birthweight infant face more than a three-fold increased risk of doing so in a subsequent pregnancy.

8. Past medical history. The taking of a medical history is an important method of detecting chronic and continuing problems in the health of the mother which may affect the outcome of her pregnancy, as well as any maternal problems that may be aggravated by the pregnancy such as:

(a) Diabetes mellitus, even with the best of care, can result in a 10% fetal mortality.

(b) Hypertension may through alterations in placental vasculature lead to growth retardation or intrauterine asphyxia due to placental separation.

(c) Cardiac disease in pregnancy is usually the result of a congenital heart defect or rheumatic fever, and may result in the mother not being able to increase her cardiac output or cope with the increased cardiac work required during pregnancy. Cardiac failure or arrhythmias may develop and increase the risk of venous and arterial thrombosis, embolism and maternal death. The severity of the disease will determine the mother's antenatal admission and modify her care in labour.

(d) Renal disease may complicate a pregnancy and produce problems related to filtration, renal blood flow and hypertension. Patients who have had renal and heart transplants, however, can be guided through a successful pregnancy with care.

(e) Anaemia and other medical problems in the mother can increase the risk to both the mother and fetus.

(f) Ulcerative colitis, which may be exacerbated by pregnancy, if severe can interfere with the absorption of important nutrients.

(g) Surgical problems, especially those that result in or have caused bony deformities in the spine, pelvis, lower limbs and chest can give rise to problems of discomfort during pregnancy and may interfere with the normal birth mechanisms. Abdominal or pelvic soft-tissue tumours, or abnormalities such as uterine fibroids or a vaginal septum, can also cause problems during pregnancy and labour.

9. Family history. The family history of the potential parents, especially that of the mother's immediate family, may also

provide definite indications as to whether the pregnancy is at risk or not. A history of diabetes mellitus in a first-degree relative would be an indication to screen the mother during pregnancy for this disorder. Where there is a family history of a chromosomal or genetic abnormality antenatal diagnosis may be indicated.

Physical examination

A thorough physical examination is the next logical step after eliciting from the history the presence or absence of any of the risk factors mentioned. It is important to determine the size of the uterus early in the pregnancy and thus confirm the estimated gestation as accurately as possible. This may involve the use of an ultrasound scan. The timing of any management of a high-risk patient may depend on an accurate estimate of fetal maturity.

2.5 RETARDED INTRAUTERINE GROWTH OF THE FETUS

Retarded intrauterine growth may occur because of abnormalities in the mother, the placenta or the fetus leading to defective nutrient transfer or a decrease in nutrients. Examples are as follows:

1. The mother
    (a) Medical conditions such as hypertension, renal disease, endocrine disease or advanced cardiovascular disease.
    (b) Toxins such as cigarette smoke.
    (c) Nutritional problems associated with poor intake (dieting, food fads and vegans) or severe malabsorption syndrome.
2. The placenta
    (a) Impaired placental transport associated with antepartum haemorrhage, placental infarction and poor implantation (such as that which results in a circumvallate placenta).
    (b) Transplacental circulation in twins.
3. The fetus
    (a) Congenital abnormalities.
    (b) Infection.
    (c) Twins.

Signs of retarded intrauterine growth

There is a small group of neonates who are born small for gestational age when there has been no detectable reason during pregnancy. Thus, while it is important to be vigilant for the risk factors associated with small-for-gestational-age infants, it is also important to observe the growth of both the uterus and the fetus so as to detect at the earliest possible opportunity any sign of fetal growth retardation.

The signs of regarded intrauterine growth include the following:

1. Uterine size smaller than expected for the period of amenorrhoea as judged by:
   (a) Symphyseal–fundal height measurement, which is in part dependent on the lie and engagement of the fetus, and
   (b) Uterine volume.
2. Fetal size. If there is any question about intrauterine growth an attempt should be made to estimate the weight of the fetus.
3. The volume of amniotic fluid. Oligohydramnios tends to be a poor sign when associated with intrauterine growth retardation and should lead to further investigations.
4. Decreased number of fetal movements may be reported by the mother.
5. Maternal weight loss or lack of weight gain during the third trimester.
6. Abnormal fetal development. Asymmetrical growth or the presence of fetal abnormality.

Investigation of suspected retarded intrauterine growth

This should be directed towards confirming its presence, attempting to estimate the severity, and eliciting the cause. Growth retardation can be confirmed and its severity estimated by:
1. Repeated clinical observation (Fig. 2.1), including:
   (a) Abdominal palpation.
   (b) Symphyseal–fundal height measurement.
   (c) Maternal weight gain.

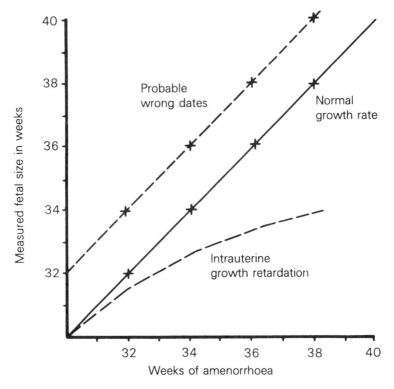

Figure 2.1 Weeks of amenorrhoea.

These repeated observations should be made by the same observer.

2.   Ancillary tests
     (a)   Ultrasound examination
           Routine ultrasound. A single ultrasound examination is now commonly performed at 18 weeks of gestation to confirm the gestational dates as well as to detect any fetal abnormalities. Repeated echograms will then give information as to whether the growth rate is normal, decreased or ceased.
           Biophysical profile. Five fetal parameters are used as a biophysical assessment of fetal well-being. These are fetal breathing movements, gross body movement, fetal tone, reactive fetal heart rate, and amniotic fluid volume (Table 2.1). A very low score is indicative of impending fetal demise. The scoring system is somewhat subjective as it does not take into account gesta-

Table 2.1 Biophysical profile scoring (adapted from Manning, F.A. et al, 1981. *Am. J. Obstet. Gynec.*, **140**: 289–294)

Biophysical parameters	Normal (score = 2)	Abnormal (score = 0)
Fetal breathing movements in 30 minutes observation	One episode of >30 seconds	Absence of fetal breathing >30 seconds
Gross fetal movement in 30 minutes observation	At least three discrete body/limb movement	Up to two episodes body/limb movements
Fetal tone	Active extension/flexion of limb(s) or trunk Opening or closing of hand	Slow extension/flexion or absent fetal movement
Reactive fetal heart rate in 30 minutes	At least 2 episodes of acceleration of >15 bpm associated with fetal movement	Fewer than two accelerations or <15 bpm
Amniotic fluid volume	At least one pocket >2 cm in two perpendicular planes	<2 cm fluid pocket in two perpendicular planes

tional age, fetal growth, and maternal obstetric history, e.g. diabetic pregnancy, premature rupture of the membranes, polyhydramnios, etc. It also does not take into account new developments such as Doppler studies.

Doppler ultrasound. The measurement of blood flow is a sharper haemodynamic assessment of fetal condition. The latest advances of colour Doppler imaging in studying flow velocity waveforms is well established in obstetric practice. Most commonly used index is the peak systolic (A)/diastolic (B) ratio of the umbilical artery. The greater the diastolic flow, the lower the A/B ratio. On the other hand, a fall in the diastolic flow due to increased placental resistance, increases the A/B ratio. If the resistance is very great there may be absent end diastolic flow or even reversed flow in diastole.

Other Doppler studies on uterine and fetal vessels may contribute information about the fetal condition that plays an important role in the management of the at risk pregnancy.

(b) Activity of the fetus

(i) **Fetal movements count**. Fetal movements can be used to evaluate the status of the fetus at risk. Normally a fetus moves at frequent intervals and these movements can be easily felt by the mother and counted. If movements are counted for four segments of a half hour each during the day. A total of more than 10 movements is reassuring. A fetal movement count of less than 10 detected movements or a progressive decrease indicates the need for closer observation and further testing.

(ii) **Cardiotocography**. This involves a continuous recording of the fetal heart rate. The machine calculates the rate from a series of fetal heart beats and graphs the result in relation to any uterine activity that may be occurring. A normal trace shows a short-term variation of greater than 5 beats, a rate between 120 and 160 beats per minute, and no slowing of the fetal heart rate in relation to contractions, movements or maternal activity. Spontaneous accelerations of the fetal heart rate with movements or contractions is a good sign. A normal cardiotocograph trace is reassuring, as the fetus is very unlikely to die in the ensuing 4–6 days in the absence of any acute insults such as an accidental haemorrhage. An abnormal result may mean the presence of fetal hypoxia and may indicate the need to deliver the fetus if the cause of the heart rate abnormality is not reversible.

2.6 SMALL-FOR-GESTATIONAL-AGE BABIES

Babies who are small for gestational age (below the 10th percentile for gestational age) may show symmetrical or asymmetrical growth retardation.

Symmetrical growth retardation (appropriate head to body ratio) occurs from an early period of gestation and is more commonly associated with primary fetal pathology such as chromosomal abnormality or fetal infection.

Asymmetrical growth. Babies who demonstrate this appear long and thin with relatively large heads. They lack subcutaneous fat and organs such as the liver, lungs and heart are smaller relative to total body weight than those of a normal infant. Neurological development is mature and brain weight is relatively greater in relation to birthweight. These changes usually result from an abnormality of placental function which may be due to reduced placental circulation, fibrin deposition or thrombotic occlusion of the arterioles in the deciduo-placental circulation. Separation of a portion of the placenta and infarction of the separated placenta (as occurs with accidental haemorrhage) reduces the functioning placenta. A circumvallate placenta is often associated with a restricted area of implantation, which may be severe enough to compromise placental function.

Chronic poor placental function leads to a reduced oxygen supply resulting in a greater demand on the less efficient anaerobic metabolic pathways. Also there is a reduction in placental transfer of nutrients, including amino acids and carbohydrates. The combination of hypoxia and nutritional deprivation results in a rapid depletion of glycogen and fat stores, and the commencement of acidosis and further hypoxia.

2.7 MANAGEMENT OF GROWTH RETARDATION

The decision that must be made whenever fetal growth retardation is detected is when to deliver the fetus. In other words, is the fetus safer in the uterus or in the nursery? As knowledge of antenatal fetal medicine advances, it may be possible in some cases to correct the problem causing retarded intrauterine growth. At the present time, most of the explored avenues have proved fruitless. The main aims at present are to limit the effect of placental inadequacy in pregnancy and to try and improve placental blood flow by resting the patient in bed with precautions to prevent postural hypotension.

If clinical evidence and investigations indicate that the fetus is compromised and growth has ceased, then delivery needs to be considered and expedited if the fetus is mature. The fetal maturity depends upon gestational age and the severity of the growth retardation. The number of infants who die from the effects of prematurity decreases markedly after 30 weeks of gestation.

However, before 34 weeks of amenorrhoea, each week of maturity gained produces a significant increase in the likelihood of the fetus surviving neonatally. Thus accurate knowledge of the last normal menstrual period, and the length of the cycle, is most important. If this information is available it should have been correlated with the size of the uterus at the first visit. If there is any discrepancy between the clinical signs, ultrasound examination can give an accurate guide to gestational age if it is performed before 24 weeks of amenorrhoea.

Regular clinical assessment of symphyseal–fundal height measurements, biophysical parameters of fetal well-being (fetal movements, fetal breathing and cardiotocography) and ultrasound assessment of fetal size, growth and liquor volume are invaluable in deciding how long to keep the pre-term growth retarded infant *in utero*. Ultrasound assessment of fetal subcutaneous fat and measurements of fetal blood flow appear at the moment to be a useful adjuvant.

It is important to individualize each case rather than make strict guidelines as to when fetuses should be delivered or remain *in utero*. Biochemical assessment of fetal lung maturity generally is not particularly helpful. If the fetus is considered to be sufficiently compromised *in utero*, then delivery will be indicated independent of fetal lung maturity. There are however, cases where delivery may be, in part, elective either to make sure the patient is delivered in a large hospital or where fetal surgery may be indicated. Assessment of fetal lung maturity in these cases may well help with the timing of delivery. If there is any doubt about fetal lung maturity, corticosteroids should be given to accelerate fetal lung maturity.

2.8 DELIVERY

The type and timing of delivery can affect the perinatal morbidity and mortality. Providing there are no complicating factors, the spontaneous onset of labour at term (38–40 weeks of amenorrhoea), with a vaginal delivery occurring 2 hours to 12 hours later, is the ideal aim.

Pre-term delivery
This carries a higher risk of respiratory distress, intracranial haemorrhage, neonatal death, jaundice, infection, low birthweight and hypoglycaemia. Prolonged stay in the intensive care nursery for the baby may lead to increased parent anxiety and problems with parent–child handling and bonding.

Pre-term delivery may be essential in the presence of marked intrauterine growth retardation. However, elective induction or induction for convenience, together with over-interpretation of signs of fatal jeopardy and incorrect or misleading estimates of gestational age, have all been implicated as causes of unnecessary pre-term deliveries.

Post-term delivery
Post-maturity (pregnancy prolonged more than 42 weeks of amenorrhoea) is not synonymous with post-dates. Post-maturity is present when the pregnancy is prolonged so far beyond term that a risk to the fetus exists. The fetus may have the features of a growth-retarded baby, except it has signs consistent with a term infant (longer finger nails, skin creases on heels and feet, joint movements, cartilage in ears), but has almost no subcutaneous fat and no glycogen stores. The post-mature baby frequently develops hypoglycaemia, and meconium is often present in the liquor. Most obstetricians advise induction before 42 weeks of gestation.

2.9 INDUCTION OF LABOUR

Labour may be induced for any of the following reasons:

1. Fetal
    (a) Signs of fetal compromise.
    (b) Intrauterine growth retardation.
    (c) Diabetes.
    (d) Rhesus incompatibility.
    (e) Infection.
2. Maternal
    (a) Pre-eclampsia, eclampsia or hypertension.
    (b) Dead or grossly abnormal fetus.
    (c) Antepartum haemorrhage.
3. Social.

Table 2.2 Bishop's pre-induction cervical scoring system

Clinical findings	Score			
	0	1	2	3
Cervix				
Dilitation (cm)	Closed	1–2	3–4	5+
Effacement (%)	0–30	40–50	60–70	80+
Position	Posterior	Central	Anterior	–
Consistency	Firm	Medium	Soft	–
Head				
Station	–3	–2	–1,0	+1,+2

Total score = 13   Favourable score = 6–13   Unfavourable score = 0–5

Suitability for induction (ripeness of the cervix)

To estimate the likely success of induction the cervix can be assessed using the modified Bishop's score (see Table 2.2). Other factors that need to be considered are parity, age of patient, condition of the fetus.

If the cervix is unfavourable for induction and there is no great urgency to deliver the fetus, the cervix may be ripened using:

1. Intravaginal prostaglandin E_2 gel 1–2 mg
2. Extra-amniotic prostaglandin $F_{2\alpha}$
3. Intracervical Foley's catheter
4. Intravenous Syntocinon
5. Stripping the membranes

Methods of induction

In most cases, induction involves an oxytocin (Syntocinon) infusion and the surgical rupture of the membranes. More recently, prostaglandin E_2 vaginal gel is commonly used for induction of labour.

1. **Surgical rupture of membranes**
   Fetal problems may arise from the following:
   (a) Prolapse of the cord. This results in cord compression and rapid onset of fetal distress, leading to death if immediate delivery (usually by Caesarean section) is not accomplished. The membranes should not be ruptured if there is malpresentation, the cord is presenting, or the presenting part is not well applied to the cervix.
   (b) Intrauterine infection. This usually only occurs when aseptic techniques are not adhered to. Membranes that have been ruptured for more than 12 hours during a labour predispose to intrauterine infection. The risk is increased after 24 hours or if the membranes have been ruptured for some time prior to the onset of labour.
   Repeated vaginal examination may increase the risk of infection.
   Fetal infection may result in pneumonia, septicaemia and meningitis. The haemolytic streptococcus group B is particularly virulent, and an intrauterine infection with these organisms results in a high risk of neonatal mortality.
   In order to shorten any delay in the onset of labour, it is now usual to combine Syntocinon with the surgical rupture of the membranes.

2. **Oxytocin infusion**
   This may cause the following problems:
   (a) Abnormally strong or prolonged contractions. These reduce the placental blood flow below that required by the fetus to maintain an aerobic form of metabolism, resulting in acidosis, fetal distress and, if prolonged and severe, fetal death. Thus it is important to monitor both the fetal heart rate and the contractions closely.
   (b) Rupture of the uterus. This is usually associated with a uterus weakened by a scar, grand multiparity, or obstructed labour. Rupture of the uterus commonly results in maternal haemorrhage, hypotension, greatly reduced or absent placental circulation, death of the fetus and a threat to the life of the mother.

3. **Oxytocin dosage.**
   Dose–response titration will result in the appropriate dose

for each individual patient. The infusion is commenced at 1.5 iu/min and doubled every 30 minutes until the patient is in established labour. Oxytocin should always be infused in a solution that contains electrolytes because of the danger of overdosage and possible water intoxication.

4. **Prostaglandin**

Prostaglandin E_2 (PGE_2) in the form of a gel is commonly used for the induction of labour. Many clinical trials have demonstrated its efficacy and safety. PGE_2 is a potent myometrial stimulant as well as a connective tissue softener. It therefore is suitable for those patients with an unfavourable cervix scheduled for induction of labour. However, the following contraindications should be observed in its use:

   (a) Grand multiparity.
   (b) Cases with high fetal presenting part or suspected cephalopelvic disproportion.
   (c) Abnormal cardiotocography or suspected fetal comprise.
   (d) Malpresentation.
   (e) History of previous scarred uterus.

Prostaglandin $F_{2\alpha}$, given by the extra-amniotic route, has also been used effectively.

Failure to achieve induction of labour

Once the membranes have been ruptured for the purpose of inducing labour, the fetus should be delivered within 24 hours. Thus a Caesarean section may be the end result of an induction of labour.

Adverse effects of Caesarean section

Caesarean section may adversely affect the baby in the following ways:

1. There may be an increased risk to the baby of respiratory distress due to hyaline membrane disease associated with prematurity. The risk must be foremost in the mind of the obstetrician planning an elective Caesarean section.
2. 'Wet lung syndrome' may be present where the baby has inhaled copious quantities of liquor. This may result in a

syndrome that is similar to hyaline membrane disease, but is usually less severe and prolonged. In a delivery by Caesarean section, 'wet lung syndrome' is more difficult to prevent.

3. Anaesthetic complications:

   (a) Postural hypotension is more prone to develop in the anaesthetized patient. Her muscles are paralysed, and the uterus presses on the inferior vena cava and the iliac veins. This reduces the venous return to the heart, impairs cardiac output, lowers the blood pressure and reduces uterine blood flow. The reduction in uterine blood flow often may be sufficient to cause severe distress or death to an already compromised fetus. The incidence and effect of postural hypotension may be reduced by shortening the time between induction of the anaesthetic and the delivery of the baby, and by tilting the patient, using a wedge under one side of her back.

   (b) Effects of the anaesthetic agents on the fetus. If time between the induction of anaesthesia and the delivery of the fetus is prolonged, then anaesthetic agents may depress the fetus, in particular its respiration. If a narcotic had been given prior to the anaesthetic or cyclopropane is used for maintenance of the anaesthetic, this effect is aggravated.

   (c) Complications occurring to the mother. In particular, the inhalation of gastric contents (Mendelson's syndrome), may result in severe hypotension and poor oxygenation.

2.10 ANAESTHESIA

General anaesthesia within the labour ward increases the risks to both the mother and child, as the anaesthetic is frequently associated with an emergency procedure and is performed in a room primarily designed for the delivery of the patient rather than the routine administration of general anaesthesia.

Epidural anaesthesia has replaced general anaesthesia for many procedures within the labour ward, because the mother is provided with pain relief and is still able to witness and cooperate in the birth of her child. Epidural anaesthesia may result in vasodilatation which is followed by hypotension; thus the position and hydration of the patient must be watched carefully to prevent reduced placental blood flow.

Local anaesthetic agents, sedatives and narcotic agents may reduce the short-term variation of the fetal heart rate. This is one of the parameters observed when monitoring an at-risk fetus in labour. Narcotic analgesics may also cause neonatal respiratory depression when they are given between 1 and 4 hours prior to the delivery.

2.11 VAGINAL DELIVERY

Vaginal delivery is not without its risks of trauma to the fetus. Intracranial haemorrhage may occur in association with a traumatic delivery, and is particularly predisposed to by hypoxia. Situations in which the fetus is particularly at risk are:

1. Breech delivery.
2. Pre-term infants, as the moulding of the head may be marked or occur over a short period of time. (With a rapid delivery, the cranial bones may spring apart when the vaginal pressure is released, resulting in the tearing of an intracranial vein.)
3. Forceful forceps delivery, where a great deal of traction is required to bring the head through the pelvis, may fracture the fetal skull. The difficult forceps delivery should be abandoned in favour of a Caesarean section, which would result in a lower morbidity and mortality.
4. Fractures of the fetal leg or arm can occasionally occur from incorrect manipulation during a breech delivery or excessive traction.
5. Internal version and breech extraction of a fetus is associated with a high perinatal morbidity and mortality and should only be performed in the management of the second twin.

3

Drug treatment in pregnancy

3.1 GENERAL INSTRUCTIONAL OBJECTIVE

The students are expected to learn the potential risk of prescription drugs in pregnancy and they should know which drugs are safe to prescribe during pregnancy and lactation.

3.2 SPECIFIC BEHAVIOURAL OBJECTIVES

1. Discuss the adverse effects of various exogenous hormones and drugs that may alter the physiological processes or cause abnormal development in a fetus.
2. Discuss the effects of analgesics and anaesthetic agents used in labour on the fetus.
3. Provide information and counselling about drug use in pregnancy and lactation.
4. Discuss the safety of drug treatment in lactating mothers.
5. Discuss the fetal and obstetric effects associated with narcotic use in pregnancy.

3.3 REASONS FOR LEARNING ABOUT DRUG TREATMENT IN PREGNANCY

One of the most frequently asked questions by pregnant women is whether certain drugs are safe for their fetus. Medical students should have knowledge about drugs that may have a harmful effect on the fetus. For some medical disorders in pregnancy, they should know the aternative treatments when there are adverse fetal effects of commonly used drugs.

Pregnant women may need assurance if they have taken or need to take drugs during their pregnancy. It is sometimes difficult to be certain about the safety of some of the newer drugs as the adverse side effects are usually noted from reports and experimental evidence accumulated over years and these may not yet be available. Under these circumstances and older and known safer drug should be used. Students should have a knowledge of which drugs are safe to use in pregnancy.

3.4 TERATOGENIC RISK

The teratogenic period in the humans is the first 10–12 weeks from the last menstrual period (LMP). The teratogenic effect of any drug is dependent on the timing of exposure as well as the teratogenic nature of the drug. If the exposure is before organogenesis (within approximately 31 days after LMP), an exposure to a teratogen may be embryocidal. If the pregnancy continues, there appears no increased risk of congenital anomalies. Exposure to a known teratogen in the early teratogenic period (<10 weeks) may result in congenital heart disease or neural tube defect. Late in the teratogenic period, i.e. about 10 weeks from LMP, exposure to a teratogenic drug will lead to malformation of the ear or palate. Although defects produced in the teratogenic period may be overt at birth, other important internal organ mal-developments or behavioural abnormalities may occur from continual exposure to drugs in other periods of pregnancy.

3.5 DRUG USE IN PREGNANCY

Drugs used by a mother may affect the developing fetus and neonate during pregnancy and lactation; therefore doctors should be able to advise a pregnant woman about the possible harmful effects of drugs in pregnancy and lactation. This chapter categorizes common drug groups and documents their known adverse effects, if any, on the developing fetus. In general, drugs that are believed to be safe in pregnancy and lactation are recommended if drug treatment needs to be instituted.

Drugs commonly used in medical conditions in pregnancy

Antibiotics

1. Penicillin and its derivatives are apparently safe in pregnancy. Newer penicillins should be used only when other alternatives are not available.

2. Cephalosporins have no known teratogenic effects. Erythromycin and nitrofurantoin are also safe when used during pregnancy as no adverse fetal effects have been reported.

3. Tetracycline may produce mottling and brown discoloration of neonatal teeth when it is used in the second or third trimester. Fetal exposure to tetracycline in the first trimester should be avoided as its safety has not been clearly established.

4. Sulphonamides are not teratogenic, but compete with bilirubin binding sites, thereby leading to increased risk of neonatal jaundice. Sulfamethoxazole with trimethoprim (Bactrim, Septrin) is safe for treatment of urinary tract infections in pregnancy and shows no increased risk of birth defects after exposure in the first trimester of pregnancy.

5. Aminoglycosides (streptomycin, kanamycin) may be ototoxic to the fetus.

6. Chloramphenicol is associated with 'grey syndrome', resulting with severe haemolytic anaemia and vascular collapse.

7. Metronidazole (Flagyl) is commonly used to treat anaerobic infections and trichomoniasis in pregnancy. There is no increase in congenital defects among the newborn. Its use at a high dose has been shown to be carcinogenic in animals, and some have recommended against its use in pregnancy. Use of metronidazole should be avoided therefore in the first trimester and the drug should only be given for clear-cut indications.

8. Antifungal creams (nystatin, chlotrimazole, miconazole) are not known to be associated with congenital anomalies.

Whenever possible, antibiotics with known adverse effects to the fetus or neonate should not be recommended. Alternative antibiotics of the same efficacy should be prescribed at a minimal effective dosage.

Anticonvulsants

Epileptic women taking anticonvulsants in pregnancy have twice the risk of having babies with a congenital abnormality than the general population. The malformation rate is about

4–6%, especially for cleft lip or palate and for congenital heart disease. However, the issue remains unresolved as to whether it is the epilepsy for which the drug is prescribed or the drug itself that has contributed to the defect.

1. Phenytoin and carbamazepine can cause fetal abnormality in up to 6% of exposed fetuses. They are associated with an increased incidence of congenital heart abnormalities, cleft lip or palate and diaphragmatic hernia. Phenytoin is also associated with an increased risk of a fetal hydantoin syndrome which consists of microcephaly, growth and mental retardation, and dysmorphic craniofacial features.
2. Sodium valproate may be associated with neural tube defects (1% risk).
3. Phenobarbitone may cause withdrawal symptoms in the neonate.
4. Diazepam (Valium) in a large dosage causes neonatal hypotonia, hypothermia, respiratory depression, lethargy, poor sucking, and diminished response to the environment.

For women who have been free from seizures for 1–2 years before pregnancy and who have normal electroencephalograms, withdrawal of anticonvulsant treatment before pregnancy should be considered. For a patient who is already pregnant, if the benefits of treatment outweigh the fetal risks, a minimal dosage monitored by therapeutic blood levels of the drug is recommended. Haemorrhagic diseases in the newborn are more common in mothers receiving anticonvulsants, because these drugs might affect vitamin K-dependent clotting factors. Intramuscular injection of vitamin K at birth for the infant is recommended.

Women on anticonvulsant therapy should start folic acid and vitamin K supplementation before conceiving and continue this throughout the pregnancy.

Antihypertensive drugs

1. Labetalol (Trandate) appears to be a good antihypertensive drug without known fetal risks. Propanolol (Inderal) had been used in the past and was thought to be associated with intrauterine growth retardation and fetal distress.

2. α-Methyldopa (Aldomet) and hydralazine (Apresoline) are safe and commonly used in pregnancy.
3. Thiazide diuretics further reduce the maternal plasma volume in pre-eclampsia without evidence of clinical improvement. They also cause fetal hyponatraemia, hypokalaemia and thrombocytopenic purpura. They should not be used.
4. Diazoxide is a fast, effective hypotensive agent. It may cause a profound and unpredictable fall in blood pressure. This should be used with caution in pregnancy. Fetal bradycardia and impaired carbohydrate metabolism have been reported.

Anti-thyroid drugs

1. Carbimazole and other anti-thyroid drugs such as propylthiouracil (PTU), methimazole (Tapazole) cross the placenta, and may cause fetal goitre, hypothyroidism in 2–5% of infants. If such conditions are severe, they lead to cretinism.
2. Radioactive ^{131}I is contraindicated in pregnancy as it may lead to neonatal goitre or complete ablation of fetal thyroid.

The goal of anti-thyroid treatment during pregnancy is to keep the mother slightly hyperthyroid to minimize drug exposure. PTU is the drug of choice in pregnancy because of its low incidence of adverse fetal effects.

Anti-asthmatic drugs

1. Bronchodilotors such as theophylline, terbutaline, salbutamol and aminophylline are all safe for treatment of asthma during pregnancy.
2. Adrenaline (epinephrine) use has been reported to cause minor fetal malformations in the first trimester of pregnancy.
3. Topical corticosteroid aerosols can be used safely during pregnancy.
4. Corticosteroid treatment for asthma during pregnancy has shown no increase in teratogenicity in humans, although cortisone may produce a minimal increase in the incidence

of cleft palates as suggested from animal studies. Prednisone and prednisolone are inactivated by the placenta and only 10% of these steroids cross the placenta. Their use is safe and their high maternal concentrations make them the drugs of choice to treat asthma during pregnancy.

Anti-psychotic drugs

1. Lithium increases the incidence of cardiovascular anomalies and causes respiratory depression, hypotonia, lethargy and poor feeding at birth. It is advisable to discontinue lithium to avoid fetal drug exposure. Tricycle antidepressants should be tried if continuous treatment is required during pregnancy.
2. Tranquilizers, including chlordiazepoxide (Librium), do not show any increased risk of anomalies. However, there are conflicting reports of the teratogenic risks of various tranquilizers.

Anticoagulants

1. Warfarin (Coumadin) if used in the first trimester may cause chondrodysplasia with nasal hypoplasia, bilateral optic atrophy and mental retardation. It occurs in about 3–5% of exposed pregnancies. In the third trimester there is a risk of haemorrhagic complications.
2. Heparin, should be used as an alternative because its large molecule does not cross the placenta. No adverse effects on the fetus have been reported.

Drugs for common colds

Although no known teratogenic effects have been reported with antihistamines and decongestants sold over the counter to treat common colds, other remedies, such as encouraging higher fluid intake and bed rest, should be recommended. If medications are necessary, a commonly used drug should be given alone for symptomatic relief because it is not known if adverse fetal effects will occur with any new preparation. Paracetamol and chlorpheniramine maleate are most often used to treat common colds in pregnancy.

Anti-cancer drugs

Alkylating agents and antimetabolites may lead to abortion and fetal abnormality. There is also a theoretical risk to the germ cells in the fetal gonads, leading to genetic damage in future generations.

Alcohol and narcotics

Despite their known deleterious effects, these drugs remain widely used by a small group of mothers with the problem of alcoholism and/or drug addiction.

1. Very small and occasional alcohol consumption is probably safe.
2. Fetal alcohol syndrome is seen in the neonates of mothers who drink heavily ($>80\,g$/day, equivalent to eight large glasses of wine or more) during pregnancy. The fetus may show growth retardation. The neonate may be mentally retarded and have characteristic facial features at birth – micrognathia, low set, unparallel ears, hypoplastic nose and short palpebral fissures.
3. Narcotics addiction has potential serious fetal complications. The associated risk of infection, social deprivation and lack of antenatal care result in an increased incidence of premature delivery, low birthweight, growth retardation and serious fetal compromise.
4. Narcotics have the effect of causing neonatal respiratory depression at birth.
5. Maternal withdrawal is rarely harmful to the mother, but neonates with severe withdrawal symptoms show hyperactivity, hypoxia, irritability, poor feeding and occasional fits.
6. The use of cocaine in pregnancy results in increased risk of congenital abnormalities like dysmorphic features and neurobehavioural abnormality.
7. Methadone, used in maintenance programmes for narcotic addicts, has not been associated with congenital anomalies in exposed fetuses. It may lead to milder withdrawal symptoms in the neonates at birth.

3.6 DRUG USE IN OBSTETRICS

Hormones

1. There appears little or no risk to the exposure of oral contraceptives in the first few weeks of pregnancy. There is a small risk that a female fetus may be virilized if exposed to an androgenic progesterone for a prolonged period in the first trimester.
2. Some synthetic progestogens (of the 19-nortestosterone group, which have mild androgenic effects) may produce clitoromegaly and labial fuson in female infants. Natural progesterone can be used with safety in some women who undergo *in vitro* fertilization and need luteal phase support in early pregnancy.
3. Oestrogen usage was once popular as a means to prevent early abortion. Diethylstilboestrol, which was once a common drug administered to the mother is known to produce vaginal adenosis leading to an increased risk of clear-cell carcinoma of the vagina in exposed adolescent girls. They may also affect normal development of the genital tract in both male and female offspring.
4. Danazol has been reported to cause clitoromegaly and labial fusion because of its androgenic effect.
5. With the introduction of very sensitive hormone pregnancy tests, i.e. a progesterone withdrawal bleed should not be used to diagnose pregnancy as progesterone may increase the risk of congenital abnormality, i.e. virilization in female fetuses (see 2 above).

Anaesthetic agents

1. Atropine was used as premedication before the induction of anaesthesia. Its anticholinergic action blocks vagal reflexes resulting in transient fetal tachycardia without beat-to-beat variability.
2. Use of ranitidine (Zantac) before Caesarean delivery helps to reduce gastric acidity. It is used in conjunction with metaclopramide, which increases the rate of gastric emptying and sodium citrate (0.3 M, 30 ml). This also helps to raise gastric pH.

3. Nitrous oxide (70%) and oxygen (30%) may result in fetal respiratory depression as a result of reduced maternal oxygen saturation. Use of pulse oximetry has minimized this risk. If the maternal O_2 saturation falls, the amount of nitrous oxide can be reduced. The longer the incision–delivery interval, the more likely it is to result in infant depression. The addition of halogenated anaesthetics (halothane, enflurane, methoxyflurane) can safety supplement 50% nitrous oxide–50% oxygen during general anaesthesia. No significant changes to maternal and neonatal conditions are noticed.

4. One research study suggested that female operating theatre personnel have a higher abortion rate than controls, though no specific causative anaesthetic agent has been named. Most operating theatres have scavaging systems to deal with anaesthetic gases.

5. Bupivacaine, mepivacaine and lidocaine epidural anaesthesia may produce a decrease in fetal motor strength and tone in some infants during the first few hours after birth if specifically tested for. No persistent neonatal neurobehavioural effects have been reported.

Analgesics

1. Aspirin may cause impaired clotting as a result of decreased platelet aggregation.

2. Acetaminophen (Tylenol, Datril) and paracetamol (Panadol) are acceptable alternative mild analgesics with no known teratogenecity. They are preferred to aspirin because they are less harmful to the newborn.

3. Excessive codeine can cause newborn withdrawal symptoms.

4. Narcotic analgesics, sedatives and tranquilizers may cause depression of the fetal respiratory centre.

Many mild analgesics are prostaglandin synthetase inhibitors which may delay the onset of spontaneous labour. There are reports of premature closure of the ductus arteriosus *in utero* associated with chronic use of aspirin.

Corticosteroids

Dexamethasone and betamethasone are minimally inactivated in placenta; therefore they cross the placenta and are used to accelerate fetal lung maturity. Teratogenic risk of using dexamethasone for this purpose has not been reported.

3.7 DRUG USE IN LACTATION

Many drugs can be detected in breast milk at a level which depends on the maternal blood levels, lipid solubility, molecular weight and protein binding. Table 3.1 shows the drugs commonly listed as contraindicated during breast-feeding. The risk of drug exposure to the neonate must be weighed against the benefit of breast-feeding. Many mothers would choose to avoid any exposure to known harmful drugs to their babies, but the use of these drugs would not in itself be considered a contraindication to breast-feeding. This is because the drug level in the milk is usually very low and no adverse effects in nursing infants have been reported with many drugs which have some theoretical risk.

Table 3.1 Drugs that are commonly contraindicated in lactating mothers

Drug	Adverse effects to the neonates
Chloramphenicol	Haemolytic anemia
Cimetidine	Suppresses gastric acidity
	CNS stimulant
Cytotoxic agents (cyclophosphamide, amethopterin)	Immune suppression
Ergotamine	Vomiting, diarrhoea, convulsion
Lithium	Lethargy, hypotonia, poor feeding
Tetracycline	Possible brown staining of teeth
Phenindione	Bleeding tendency

Table 3.2 Drugs that are known teratogens and have adverse fetal effects during pregnancy

Drug	Adverse fetal effects
A. In the first trimester	
Alcohol (chronic)	Fetal alcohol syndrome
Cytotoxic drug	Greatest risk with alkylating agents and anti-metabolites
Lithium	Cardiovascular anomalies
Phenytoin	Fetal phenytoin syndrome
Synthetic progestogens	Virilization of female fetus
Thalidomide	Phocomelia
Valproate	Neural tube defects
Warfarin	Limb defects, optic atrophy, deafness
B. In the second and third trimester	
Alcohol (large chronic dose)	Fetal alcohol syndrome
Analgesics	
Aspirin	Closure of ductus
Indomethacin	Closure of ductus
Narcotic analgesics	Respiratory depression and withdrawal syndrome
Antibiotics	
Streptomycin	Auditory and vestibular nerve damage
Chloramphenicol	'Grey' syndrome, vascular collapse
Tetracycline	Discolouring of primary and secondary dentition
Sulphonamide	Neonatal jaundice, kernicterus
Dapsone	Neonatal haemolysis
Anticoagulant drugs	
Warfarin	Neonatal haemorrhage
Anticonvulsive drugs	
Barbiturates	Prolonged depressant effects
Antihypertensive drugs	
Diazoxide	Fetal distress and impaired carbohydrate metabolism
Propranolol	Hyperglycaemia
Anti-psychotics	
Tricyclic antidepressants	Neonatal irritability, fits
Benzodiazepines	Hypotonia/hypothermia
Anti-thyroid drugs	
Iodides	Neonatal goitre and hypothyroidism
Diuretics	
Thiazides	Fetal hyponatraemia, hypokalaemia, thrombocytopenia
Hormones	
Progestogens	May produce virilization of the female fetus

3.8 SUMMARY

Care should be taken with the use of any drugs in pregnancy as long-term effects of drug exposure *in utero* may not be revealed until many years after birth. Doctors should possess an adequate knowledge about the use of drugs to cope with various disorders during pregnancy. Drugs that are known teratogens and have adverse fetal effects during pregnancy are listed in Table 3.2. No drug should be considered safe in early pregnancy. As always, the management should be directed toward prevention.

1. Drugs should be used only when necessary.
2. A risk–benefit ratio should be justified for any drug use.
3. A minimal effective dose should be employed.
4. If possible, drug treatment should be postponed until after the first trimester.
5. If in doubt, it is advisable to avoid the use of the drug and refer to specialists in that field.

4

Normal pregnancy

4.1 GENERAL INSTRUCTIONAL OBJECTIVE

The students should understand the anatomical, physiological and psychological changes consequent upon conception, so that they can diagnose and manage a normal pregnancy.

4.2 SPECIFIC BEHAVIOURAL OBJECTIVES

1. Discuss the physiological changes associated with normal implantation of a fertilized ovum.
2. Discuss the changes in female anatomy occurring during a normal pregnancy.
3. Discuss the symptoms that are presumptive of early pregnancy.
4. Perform a vaginal examination on a patient who is less than 14 weeks pregnant and describe the findings.
5. Correlate the uterine size with the period of gestation.
6. Specify the problems in determining the time of conception in relation to the date of the last menstrual period.
7. Discuss the origin and the effects of the endogenous hormones (oestrogen, progesterone, human placental lactogen, oxytocin, prostaglandins and chorionic gonadotrophin) in relation to the materno–fetal unit.
8. Discuss investigations and tests that are used to assess fetal well-being.
9. Palpate the abdomen of a patient after 28 weeks of gestation and accurately describe the lie, presentation, position and engagement of the fetus.
10. Discuss the relevance of specific antenatal investigations.
11. Take a history, examine a pregnant patient attending for a routine visit to the antenatal clinic, and discuss the findings.

12. Discuss physiological and emotional changes that may occur in pregnancy.
13. Discuss the relevance of nutrition and supplements during pregnancy.
14. Discuss counselling of patients on breast care, posture, diet, smoking, exercise, intercourse and drugs during pregnancy.
15. Identify and demonstrate an ability to manage the minor discomforts in pregnancy.
16. Discuss the counselling of a woman about her normal pregnancy.

4.3 REASONS FOR UNDERSTANDING THE NORMAL PREGNANCY

The most important concepts to be understood about the management of a normal pregnancy are the following:

1. It is a process that involves normal people who undergo numerous physical, physiological and psychological changes.
2. Medically speaking, the management of such a pregnancy is an exercise in preventive medicine.

Each piece of information gained during the pregnancy, either offered voluntarily by the patient or by specific interrogation or physical examination, should be evaluated with

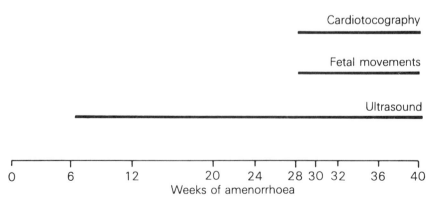

Figure 4.1 Ideal times to perform placental function tests.

these concepts in mind. There may not be an immediate use for this information; however, it may be invaluable later in pregnancy when a complication may arise or when labour commences (Fig. 4.1).

Failure to grasp these concepts can lead to uncertainty in the mind of the practitioner and in some instances, decisions may be made that will have adverse effects on the mother and her child.

The material in this chapter will provide information about the changes that occur in a woman during the course of her pregnancy and how this information can be applied to the advantage of all concerned.

4.4 PHYSIOLOGICAL CHANGES IN THE MOTHER

Blood and its components

In the course of a pregnancy, there is an increase in the total blood volume, the plasma volume and red cell mass (Table 4.1). The total blood volume increases by 30–40% by about 34 weeks. This is largely due to an increase in plasma volume (45%), while the red cell mass increases by 18%. This results in haemodilution, often incorrectly called a physiological anaemia (Fig. 4.2).

The white cell count increases from approximately 7000/mm^3 before pregnancy to 10 000–15 000/mm^3. This is due to an increase in neutrophils – the other cells do not increase. Platelets rise considerably from 180 000/mm^3 to over 300 000/mm^3, and this rise is doubled again in the puerperium.

The erythrocyte sedimentation rate (ESR) rises due to

Table 4.1 Blood volume changes

	Non-pregnant	*34 weeks*
Total blood volume (ml)	4000	5500
Plasma volume (ml)	2500	3750
Red cell volume (ml)	1500	1750
Haemoglobin (g)	492	597

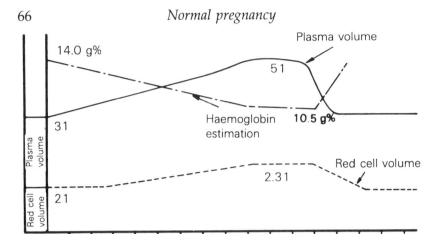

Figure 4.2 Showing that as the pregnancy advances both the circulating red cell mass and the plasma volume increase, but as the plasma volume increases by up to 50%, the haemoglobin concentration appears to fall.

increased fibrinogen and globulin levels. The plasma protein changes are shown in Table 4.2. All lipid fractions increase, while there is a fall in the levels of all electrolytes associated with haemodilution.

Table 4.2 Plasma protein alterations during pregnancy

Protein	Change
Total protein	Rises
Total protein concentration	Falls (due to haemodilution)
Albumin: globulin ratio	Falls
Albumin: α, α2 and β	Falls
Globulins: α, α2 and β	Rise (transport globulins)
Gamma globulins	No change
Fibrinogen	Rises (25–50% increases)
Clotting Factors 1,2,5,7,8,9,10,12	Rise

Table 4.3 Cardiac blood output

Condition	Output (l/min)
Non-pregnant	4.5
Pregnant	6.7
1st stage of labour	8.0
2nd stage of labour	9.0

Cardiovascular system

The main changes relate to increased cardiac output, which is produced by an increase in both heart rate and stroke volume. Peripheral resistance falls and as a result blood pressure usually remains steady throughout pregnancy, or frequently it may fall below pre-pregnancy levels during midpregnancy.

The cardiac output increases by 30–60% during pregnancy. Most of this increase occurs by the end of the first trimester, then slowly rising to 28 weeks, and is maintained to term. Further increases in cardiac output occur during labour (Table 4.3). During the first stage, a 30% increase occurs, while in the second stage an even greater output can be measured during bearing down.

Supine hypotension

During late pregnancy, a fall in blood pressure and a feeling of faintness occurs in some 10% of women who lie supine. This is due to vena caval compression by the enlarging uterus in the presence of a poor paravertebral collateral circulation. The resultant fall in venous return reduces the cardiac output, and thus also a fall in blood pressure. Women in late pregnancy and labour should **never** be flat on their backs.

Regional blood flow changes

The regional blood flow to the liver and brain does not significantly alter during pregnancy, but the uterine blood flow increases ten-fold: from 50 ml/min in early pregnancy to 500 ml/min at term. The renal blood flow increases by 30%,

renal plasma flow by 45% and glomerular filtration rate by up
to 50%. However, because tubular reabsorption is unaltered,
the clearance of many solutes (for example, urea, uric acid and
glucose) is increased.

Metabolic changes

Metabolic changes in pregnancy are complex, and currently
under much investigation. There is a general increase in the
metabolic rate, largely due to fetal demands. Oxygen consumption rises by 20%, and the thyroid gland hypertrophies in
perhaps 70% of patients.

Carbohydrate metabolism is affected by human placental lactogen during pregnancy. This hormone antagonizes the action
of insulin, breaks down body fat, and thus acts towards the
elevation of blood glucose levels. As a result, insulin rises to

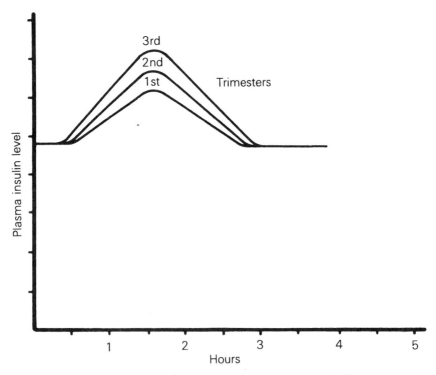

Figure 4.3 Plasma insulin level to a glucose test meal. Pancreatic stimulation by glucose during the third trimester is maximal due to the
inhibiting effect of placental lactogen.

even higher levels, so increasing glucose utilization but restricting any abnormal blood levels (Fig. 4.3). The increased demand on the pancreas may at this stage uncover a latent diabetic.

Protein metabolism shows an overall positive nitrogen balance, and about 500 g of protein are retained by term. Thus a high protein diet is required during pregnancy.

Fat is the main form of maternal energy store during pregnancy, mostly in the form of depot fat. Blood lipid also increases significantly. It is important to note that because glycogen stores are low, any major stress will draw quickly on fat for energy and so ketosis may occur.

The average total body weight gain should be about 12.5 kg (28 lb), the main increase being in the second half of the pregnancy.

4.5 FERTILIZATION

Pregnancy occurs following the fertilization of an ovum by a sperm. The ovum usually survives for no longer than 24 hours. Sperm can survive for up to 48–72 hours. Thus conception is unlikely to occur unless coitus occurs within 1–2 days of ovulation.

The sex of a child is determined at fertilization, and depends on whether the ovum is fertilized by an X sperm or a Y sperm. Some workers believe that the sex of the child can be predetermined by the timing of coitus: X sperms live longer than Y sperms, and it is said that intercourse prior to ovulation is likely to produce a female, while intercourse at the time of ovulation favours a male. However, this remains unproven.

Following fertilization, cell division ensues within 24 hours. Each daughter cell contains genetic material from both parents. By the third or fourth day the morula is formed, which then becomes partly cystic. By the seventh day a single layered, fluid-filled cyst, with a solid collection of cells in one area of its wall, is formed – this is the blastocyst. The solid area (the inner cell mass) forms the fetus, while the cyst wall becomes the trophoblast. This trophoblast differentiates into an inner layer (cytotrophoblast) and an outer layer (syncytiotrophoblast) (Figs 4.4 and 4.5), after which the blastocyst can attach to the endometrium and gain nourishment from it.

Proliferation continues to occur in the inner cell mass and

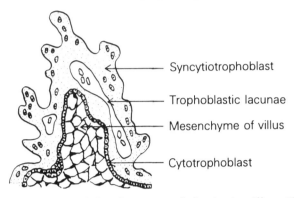

Figure 4.4 Early stage of development of chorionic villus. The trophoblast has separated into two cellular layers – the syncytiotrophoblast and the cytotrophoblast. There is a coalescence of lacunae which contain a few red cells. A mesenchymal core is beginning to form.

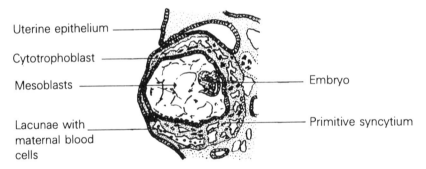

Figure 4.5 An early human embryo which is differentiating into syncytial cytotrophoblastic and mesoblastic tissue. Lacunae are forming in the syncytium and maternal red cells can be identified in the tissue which will form the placenta.

two further cysts are derived from it. The cyst lying peripherally and adjacent to the trophoblast becomes the amniotic cavity, while that lying centrally becomes the yolk sac. Separating these two structures is a cellular layer containing ectoderm and mesoderm, derived from the amnion and endoderm of the yolk sac. From these primitive cells (present by the seventh day) the fetus and umbilical cord will develop.

Simultaneously, the trophoblast has developed villous tufts on its outer surface, which give it a fluffy appearance. Each villus is penetrated by a central core of mesenchyme – the tro-

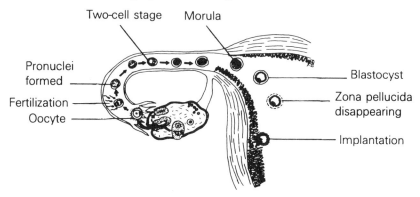

Figure 4.6 Passage of the fertilized egg through tube to implantation in decidua (6 days).

phoblast becomes the chorion and the villi are now chorionic villi. This occurs by the 14th day. By the 21st day blood vessels have formed in the mesenchyme of the villi, body stalk (cord) and embryo. The villi eventually disappear from the surface of the blastocyst, with the exception of the area adjacent to the endometrium; this will form the placenta.

The blastocyst is usually embedded in the endometrium by the sixth and seventh day following fertilization (Fig. 4.6), and commences to secrete minute quantities of human chorionic gonadotrophin (HCG), which is both luteinizing and luteo-trophic. This maintains the corpus luteum, producing oestrogen and progesterone; the endometrium becomes decidua and ame-norrhoea begins.

4.6 SYMPTOMS AND SIGNS DETECTED DURING PREGNANCY

Rise in basal temperature

Progesterone, released from the follicle after ovulation, is ther-mogenic. A persistent elevation of basal temperature for longer than 14 days is presumptive evidence of pregnancy.

Pregnancy test

When performed on early-morning samples of urine, the tests can indicate the presence of HCG as early as 14 days after ferti-lization. However, false negative results may occur if the urine is dilute. False positive results can occur due to cross-reaction with luteinizing hormone (LH). A more specific and reliable test is by means of radioimmunoassay of the beta subunit of the HCG molecule in the serum, usually present by the 10–14th day after fertilization.

Amenorrhoea

This occurs secondary to the luteotrophic and luteinizing effects of HCG which leads to the continuing production of progesterone. However, bleeding can occur from the decidua in very early pregnancy, as the gestation sac does not completely fill the uterus until 12 weeks of amenorrhoea.

Nausea

Although nausea during pregnancy is traditionally called 'morning sickness', it may occur at any time during the day or night – and may, in fact, occur throughout both. It usually disappears by 12 weeks of amenorrhoea, but may persist longer, even throughout pregnancy. Occasionally it can recur in late pregnancy. The nausea experienced by some pregnant women is presumably associated with the appearance of new hormones, or the increased levels of hormones, that occur during pregnancy. It can occur in the absence of a fetus, as for example in the presence of a hydatidiform mole or an anembryonic pregnancy. Occasionally, severe vomiting may occur, and hospitalization and rehydration are then indicated. Both multiple pregnancies and hydatiform moles are associated with exaggerated nausea and vomiting.

Breast changes

Increases in size, vascularity and heaviness may all be early symptoms of pregnancy. The breasts, especially the nipples, many become sensitive or even painful to touch or pressure. These changes are presumed to be due to the effects of oestrogen, progesterone and possibly human placental lactogen (HPL). The areola enlarges and becomes darker, as does the nipple. Montgomery's tubercles become prominent. Colostrum usually appears spontaneously by the 28th week, but may be expressed as early as the 16th week of amenorrhoea.

Bladder symptoms

Frequency, both diurnal and nocturnal, usually commences in about the sixth week and subsides in the middle trimester. These symptoms are due to bladder hyperaemia and irritation of the bladder by the pressure from the enlarging uterus.

Frequency commonly recurs late in pregnancy and is due to bladder compression by the uterus and the presenting part of the fetus. Urinary stress incontinence is a common symptom during pregnancy, which almost always subsides during the puerperium.

Uterine changes

The cervix softens and may become bluish, secondary to oestrogen-induced increased vascularity. The normal cervical and vaginal discharge increases in amount. The uterus enlarges steadily, but its shape may be irregular in early pregnancy due to implantation in one particular site in the uterus.

Palpable uterine enlargement is best compared with everyday objects:

- Small lemon size: 6–8 weeks
- Orange size: 8–10 weeks
- Grapefruit size: 12–14 weeks

Hegar's sign is difficult to elicit and uncomfortable for the patient; it should not be used.

At about 12 weeks the uterus is usually palpable above the symphysis pubis in a woman of average build whose uterus is anteverted or anteflexed. Thereafter, the uterus enlarges rapidly and reaches the umbilicus at about 22–24 weeks of amenorrhoea.

Vaginal and vulval changes

Due to increased vascularity, the vaginal epithelium becomes darker and vaginal secretion increases.

Abdominal discomfort

This may take a variety of forms. In early pregnancy the woman may experience the feelings she normally has with the menstruation but, of course, there is no bleeding. A feeling of distension and tightness of clothing is common, even in the absence of obvious abdominal enlargement.

Brief sharp pains are often experienced in one of the iliac fossae, and may continue during pregnancy. In early pregnancy they may be due to the presence of the corpus luteum. The reason for these pains in late pregnancy is not clearly understood, but they are usually explained as being due to 'pressure', 'uterine enlargement', and other such general causes.

Fetal movement (quickening)

Fetal heart movements can be detected using ultrasound at 7 weeks. Fetal body movements can also be seen at 8/9 weeks on ultrasound. In a primigravid patient, movement is first felt as a 'fluttering' or 'wind' at about 18–20 weeks. After that time, definite movements are noticed. In the multigravida who is familiar with the sensation, movements are commonly noticed from about the 16–18th week onwards.

The most common form of antenatal fetal monitoring is by charting the fetal movements perceived by the mother.

Audible fetal heart sounds

These may be detected as early as 24 weeks with a monaural stethoscope – of course, with a Doppler they can be detected at 14 weeks or even earlier.

Palpable fetal parts

Depending on the thickness of the patient's anterior abdominal wall and the position of the placenta, fetal parts may be palpable abdominally from the 22–24th week onwards.

Changes in the skin and subcutaneous tissues

Brownish pigmentation of the nipples and areola occur early in pregnancy. Later, the linea nigra develops in the midline between the umbilicus and pubic hair. Patchy brown discoloration of the facial skin – known as chloasma – may also develop in some women.

Fat deposition occurs, especially over the buttocks, thighs and upper arms. Sebaceous secretion may increase and skin lesions, especially acne-form types, may curiously be either exacerbated or diminished. Cutaneous haemangiomas may develop; presumably these are secondary to high oestrogen levels.

Striae gravidarum may develop on the skin of the abdomen, buttocks, thighs and breasts. Their formation is frequently preceded and accompanied by pruritus. Striae are due to changes in the deeper layers of the skin and initially are red or purple in colour. However, they fade with time to a silver colour, and are then relatively inconspicuous.

Other symptoms

Giddiness and faintness, and at times even fainting, may occur during pregnancy, especially in crowded, stuffy rooms. Epistaxis and bleeding from the gums may occur in late pregnancy. The gums may hypertrophy to a small extent. Headaches (usually 'tension' headaches) are not uncommon in the first half of pregnancy. Although they do not respond to commonly used analgesics, diazepam (Valium) is effective.

Muscular cramps are reasonably common after the 24th week, and may respond to muscle stretching exercises or calcium lactate (300 mg t.i.d.) or diazepam. The cause of these cramps is unknown. Backache, especially sacroiliac pain, is common in late pregnancy, particularly in multigravidas. This is attributed to altered posture and the softening of the pelvic ligaments that occurs in late pregnancy. A maternity girdle may be helpful.

Constipation is a common occurrence during pregnancy due to the effect of progesterone on the smooth muscle of the colon. A diet containing fruit, bran and cereals may be helpful.

Varicose veins and haemorrhoids may also occur, especially where there is a family history of these complaints. They are due to the effect of progesterone on the musuclaris coat of veins, and the increased venous pressure in the lower part of the body as the uterus enlarges and compresses the inferior vena cave. Supportive stockings are most helpful in relieving any discomfort, and their prophylactic use should be recommended to women with positive family history.

Psychological changes

A variety of psychological changes also occurs. In the early stages of pregnancy a feeling of dejection may occur, especially if the discomforts of pregnancy are great – a 'cheated' feeling is not uncommon. As pregnancy progresses, a number of women feel extremely well and active.

In late pregnancy, when it is more difficult to move quickly or to bend and stoop, the woman feels cumbersome. As her abdomen enlarges and her weight increases, she may feel unattractive. The patient finds it difficult to become comfortable, especially at night, so that sleeping is disrupted. These problems often provoke a feeling of 'I wish it were all over'. The expression of such feelings must never be seen by obstetricians as an opportunity to offer elective induction.

Sexuality may also alter during pregnancy: for some women libido increases, while for others it may decrease. Provided there is no vaginal bleeding or other contraindication like a cervical suture, intercourse need not be restricted.

During pregnancy a woman will undergo a tremendous number of physical, physiological and psychological changes. She may be able to cope with all of them or very few. The obstetrician must always be willing to answer any questions the couple may have and, when necessary, to offer help and reassurance. Patient education is very important, for both the patient and the doctor, because a lot of time is saved by answering questions fully and by explaining what is likely to occur.

4.7 THE FIRST ANTENATAL VISIT

The routine for taking the history is described in Chapter 1. Remember that this is the best time to establish rapport with the patient. On the first visit the diagnosis of pregnancy is usually established: and the patient's memory is then also most clear as to recent events, especially her last normal menstrual period. This is the time to recognize current or previous illness, or other factors that could influence the course of the pregnancy and labour.

The majority of risk factors related to a pregnancy can be established at this first visit. These factors include:

1. Age: younger than 16 or older than 35.
2. Parity: grand multiparity (fifth or subsequent pregnancy).
3. Poor economic circumstances.
4. Drug taking: smoking, salicylates, methadone, amphetamines, heroin and alcohol.
5. Poor obstetric history: infertility, recurrent abortion, premature labour, stillbirths and neonatal deaths.
6. Previous postpartum or antepartum haemorrhage.
7. Previous Caesarean section or difficult delivery.
8. Chronic maternal disease: hypertension, renal disease, cardiac disease, anaemia, diabetes mellitus and other endocrine disorders.
9. Short stature: problems with cephalopelvic disproportion if 152 cm or less.
10. Rhesus iso-immunization.

A general physical and pelvic examination are performed at the first visit. The uterine size is assessed and correlated with the stated period of amenorrhoea. The presence of other pelvic tumours is sought, as these may produce problems during a pregnancy or obstruction during labour. Their detection and removal (if they are ovarian tumours) can forestall many complications. Pelvimetry is not performed at this stage. The cervix is inspected and a cervical smear taken.

Advice should be given at this stage about obvious avoidable factors:

1. Obesity. The overweight woman should be given a low-kilojoule (calorie) diet when seen early in pregnancy, as obesity is a risk factor of pregnancy.
2. Smoking. Women who smoke more than ten cigarettes per day are more likely to produce babies of lower birthweight than women who do not smoke at all. They are also more likely to come into labour pre-term, and statistically are more likely to have a stillborn baby or neonatal death.
3. Medications. The pregnant woman should be told that all drugs cross the placenta, so medications should only be taken after ensuring their lack of harmful effect on the fetus. She should be warned about taking excessive amounts of analgesic or tranquilizing drugs.
4. Alcohol should be avoided during pregnancy. Fortunately many women become intolerant to alcohol while pregnant.

4.8 SUBSEQUENT VISITS

A healthy primigravida should be seen every 4 weeks until 28 weeks, then fortnightly until 36 weeks and thereafter weekly until confinement. The visits between 28 and 32 weeks are especially important because at this stage multiple pregnancy is most likely to be diagnosed, and pre-eclampsia can be detected.

During antenatal visits:

1. All her questions should be satisfactorily answered.
2. General enquiries should be made about health, fetal movement, vaginal discharge, bleeding or pain.
3. Weight, blood pressure and fundal height should be recorded. After 28 weeks the lie, presentation and position of the fetus are checked, as are the fetal heart sounds.
4. Oedema is looked for.
5. Urinalaysis is performed.

If after 38 weeks the head is not engaged in a primigravid and doubt exists regarding the capacity of the pelvis, or if a breech presentation persists after 36 weeks, X-ray pelvimetry may be ordered but rarely contributes to the management.

4.9 GENERAL ADVICE

The woman should be encouraged to pursue her normal activities, but to avoid obviously hazardous activities such as water-skiing, horse-riding or body surfing. Sexual intercourse is permissible up to the onset of labour if there are no contra-indications such as antepartum haemorrhage and/or premature labour. Achieving orgasm during pregnancy is not harmful, and this can be done in late pregnancy by oral sex or masturbation if so desired.

Advice should also be given about diet, iron and vitamin supplements and what facilities are available for childbirth education and breast care. Iron supplement should be given to all pregnant women from the beginning of the second trimester until they cease breast feeding.

Diet

Extra nutrition is required during pregnancy, as the mother's

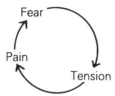

Figure 4.7 Illustrating how fear, pain and tension produce a vicious circle of activity.

basal metabolic rate rises and the needs of the fetus and mother increase.

The usual nutritional requirement in pregnancy is about 10 500 kilojoules (2500 calories) daily, with a distribution of approximately 100 g protein, 100 g fat and 300 g carbohydrate. More specific diets can be found in booklets which are easily accessible. Calcium supplements are necessary. If the woman dislikes dairy products, calcium tablets can be taken. Fluoride unless present in drinking water should be taken during the second half of pregnancy.

Childbirth education

In more recent times, the concept put forward by Grantley Dick-Read (Fig. 4.7) has gained wide acceptance. Programmes aimed at educating parents about pregnancy and labour, coupled with the teaching of relaxation techniques, have done much to allay the anxiety of pregnant women. Apart from the more conventional programmes offered by hospitals, alternative methods of education and relaxation by methods such as psychoprophylaxis have much to offer.

4.10 ESTIMATION OF THE DATE OF CONFINEMENT

Over the last 150 years the method mostly used to determine the estimated date of confinement (EDC) is Naegel's method, which allows for an average pregnancy of 280 days from the commencement of the last menstrual period (LMP).

A quick calculation can be made of the expected date of confinement, by adding 7 days and 9 months to the first day of the LMP. This assumes, however, that every woman has a regular cycle and ovulates on the 14th day of her cycle. Allowance must be made for cycle length, e.g.

28-day cycle	LNMP 10-5-94	EDC 17-2-95
24-day cycle	LNMP 10-5-94	EDC 13-2-95
35-day cycle	LNMP 10-5-94	EDC 24-2-95
42-day cycle	LNMP 10-5-94	EDC 3-3-95

One must also be cautious when the LMP is a withdrawal bleed associated with an oral contraceptive as ovulation is frequently delayed in such an instance. Bleeding at the time of implantation and early threatened abortion is also a source of confusion, and so the duration of amenorrhoea must always be compared to the uterine size. If there is any doubt about the LMP, then an ultrasound examination is indicated.

4.11 INVESTIGATIONS PERFORMED DURING PREGNANCY

At the initial visit the following tests are made:

1. Blood tests
    (a) Haemoglobin: an initial screening to detect anaemia. If it is found, further investigations should ensue to determine the nature of the anaemia. Anaemic women are more likely to produce babies of low birthweight and they tolerate antepartum and postpartum haemorrhages poorly.
    (b) Blood grouping: ABO and Rhesus (Rh) grouping.
    (c) Antibody screen: all patients (both Rh +ve and Rh –ve) should be screened. Antibodies that can cause haemolytic disease may occur in Rh +ve women (e.g. Kell). In addition, antibodies such as anti-Lewis may be detected, which may produce difficulties with the crossmatching of blood.
    (d) Rubella antibody titre: a titre of 1 in 20 or greater is evidence of previous rubella infection. The test also provides a baseline for future comparison in the unprotected if infection is suspected.
    (e) VDRL: a screening test for syphilis. Untreated syphilis can cause congenital infection of the fetus which, if recognized antenatally is readily treated. If a positive VDRL is found, further investigations should be performed to ensure that it is not a false positive.

    (f) Hepatitis B is screened for since antigen-positive women are a risk not only to those involved in their care, but also their newborn.

    (g) Hepatitis C: This is highly infectious and staff coming in contact with body fluids may be at risk.

2. Urine tests

    (a) Routine urinalaysis: traditionally an early-morning specimen of urine tested to exclude orthostatic proteinuria. If protein is found, a midstream specimen of urine should be tested to exclude contamination by vaginal secretions.

    (b) Bacilluria screening test: 6% of pregnant women have asymptomatic bacilluria. If untreated, up to one-third of these women may develop acute pyelonephritis during pregnancy. This can be prevented by detection and treatment. Some workers claim a higher incidence of low birthweight babies and pre-term labours among women with untreated asymptomatic bacilluria.

3. Cervical smear. This will ensure that any overt cervical lesion is noted.

At 28 and 36 weeks a haemoglobin estimation, and Rhesus screen should be performed.

Tests of fetal well-being

Even in a normal pregnancy, obstetricians may wish to perform investigations to ensure that all is well. Often, the uterus appears to be either too large or too small for the period of amenorrhoea. The best investigation to perform is an ultrasound examination, which can measure fetal size, confirm or deny the presence of a multiple pregnancy, and give information about the placental site and amniotic fluid volume.

Fundal height

It is also helpful to regularly measure the symphysial fundal height at each antenatal visit. Less than expected growth may indicate intrauterine growth retardation and is an indication for a further ultrasound examination.

Cardiotocography

During late pregnancy, the fetal heart rate (FHR) can be monitored by using an ultrasonic transducer applied to the mother's abdominal wall, and uterine contractions can be recorded by an external transducer. Variations in the FHR may be noted in response to Braxton–Hicks contractions if the ability of the fetal cardiovascular system to compensate is diminished, such as a prolonged pregnancy, hypertension or antepartum haemorrhage.

The information obtained from measurements of FHR can be used, in conjunction with clinical findings and other measurements of fetal well-being, to determine the optimal time for delivery in certain situations where the fetus may be at risk.

4.12 PLACENTAL FUNCTION

1. Respiratory exchange.
2. Nutrition.
3. Hormone production.
4. In certain situations, it acts as a barrier to abnormal environmental agents.

The first two functions require transport of substances to and fro across the placenta, and to achieve this four types of transport mechanisms have been described: simple diffusion (e.g. of oxygen); facilitated diffusion (e.g. of glucose); active transport (e.g. of amino acids); and special processes, such as pinocytosis (e.g. leakage of large molecules up to cellular size) and iron transport.

The concept that the placenta acts as a barrier to protect the fetus from damaging agents has been shown to be largely incorrect. Apart from the rubella virus, vaccinia, Cytomegalovirus (CMV) and Cendehill virus have all been shown to cross the placenta. In addition, *Toxoplasma gondii*, *Mycobacterium tuberculosis*, *Treponema pallidum* and malarial parasites may also reach the fetus. In the case of *Treponema*, however, there is protection up to the 16th week, before which time no case of congenital syphilis has been reported.

All drugs, except heparin, some muscle relaxants and a small proportion of insulin cross the placenta. Drugs such as thalido-

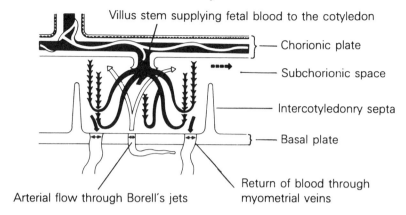

Figure 4.8 Haemodynamics of the placenta. Approximately 500–700 ml of maternal blood enter the placental 'lake' each minute, spurting like an intermittent fountain to reach the chorionic plate before diffusing back past fetal villi and finally out through maternal sinuses in the decidua.

mide have been proven to produce fetal malformations, while several other drugs have been linked by strong circumstantial evidence. Although it is possible that the placenta may prevent potential teratogens from reaching the fetus, it is probably wiser to exclude fetal protection as a placental function.

Haemodynamics of placental blood flow (Fig. 4.8)

There is a gradually increasing flow of blood through the utero-placental unit until, by the 32nd week, the amount of blood passing through the placenta each minute reaches 500–700ml. Any reduction in this placental blood flow (exercise, spasm of arteries or fibrin deposition) may interfere with the nutritional transfer mechanisms of the placenta. Thus, infants born to mothers who suffer from a reduced placental blood flow will have reduced levels of glucose and glycogen, amino acids and protein, and fatty acids. These infants are often described as being dysmature and have reduced chances of survival.

Hormonal functions of the placenta

Two types of hormones are associated with the placenta:

1. Protein hormones
   (a) Human chorionic gonadotrophin (HCG).
   (b) Human placental lactogen (HPL)
   (c) Other, less well-understood hormones such as human chorionic thyrotrophin and pregnancy-specific β-globulin.

These hormones are never found in the absence of trophoblastic tissue and they are transferred directly to the maternal circulation; very small amounts are found in fetal blood. They consist of two basic units, alpha and beta, the latter giving the hormone its specificity.

2. Steroid hormones
   (a) Progesterone
   (b) Oestrogens

Although progesterone is produced by the placenta, the oestrogens are not. In pregnancy the major oestrogen is oestriol. The placenta does not possess all the enzymes necessary to synthesize oestriol, but suitable enzymes in the fetal liver and adrenals enable this synthesis to occur. Because of the contributions from both the fetus and placenta, the concept of the feto–placental unit was put forward in relation to estriol biosynthesis.

Human chorionic gonadotrophin

HCG is a glycoprotein, and its exact site of formation within the placenta is still uncertain. Similar HCG concentrations are found in the placenta, maternal blood and urine from the 11th day after ovulation, and urinary excretion reaches a peak level between 11 and 12 weeks of amenorrhoea, and then declines.

The main action of HCG is maintenance of the corpus luteum (luteotrophic action), until the placenta produces sufficient progesterone after the 10th week of pregnancy. Higher than normal levels of HCG are found when more trophoblast is present (e.g. in multiple pregnancy or hydatidiform mole).

The main clinical use of HCG is in the diagnosis of pregnancy and trophoblastic tumours, and in monitoring the response of the latter to treatment. HCG determinations in the management of threatened abortion is of no use, as levels will persist while there is retained placental tissue and for many days after its removal.

Human placental lactogen

HPL is a polypeptide, and is immunologically and chemically similar to human growth hormone (HGH). It is produced by the syncytiotrophoblast and levels increase steadily to term. After labour, the HPL level falls rapidly. The major functions of HPL include:

1. Diversion of glucose from the mother to the fetus.
2. Mobilization of fat stores in the mother.
3. Nitrogen retention.
4. Effects on the breast and a role in the initiation of lactation.
5. Antagonistic action to maternal insulin.

There is virtually no clinical application for HPL assays.

Progesterone

Plasma concentrations of progesterone rise rapidly after conception. Although progesterone is initially produced by the corpus luteum, the placenta soon becomes the sole source. The effects of progesterone include:

1. Reduction of uterine activity.
2. Reduction of smooth muscle tone generally (e.g. of the stomach, colon, ureter and blood vessels).
3. Thermogenic. The basal temperature is raised after ovulation and thereafter.
4. Stimulation of growth of breast alveoli.
5. There is some evidence to show that a fall in progesterone precedes the spontaneous onset of labour.

There is no practical value currently in estimating progesterone levels during pregnancy.

Oestrogens

The three major oestrogens found during pregnancy are oestriol, oestradiol and oestrone – and of these, oestriol is the most important quantitatively. Precursors from the fetal adrenals undergo changes in the fetal liver and in the placenta, and ultimately are excreted in the mother's urine as oestriol.

Urinary oestriol excretion has been exhaustively studied, and plasma oestriols have recently been found to have a similar significance. Oestriol levels rise steadily after the 10th week to term. The actions of oestrogens during pregnancy are considered to be:

1. Stimulation of protein synthesis at a cellular level.
2. Myometrial hypertrophy, to accommodate the enlarging conceptus.
3. Fluid retention, especially by increasing the hygroscopic properties of collagen and other connective tissues.
4. Alteration of serum protein levels.
5. Stimulation of growth of the breast duct system.
6. Increase in uterine blood vessel diameter.

There is no practical value currently in estimating oestrogen levels during pregnancy.

5

Deviations from normal
pregnancy

5.1 GENERAL INSTRUCTIONAL OBJECTIVE

The students should recognize deviations from normal pregnancy and understand their effects on mother and fetus so that they can initiate management.

5.2 SPECIFIC BEHAVIOURAL OBJECTIVES

1. Identify abnormalities of uterine size and shape, or lie and presentation of the fetus, by clinical examination of the abdomen of a pregnant patient, and discuss their significance.
2. Identify by history and examination the causes of vaginal bleeding in early pregnancy and discuss their significance.
3. Examine and counsel a patient with vaginal bleeding in early pregnancy.
4. Identify by history and clinical examination the differences between placenta praevia, accidental haemorrhage and bleeding due to other causes.
5. Discuss the principles of the immediate management of the patient with antepartum haemorrhage.
6. Identify hypertension, proteinuria, oedema and abnormal weight gain in a pregnant patient and discuss their significance.
7. Discuss the investigation of suspected fetal growth retardation.
8. Describe the application, risks and information to be derived from the use of amniocentesis, radiology and ultrasound in pregnancy.

9. Discuss the significance and management of urinary tract infection in pregnancy.
10. Discuss the significance of heart disease in pregnancy.
11. Discuss the significance of glycosuria and diabetes in pregnancy.
12. Diagnose clinically, and with the aid of laboratory studies, the presence of anaemia in pregnancy and indicate appropriate therapy.
13. Discuss the management of rhesus iso-immunization in pregnancy and stress the prophylaxis.
14. Discuss the symptoms, signs, significance and management of convulsions and their prodromata in pregnancy and the puerperium.
15. Describe the causes of threatened premature labour in a patient and discuss her management.
16. Counsel and provide emotional support where necessary to a patient with an abnormal pregnancy.
17. Identify medical and psychiatric conditions in pregnant patients that necessitate specialist care.

5.3 REASONS FOR STUDYING DEVIATIONS FROM NORMAL PREGNANCY

Two factors should be borne in mind:

1. Deviations from normal may occur due to disease processes present in the mother before conception. Knowledge of these conditions will enable the practitioner to seek advice early and form a plan of management. As with normal pregnancies, the aim should be the prevention of complications.
2. The majority of problems that occur, however, are *not* associated with pre-existing conditions. Once again, their incidence can be reduced by thoughtful observation of and advice to the pregnant patient.

Most complications that occur during pregnancy can either be eliminated or at least minimized by careful antenatal care. Where complications do arise, they should be recognized **because** they are deviations from normal. If this concept (i.e. deviation from normal) is followed, complications will be detected earlier and so risks to the mother and fetus can be minimized.

Remember, obstetrics is an exercise in preventive medicine.

5.4 BLEEDING IN LATE PREGNANCY

Bleeding from the genital tract after the 20th week of pregnancy is referred to as antepartum haemorrhage (APH). The significance of this condition lies in its importance as a cause of maternal mortality and morbidity, and in its contribution to perinatal mortality.

Classification of APH

1. Abruptio placentae or accidental haemorrhage (Fig. 5.1). The word 'accidental' refers to bleeding occurring by chance (or by accident) and refers to bleeding related to a placenta that is normally situated in the upper segment of the uterus. Accidental haemorrhage (abruptio placentae) is the condition present when bleeding occurs from the decidua, behind the placenta, i.e. from the mother. If the

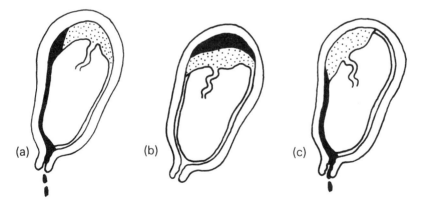

Figure 5.1 (a) Partial detachment following retroplacental haemorrhage followed by external blood loss; (b) Complete detachment following retroplacental haemorrhage near the centre of the placental attachment site – no external blood loss; (c) Marginal blood with little detachment of the placenta, but early bleeding seen externally.

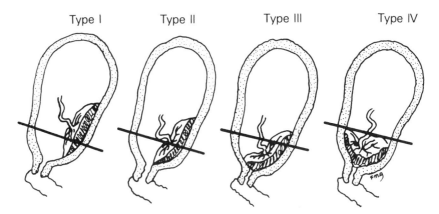

Figure 5.2 Anatomical classification of placenta praevia. Type I, a minor portion of the placenta lies below the lower uterine segment. Type II, most of the placenta lies below the lower uterine segment, but the placenta does not cover the internal os. Type III, the placenta covers the internal os when the os is closed but not when dilated. Type IV, the placenta completely covers the internal os, even when dilated.

blood tracks down behind the membranes and appears through the cervix it may be described as 'revealed', but if it remains retroplacental it is described as 'concealed'. Occasionally it may be mixed, when there is retroplacental bleeding and some tracks down through the cervix to be revealed.

APH may also occur from the edge of the placenta (marginal haemorrhage), and in this instance the bleeding is always 'revealed'.

2. Placenta praevia (Fig. 5.2) refers to a placenta that is lying partially or wholly within the lower uterine segment and, according to the extent to which it intrudes into the lower segment, the degree of placenta praevia is classified into four types, I–IV.

3. 'Of uncertain origin' is the third major category of APH. This group covers marginal haemorrhage, vasa praevia and those cases that cannot be confidently diagnosed as either abruptio placentae or placenta praevia and accounts for the largest proportion of APH.

Incidence: APH occurs in about 4% of all pregnancies, with an almost equal occurrence of all three categories – abruptio, placenta praevia and the uncertain group.

Placenta praevia

Incidence: it occurs in up to 1% of all pregnancies after 28 weeks, and accounts for 15–20% of cases of antepartum haemorrhage.
Aetiology: uncertain, but it may be due to low implantation of the blastocyst or fusion or the decidua capsularis with the decidua vera.
Association: it occurs more often in uteri that have had previous surgery, particularly Caesarean sections.

Clinical symptoms and signs

Painless, recurrent, bright red bleeding.

Usually this occurs after 28–30 weeks, but may occur earlier. Any antepartum bleeding should be viewed with suspicion. The bleeding may be of small or large volume, and the patient's condition will reflect the amount of blood lost.

Uterine contractions result in the shearing off of the placenta from the myometrium and decidua.

Placenta praevia is often associated with an unstable lie, an abnormal presentation or a high presenting part.

Diagnosis

1. History (painless, bright red bleeding).
2. Soft uterus without areas of tenderness.
3. Usually no associated hypertension.
4. Unengaged presenting part.
5. Malpresentation

Do not perform a vaginal examination
Confirmation of the diagnosis can be made by the use of an ultrasound examination.

Management

1. Admission to a hospital that is equipped to deal with such an emergency.

2. Bed rest.
3. Blood should be cross-matched and kept available.
4. Perform ultrasound examination to confirm diagnosis.
5. If bleeding occurs before 30 weeks inappropriate uterine activity may be present. Careful use of tocolytic agents such as indomethacin may be used in the short term to suppress uterine activity and reduce bleeding. Beta-adrenergic agents should be used with great caution in the presence of vaginal bleeding.

The main aim is to prolong the pregnancy until the fetus is mature (37–38 weeks), but heavy bleeding may force delivery much sooner.

Repeated minor bleeding as well as more severe bleeding, may produce anaemia, thus transfusion may be indicated.

Where a major degree of placenta praevia is diagnosed delivery should be by Caesarean section.

Postpartum haemorrhage is more common with placenta praevia because of the poor ability of the lower segment to retract.

Accidental haemorrhage (abruptio placentae)

Associated factors occur in a small number of cases:

1. Hypertension and proteinuria.
2. Trauma.

Bleeding occurs from the decidua basalis separating the placenta from its attachment. As the volume of blood increases, placental separation occurs. After delivery, a clot may be found adhering to the maternal surface of the placenta. In severe forms of abruptions, the uterine muscle is suffused with blood and presents a very dark congested appearance (Couvelaire uterus).

Clinical features

These vary depending on the site and extent of bleeding and, as described previously, bleeding may be: revealed, concealed, or mixed. Cardiotocography may show frequent small contractions.

Three grades of accidental haemorrhage are described: mild, moderate, or severe:

1. **Mild**

Only a small area of placental separation occurs and blood loss is usually less than 500 ml. There may be some abdominal discomfort or pain. Occasionally the uterus may be tender.

Management

1. Admission to hospital.
2. Bed rest.
3. Cross-match blood.
4. Localize placenta by ultrasound.
5. Inspect cervix.

If bleeding settles and does not recur, the patient may be discharged after 4–5 days. Intercourse should be avoided. The pregnancy should be followed thereafter using regular ultrasound examination, fetal growth patterns and fetal movement and cardiac monitoring.

2. **Moderate**

A greater area of the placenta separates (up to one-third) and the bleeding is more severe (>1000 ml). Pain is always present and the uterus will be locally tender. The patient does not usually have symptoms and signs of hypovolaemia, but will have a tachycardia and be understandably anxious. Fetal heart sounds are present and the uterus is frequently irritable. Abruptions can kill the baby either as the result of hypoxia or from the effects of prematurity if the baby has to be delivered or if premature labour ensues.

Management

Premature labour can often follow a bleed of this magnitude. Placental localization is indicated with ultrasound. A decision needs to be made whether the danger of possible hypoxia from the abruption is a greater threat to the fetus than the risk of prematurity. If there is clinical evidence of an abruption and the baby is mature and alive then an emergency Caesarean section should be done. If the fetal condition allows it and the fetus is immature, corticosteroids should be given to accelerate fetal lung maturity before delivery.

Where there is doubt about the diagnosis, and the bleeding settles, labour should be induced no later than term, or earlier if the fetus appears to be endangered. Delivery should be undertaken when either mother or fetus demonstrate evidence of compromise.

3. Severe

More than half the placenta separates. Abdominal pain is more severe and the uterus is tender and rigid. Fetal heart sounds are muffled or often absent. Fetal movements may have ceased.

The patient is shocked, and is often in a worse condition than expected from the observed blood loss.

Management

Remember the two major complications-coagulation disorders and renal failure:

1. Withdraw blood for cross-matching and estimation of clotting time.
2. Insert central venous pressure (CVP) catheter.
3. Administer morphine (10 mg intravenously).
4. Give blood and fluids according to CVP reading.
5. Insert indwelling catheter into bladder.
6. If fetal heart sounds are present, assess the cervix and if delivery is imminent, perform an amniotomy: if there is likely to be a delay in delivery, perform a Caesarean section **after** restoring central venous pressure and ensuring that clotting time is normal.
7. If the fetus is dead, the mother's condition must be stabilized before labour is induced.

Beware of postpartum haemorrhage, as the uterine muscle cannot retract efficiently.

If the correct steps in management are taken, the maternal mortality will be minimal. Fetal mortality may be as high as 75%, mainly due to immaturity and hypoxia.

Uncertain APH

This includes bleeding from a marginal placental sinus, circumvallate placenta where the trophoblast extends beyond the major placental mass, and vasa praevia. Vasa praevia is associated with a velamentous insertion of the cord, so that fetal blood is lost.

The bleeding may be due to local causes, such as ectopic columnar epithelium, cervical polyps and carcinoma of the cervix. However, bleeding should not be attributed to these conditions unless they are actually found to be bleeding on inspection.

5.5 RENAL DISEASES ASSOCIATED WITH PREGNANCY

Renal infection

Of the various forms of renal disease occurring in pregnancy, renal infection is by far the most common. It is mostly thought of as an acute pyelonephritis, but may in fact be a subclinical renal infection which, because it is asymptomatic, is not often diagnosed unless special screening tests are performed. The significance of renal infection in pregnancy lies not so much with the pyrexia, nausea, vomiting and dehydration of acute infection, nor with the chronic lethargy and bone marrow depression of subclinical renal infection, but with the effect the renal infection has on the outcome of the pregnancy.

Renal infection is associated with an increased risk of abruptio placentae, pre-term labour and increased perinatal loss. Elimination of kidney infection will assist in reducing this morbidity and mortality.

Types of urinary infection

There are three major groups of urinary infection seen in pregnancy:

1. Asymptomatic bacteriuria (incidence 5–10%). This condition is the presence of significant numbers ($>100\,000$) of organisms in urine without any associated symptoms. Although about 5–10% of pregnant women have asymptomatic bacteriuria, this condition is not a disease of pregnancy – the same incidence of the disease is found among non-pregnant women who may have associated conditions, such as chronic interstitial fibrosis in the kidney, stones, obstruction, reflux or diverticulae, to explain the persistent presence of organisms.

2. Acute cystitis (incidence 2–3%). In pregnancy, the
    changes in the anatomy, physiology and biochemistry of
    the urinary tract and urine predispose to retention of urine
    and to the rapid growth of organisms. If these organisms
    multiply at a rate greater than the bladder wall has the
    capacity to reject them, then acute inflammation occurs,
    particularly of the trigone and urethra, and leads to the
    symptoms of frequency and dysuria. The major reason for
    the increase in number of organisms is the increased nutri-
    ents (glucose, amino acids) found in the urine of pregnant
    women.

    The physiological stasis and dilatation of the urinary
    tract, the anatomical changes in the position of the trigone
    and the ureters, and hyperaemia and softening of the pelvic
    fascia predispose to infection. Trauma and introduction of
    bacteria to the bladder are more frequent, so that even-
    tually the natural defences (complete emptying of the
    bladder, vesical antibacterial activity) are overcome.

    The organisms producing cystitis may have been present
    in the bladder as asymptomatic bacteriuria or may have
    been introduced during such activity as intercourse, a
    gynaecological examination or catheterization.

3. Pyelonephritis (incidence 1–2%). Once organisms enter the
    bladder, they will ascend to the kidney if there is reflux of
    urine. Reflux may be associated with congenital abnorm-
    ality of the uretero-vesical junction, with anatomical
    changes as in pregnancy, or with infection in the bladder
    causing oedema and fibrosis of the ureteric opening. Once
    reflux occurs in pregnancy, the hydroureters and urinary
    stasis then increase the risk of the infection in the calyceal
    region of the kidney.

Clinical and laboratory evidence of urinary infection

Patients with asymptomatic bacteriuria have no symptoms
related to the urinary tract. Urine examination will disclose a
bacteriuria of more than 100 000 organisms/ml.

Cystitis will produce frequency and dysuria, associated with
a positive urine culture and an increase in urinary white cell
count, epithelial cells, occasionally red cells and mucous secretions. Acute pyelonephritis may present with fever, nausea,

vomiting, loin pain and tenderness. Laboratory investigations will demonstrate a positive urinary culture.

Detection of subclinical renal infection

Asymptomatic bacteriuria and cystitis account for about 80% of all cases of urinary infection in pregnancy and when present should be appropriately treated with antibiotics.

Treatment

1. Asymptomatic bacteriuria. This should be initially managed as for cystitis.
2. Cystitis. This should be treated by using a chemotherapeutic agent that is specifically concentrated in urine and renders the urine sterile. The most common used agents are amoxycillin, trimethoprim–sulphamethoxazole (Bactrim, Septrin), nitrofurantoin (Macrodantin), nalidixic acid (Negram). All are given for 10–14 days, and after cessation of treatment the urine is re-cultured for organisms.
3. Pyelonephritis. When renal infection is present, the chemotherapeutic agents of choice are indicated by *in vitro* testing. If nausea, vomiting and dehydration require admission to hospital, then the appropriate antibiotics may be administered by the parenteral route. However, care must be taken that renal function is adequate and that the dosage and extent of therapy is not so great as to cause harm to the fetus or the mother.

Length of treatment course

If the initial 1–2-week course of chemotherapy clears the urine of organisms, and there is no further evidence of infection, then the antibiotics should be ceased.

However, if further urine cultures show a recurrence of infection or persistence of casts and red cells, then continuation of chemotherapy is indicated. It may be necessary to maintain antibiotics throughout the whole of the antenatal period. If this is indicated, then the various chemotherapeutic agents should be alternated and the urine checked regularly for organisms and leucocytes.

Following delivery

All patients who have developed urinary infection in pregnancy should be followed-up at 8–12 weeks after delivery. At this time a full urine culture and examination should be performed. Any persistent abnormality merits further investigation. Approximately 20% of women with persistent renal infection in pregnancy will be found to have some evidence of an abnormality by pyelography and a large number of these women will have a surgically correctable lesion.

Conclusion

Approximately 5–10% of pregnant women will be found to have urinary infection in pregnancy due to pyelonephritis, cystitis or asymptomatic bacteriuria.

Treatment can eliminate the infection and reduce the risk to the fetus. Thus investigation and management of all pregnant women should include an adequate screening test to detect organisms in the urine.

Acute glomerulonephritis in pregnancy

This is relatively rare compared with renal infection, but should be suspected when hypertension, oedema, proteinuria and haematuria occur about 10–12 days following an acute streptococcal sore throat. It is more common in early pregnancy, but may be confused with severe pre-eclampsia. However, microscopy to show red cells, granular casts and increased white cell count, together with a high antistreptolysin titre, should confirm the diagnosis. Acute glomerulonephritis is often associated with spontaneous abortion and pre-term labour, as well as an increased incidence of fetal loss. The maternal mortality may be as high as 2–3% and if the renal problem appears to be severe, it is advisable to consider terminating the pregnancy.

Chronic glomerulonephritis

In pregnancy, this usually presents with hypertension, occasionally cardiovascular problems and renal insufficiency.

Although pregnancy does not appear to make the disease process worse, it has a poor prognosis for the fetus, in the presence of abnormal renal function. There is a high risk of intrauterine death, growth-retarded infants, prematurity and severe hypertensive problems. It is wise to involve a renal physician in the management of these patients.

Nephrotic syndrome in pregnancy

This is due to such diseases as diabetes, amyloidosis and lupus erythematosus. It is very rare, and the general effect on mother and fetus is to increase mortality. Unless the disease is well controlled and managed, it is often advisable to terminate the pregnancy early.

Surgical problems

Such problems as large calculi, polycystic kidney or congenital abnormalities should not be treated in pregnancy unless they actually obstruct or interfere with the normal delivery process or are causing acute problems (renal calculi in a ureter). Calculi can be sometimes detected using ultrasound. Occasionally a single film intravenous pyelogram (IVP) needs to be done in pregnancy.

Acute renal failure

This is seen when less than 500 ml of urine are passed in 24 hours. It may follow obstetric, medical or traumatic conditions. It is common in association with Gram-negative infection (endotoxic shock), blood loss, trauma and drugs. The maternal and fetal prognosis is often poor, but is improved when the mother is transferred early to a renal unit to receive highly specialized therapy. Care must be taken in the anuric or oliguric phase that fluid requirements are carefully monitored and maintained, that diuretics are not used and that electrolyte balance is maintained. The prognosis for cases treated by inexperienced medical practitioners is very poor. The ideal management is in specially equipped renal units.

5.6 ANAEMIA IN PREGNANCY

Anaemia in pregnancy is significant because of increased risk to both mother and fetus:

1. Maternal
   (a) Inability to withstand haemorrhage.
   (b) Susceptibility to infection.
   (c) Developing heart failure if the anaemia is severe.
2. Fetal
   (a) Hypoxia – less oxygen is carried to the placenta by maternal blood.
   (b) Premature labour is more common.

Anaemia is present when the circulating haemoglobin mass is reduced. An arbitrary figure of 10.5 gm/dl is often used as an indication that investigation for anaemia should be undertaken.

Changes seen during pregnancy

Both the plasma volume and red cell mass increase during pregnancy, but the rise in plasma volume (45%) greatly exceeds that of the red cell mass (18%). The resulting haemodilution allows for easier blood flow. It follows that the red cell count and packed cell volume fall during pregnancy and the haemoglobin will appear to be low.

Red cell size and haemoglobin content are unaffected and so the MCV and MCHC remain constant. Serum iron levels rise because the amount of iron-binding protein, like all plasma proteins, increases.

Types of anaemia

1. Iron deficiency. The patient may enter pregnancy with iron deficiency due to:
   (a) Inadequate intake.
   (b) Poor absorption.
   (c) Excessive losses from too frequent pregnancies, menorrhagia.

This initial deficiency may be aggravated by the extra

demands for iron imposed by the pregnancy. Iron-deficiency anaemia is the most common type seen in Australia.

2. Thalassaemia minor. This is the second most common anaemia seen in pregnancy – 6% of Greek-born and 4% of Italian-born patients carry this trait. There is a genetically determined abnormality in β-chain production, resulting in fewer red cells whose life span is reduced. Alpha-thalassaemia is much rarer and occurs among South-east Asian people.
3. Folic acid deficiency. This is no longer common. Folic acid is necessary for amino acid metabolism, and increased amounts are needed for dividing cells. It usually manifests itself late in pregnancy. This is the most common anaemia seen in multiple pregnancies.
4. Renal disease. This is a rare cause of anaemia, but when no obvious cause is found for a normochromic, normocytic anaemia, it may well be present.

Symptoms and signs

As in the non-pregnant state, the symptoms are non-specific and include lassitude, dyspnoea, palpitations, giddiness, fainting and oedema. These symptoms may have a gradual onset (iron deficiency) or a rapid onset (folic acid deficiency). Iron deficiency or β-thalassaemia can produce symptoms at any time during the pregnancy, but it is rare for folic acid deficiency to cause symptoms before 26 weeks – symptoms are usually first seen after 30 weeks.

Management

Prophylaxis: iron and folic acid supplements should be given routinely during pregnancy. FGF or Fefol given daily provides 270 mg of ferrous sulphate and 300 μg of folic acid.

Increased amounts of folic acid should be given in multiple pregnancy and to women taking phenytoin.

Investigations

1. Haemoglobin estimation. This should be done routinely at the first antenatal visit, and again at 28–36 weeks. If this

value is below acceptable limits, further investigations are performed.

2. Blood film. Abnormal red cell size, shape and haemoglobin content can be readily observed.
3. Packed cell volume. This is an unreliable test during pregnancy, but its determination is necessary in order to calculate red cell indices:
   (a) Mean corpuscular volume (packed cell volume (PCV)/ red cell count). This is diminished in iron deficiency.
   (b) Mean corpuscular haemoglobin (haemoglobin concentration/red cell count). This is diminished in iron deficiency.
   (c) Mean corpuscular haemoglobin concentration (haemoglobin concentration/packed cell volume). This is decreased in iron deficiency, and is probably the most significant test for iron-deficiency anaemia in pregnancy.
4. Serum iron and iron-binding capacity. The serum iron levels fall and the iron-binding capacity rises.
5. Serum ferritin. This provides some measure of iron stores.
6. Serum folate and red cell folate. Levels fall with folic acid anaemia.
7. Haemoglobin electrophoresis. This will detect elevated levels of HbA_2 and HbF in thalassaemia minor.
8. Bone marrow examination. This is indicated in unresponsive cases or where blood studies are non-specific or suggest leukaemia.

Treatment

1. Iron deficiency. Either oral iron or total dose infusion with iron dextran (Imferon).
2. Packed cells. These may be given before or in labour if haemoglobin levels are below 8 g% and a rapid rise is needed. Provided the cells are infused slowly with added frusemide, no complications should occur.
3. Folic acid anaemia. Folic acid (5–15 mg daily by mouth) will produce a fairly rapid rise in haemoglobin levels.
4. Thalassaemia minor. Usually these patients are not iron-deficient, but iron therapy may be indicated in certain cases. Ensure that folic acid is being taken (5 mg/day). Blood should only be given for acute blood loss.

In addition to specific measures, the importance of a well-balanced diet should be stressed to the mother. This measure, together with routine iron and folic acid supplements, has served to diminish the incidence of anaemia in pregnancy.

5.7 HEART DISEASE IN PREGNANCY

Deaths due to heart disease are the fourth most common cause of maternal mortality, and are the most common cause of death not due solely to obstetrical factors. Additionally, the perinatal mortality is at least doubled and in the most severe forms can be as high as 33%.

Incidence

Less than 1% of pregnancies occur in patients with heart disease or who have previously had cardiac surgery.

Previously, rheumatic heart disease was by far the most common form seen, but its incidence in Australia has declined to a level below that of congenital heart disease. Other types of heart disease encountered are cardiomyopathy, ischaemic and hypertensive heart disease.

Assessment

The severity of heart disease is commonly assessed by grading of symptoms, according to the New York Heart Association (NYHA) categories:

Grade I   The patient has no symptoms and can undertake all physical activities.

Grade II   The patient is comfortable at rest and can manage the usual physical activities of domestic work. Any more exertion than usual, however, will result in fatigue and dyspnoea.

Grade III   The patient is comfortable at rest but quickly becomes dyspnoeic when attempting any domestic activity about the house.

Grade IV   The patient is breathless at rest and is probably in cardiac failure. She requires urgent admission to hospital.

In addition, the following points should be determined from history and examination:

1. Outcome of any previous pregnancy.
2. Previous episodes of heart failure.
3. The precise nature of the cardiac lesion.
4. Presence of arrhythmias.

In almost all cases, the cooperation of a cardiologist is desirable in both initial assessment and subsequent management through pregnancy, labour and the puerperium.

Effect of pregnancy on heart disease

Cardiac output rises by up to 40% during pregnancy, the greater part of this rise occurring in the first 20 weeks. There is an increased blood flow to all areas of the body except the liver. Cardiac output remains at this elevated level until the commencement of labour, and increases even further during the first and second stages of labour. The increase in cardiac output increases the amount of cardiac work, and also the risk of women developing left ventricular heart failure.

Antenatal care is largely devoted to avoiding complications that may lead to heart failure, and to improving the grade of disability.

Obesity, hypertension, anaemia and multiple pregnancy may be deleterious factors, as can the development of a cardiac arrhythmia, especially atrial fibrillation. If any signs of heart decompensation develop, immediate admission to hospital and conventional management are indicated.

Patients on prophylactic anticoagulants following cardiac surgery should continue with this treatment. Warfarin sodium (Coumadin) however, may be teratogenic – so heparin should be substituted in the first trimester and in the last 6 weeks of pregnancy, as it does not cross the placenta.

Labour should not be induced, nor Caesarean section undertaken, unless there is an obstetric indication. If heart failure develops, it should be controlled before there is any obstetric interference.

Management during labour

Endocarditis: women with structural heart disease or anomaly are exposed to infection during labour. Antibiotic cover should be given during labour and for at least 4 days afterwards.

The patient's head and shoulders should be kept propped up and it is best to avoid delivery in the conventional lithotomy position.

For patients with minor degrees of heart disease, lumbar epidural block is helpful as it will greatly diminish the additional increase in cardiac output during labour. With the more severe types of heart disease where patients are likely to develop left ventricular heart failure, this form of pain relief is contraindicated.

If acute pulmonary oedema develops, it is treated by conventional methods; the patient is propped up, 80–120 mg of frusemide (Lasix) are given intravenously, and digitalization may also be necessary.

Delivery

With minor degrees of heart disease, there is no reason why a normal vaginal delivery cannot be achieved; however, a prolonged second stage should be avoided. With more severe forms of heart disease, forceps delivery is indicated to minimize maternal effort.

Caesarean section is only performed for obstetric reasons.

Oxytocic agents

Normally these drugs are given prophylactically to prevent postpartum haemorrhage. Following the third stage of labour, there is an injection of up to 500 ml of blood into the circulation from the uterus. In certain instances the use of oxytocic agents is contraindicated (e.g. in women with incipient left ventricular heart failure).

Active management of the third stage of labour should be unchanged in NYHA Grade I and II cardiacs as the risk of postpartum haemorrhage is greater than the risk of precipitating cardiac failure. In more severe cases however, decisions are made on an individual patient basis and specialist obstetric and specialist anaesthetic staff must be present at this time, in case acute cardiac failure occurs, threatening the patient's life.

Following delivery, the patient must be closely watched during the first 24 hours for the development of heart failure. However, after this time the blood volume commences to fall and as the return towards pre-pregnancy levels continues, the likelihood of heart failure diminishes.

Breast feeding is only contraindicated in women with severe forms of heart failure.

5.8 PRE-TERM LABOUR

Pre-term labour is commencing before the 37th week of amenorrhoea. The onset of pre-term labour may be either spontaneous or induced – pre-term delivery occurs in approximately 6% of all pregnancies.

Causes

1. Idiopathic – by far the largest group.
2. Secondary to premature rupture of membranes.
3. Overdistention of the uterus – multiple pregnancy, polyhydramnios.
4. Placental abruption.
5. Severe hypertension, and other situations where the fetus is at risk.
6. Cervical incompetence – where the sphincteric action of the cervix is lost, either congenital or due to previous trauma.
7. Uterine malformations.
8. Acute febrile illnesses in the mother.
9. Intrauterine fetal death.

Management

In some instances labour should be allowed to proceed normally without any interference. These include severe antepartum haemorrhage, severe maternal hypertension, and intrauterine fetal death. Excluding these situations, an attempt should be made to arrest the progress of labour so that therapy can be instituted in an attempt to mature the fetal lungs.

If the period of amenorrhoea exceeds 20 weeks and

the uterine size is either commensurate with, or larger than, dates:

1. Ascertain that the fetal heart beat is present.
2. Distinguish between true and false labour. If labour is false, there will not be any 'show', nor will the cervix be effaced or dilated.
3. Determine whether or not there are uterine contractions, either by palpation or an external pressure transducer attached to a fetal monitor.
4. If the membranes are ruptured, take a high vaginal swab for culture.

If painful contractions are occurring at a rate of one or more every 10 minutes and the cervix is dilated:

1. Commence an intravenous infusion of salbutamol (25 mg/l) and titrate the dose according to the maternal and fetal responses.
2. Providing the pregnancy has not exceeded 34 weeks, corticosteroids are given to speed up the fetal lung maturation. For instance, 1 g of betamethasone (Celestone Chronodose) is given intramuscularly, and then once more 24 hours later to assist in maturing fetal lungs.
3. If the membranes are ruptured, the mother may be given antibiotics. For instance, 1 g of cephalexin (Keflex) is given intravenously, and then 6-hourly while the infusion is running. Continue a similar oral dosage after the infusion is removed for a further 4 days.

Such a regime will inhibit 'labour' in approximately 80% of cases where cervical dilatation does not exceed 4 cm before the commencement of treatment. The success rate is poor when dilatation is greater than 4 cm or when the membranes are ruptured.

False labour occurs when uterine contractions are distressing to the mother in the absence of cervical effacement or dilatation.

In most instances explanation of what is occurring will be sufficient to allay symptoms and if not, sedation with 20 mg temazepam orally is often effective.

5.9 COUNSELLING IN RELATION TO AN ABNORMAL PREGNANCY

When a pregnancy deviates from its normal course, a great responsibility falls on the obstetrician to explain to the patient and her husband the exact situation, with regard to both the mother and baby.

Where induction of labour is planned on behalf of either mother or the fetus, care should be taken to explain:

1. Why induction is necessary.
2. What may happen if the pregnancy is prolonged.
3. How induction will be undertaken.
4. What will happen if it is unsuccessful.
5. What will happen to the baby following delivery.

While many people will take advice uncritically and unhesitatingly, with a response such as 'do whatever you think best', some will question methods of management, and a frank and simple explanation must be given.

Fetal malformation

Occasionally a fetal malformation may be diagnosed in late pregnancy. Usually these are gross malformations incompatible with life, such as anencephaly.

The parents should be told and offered the alternative forms of management. In such a situation this will consist of either induction of labour, or awaiting its spontaneous onset. A great number of women find the second alternative intolerable and wish to have labour induced.

When the baby is delivered, the parents should be asked if they wish to see the baby or if they would like it baptized. Most parents will see the baby if given the choice, thereby ascertaining for themselves what the abnormality is. On no account should parents be dissuaded from looking at their baby in such a situation.

Intrauterine fetal death

The basic principles of counselling should be followed. The baby should be given to the parents to see or touch if they wish. In all instances, the cause of death should be explained to the parents. The risk of recurrence should also be ascertained and told to the parents. In most instances a post-mortem examination is indicated.

Establishing the exact diagnosis

In all instances of stillbirth or neonatal death, an exact diagnosis should be made if possible, especially if there is any fetal malformation.

It is only by establishing a precise diagnosis that you can answer such questions as: 'Will it occur again'? 'If so, what are the chances of recurrence'? 'Can the condition be diagnosed antenatally'? Such information is not only important to the parents, but also to their siblings who may be contemplating having children, and to future generations of their family.

5.10 CONVULSIONS IN PREGNANCY AND THE PUERPERIUM

Generalized convulsions may occur at any time during pregnancy and the puerperium, and may be caused by specific disorders of pregnancy (by far the most common) or by disorders unassociated with pregnancy.

Specific disorders of pregnancy

1. Hypertensive encephalopathy, associated with hypertension of pregnancy. Usually seen in late pregnancy, associated with fluid retention and proteinuria. It may, however, occur during labour or postnatally, especially in the first 24 hours following delivery.
2. Generalized convulsions can occur for the first time during pregnancy, and may be apparently precipitated by pregnancy in the absence of severe hypertension. This is much less common than hypertensive encephalopathy.

Convulsions specifically associated with pregnancy are known as eclamptic convulsions. The frequency of these convulsions is equally distributed between antepartum, intrapartum and postpartum periods.

Disorders unassociated with pregnancy

1. Idiopathic epilepsy. Anticonvulsant metabolism may be altered considerably during pregnancy, and increasing amounts are needed as pregnancy progresses to maintain therapeutic levels in the plasma. Consequently sub-therapeutic levels are more commonly found and the tendency for convulsions increases.
2. Hypoxic encephalopathy. Fainting is a common symptom of pregnancy and unless the person who faints is laid down, an hypoxic convulsion may ensue.
3. Water intoxication and hyponatraemia. This is a rare complication of high-concentration oxytocin infusions, such as with the induction of a mid-trimester abortion, or induction of labour following intrauterine fetal death. Such conclusions are wholly preventable.
4. Associated with hypoglycaemia. This is mostly seen in cases of diabetes mellitus, where the insulin dosage is increased according to blood glucose levels. It can occur in early pregnancy when nausea prevents an adequate intake of nourishment.
5. Rupture of a cerebral artery aneurysm. This is usually seen postnatally, and does not always produce a convulsion.
6. Barbiturate and alcohol withdrawal.
7. Cerebral tumour. Problems in this instance are again usually seen postnatally, associated with haemorrhage into the tumour.

Symptoms and signs

1. Sudden loss of consciousness.
2. Crying out.
3. Falling, if the patient is upright.
4. Tonic movements of the tongue and limbs.
5. Clonic movements of the tongue and limbs.
6. Occasional sphincteric incontinence.

When there has been cerebral damage, localizing signs can be demonstrated in addition to coma or altered levels of consciousness. When there is no damage, the most common sign (apart from alteration of the levels of consciousness) is bilateral upgoing plantar reflexes.

Treatment (see also the section on pre-eclampsia, section 5.19)

1. Maintain the airway.
2. Ensure adequate oxygenation.
3. If status epilepticus is present, give intravenous diazepam (Valium). The most common cause is hypertensive encephalopathy, thus the following treatment is given.
4. The level of hypertension is reduced, for example by drugs such as hydralazine or diazoxide (Hyperstat-IV, 300 mg intravenously in slow, small bolus doses). Magnesium sulphate as an intravenous infusion reduces both the blood pressure and the level of cerebral irritability.
5. If the convulsion has occurred antepartum or intrapartum, the baby may need to be delivered in order to minimize the risk to both mother and baby.
6. When clinical examination confirms an intracranial lesion, dexamethasone such as dexamethasone sodium phosphate (Decadron, 8 mg intravenously) should be given to reduce intracranial pressure.

When an intracranial lesion is suspected or where a convulsion has occurred *de novo* during pregnancy, further investigations should be undertaken to exclude life-threatening lesions.

5.11 CHRONIC ILLNESS

The obstetrician should identify medical and psychiatric conditions in pregnant patients that necessitate specialist care. As a good general principle, patients with a chronic illness (either physical or psychological) should seek advice before embarking on a pregnancy. Advice should be given relating to:

1. The likely effect of pregnancy on the mother in both the short and long term.
2. The effect of the mother's condition on the fetus, and the likelihood of any disabling disorder occurring.
3. The effects on the fetus of any medication needed by the mother.

Any decisions regarding the patient's management should only be made after discussion with the woman and her medical attendant. Frequently more specialized knowledge is required and a consultation should be sought.

Women with chronic illness who embark upon a pregnancy as a rule should be managed in a large centre, and close cooperation between the obstetrician and other physicians is essential.

5.12 RHESUS ISO-IMMUNIZATION AND HAEMOLYTIC DISEASE

The Rhesus (Rh) factor was first described by Landsteiner and Winer in 1940. Fisher (1944) discovered that individual antigens made up the Rh factor.

There are three pairs of Rh antigens inherited by six separate genes (C, c, D, d, E, e), three from each parent. It is the presence or absence of D antigen that alone determines if a person is Rh-positive or Rh-negative.

Of Europeans, 83% are Rh-positive, 50% are heterozygous (Dd), and 33% are homozygous (DD) for the D antigen. Rh-negative persons are uncommon in Asians and Polynesians.

Rh iso-immunization accounts for 98% of haemolytic disease of the newborn and of these 95% are due to D antigen.

Immunization may occur:

1. When a Rh-negative woman is pregnant with a Rh-positive fetus.
2. Following an incompatible blood transfusion.

Feto-maternal haemorrhage is most likely to occur during labour when the placenta separates. It may also occur following therapeutic abortion, spontaneous abortion, placental abruption or Caesarean section, chorionic villus sampling, amniocentesis, or spontaneously.

Maternal antibody formation depends on the size of the feto-maternal haemorrhage, the stage of pregnancy at which it occurs, the individual sensitivity of the mother and not the ABO blood grouping. If there is ABO incompatibility between the mother and fetus, the fetal cells are rapidly destroyed by the mother's anti-A and/or anti-B antibodies.

It is rare for a first pregnancy to sensitize a woman. Previously, one in ten Rh-negative women were sensitized by two such pregnancies. In recent years, the incidence of Rh iso-immunization has declined markedly due to the introduction of anti-D globulin (see Prophylaxis, page 113).

When sensitization occurs, two major types of antibody

appear in the maternal blood:

1. Immunoglobulin M (IgM) – does not cross the placenta.
2. Immunoglobulin G (IgG) – does cross the placenta. Detected by indirect Coombs' test.

Effects on the fetus

When IgG crosses the placenta, it attaches to the fetal red cells and enables them to be broken down. Anaemia results, and the fetus compensates by increasing haemopoiesis. This results in fetal hepatosplenomegaly. Red cell breakdown occurs mainly in the spleen, and accentuates splenomegaly.

There is increased bilirubin production – some bilirubin crosses the placenta and is metabolized by the mother, and some enters the amniotic fluid to give increased bilirubin levels in the fluid. These increased levels are detected by light-absorption studies, which helps assessment in the management of haemolytic disease.

If anaemia is mild, the fetus can compensate. However, imbalance may occur and increasingly severe anaemia develops. In the most severe forms, anaemia leads to hypoxia, with ultimate fetal death due to heart failure (hydrops fetalis).

Management

Prophylaxis

At the first antenatal visit, blood group and antibody screen must be ordered in all instances. Where the patient is Rh-negative, antibodies should be looked for again at 28 weeks and if absent, she should receive 250 or 300 µg of anti-D globulin.

If no antibodies are found in Rh-negative women during pregnancy, then two samples of cord blood should be collected following delivery. Fig. 5.3 shows the sequence of determinations to be followed.

If the cord blood tests indicate haemolytic disease due to Rh iso-immunization (Fig. 5.4), the baby should be assessed for the severity of its effects by haemoglobin and plasma bilirubin estimations, and then managed accordingly.

Anti-D globulin should also be given to Rh-negative women

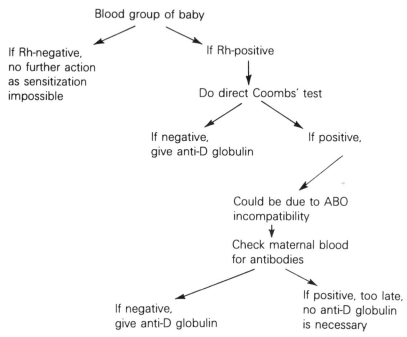

Figure 5.3 Sequence of steps to be taken following delivery of infant to Rhesus-negative mother.

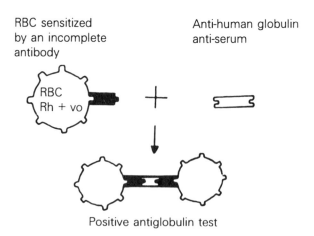

Figure 5.4 The direct Coombs' test. The fetal red cells carrying Rh-positive antigens are coated with maternal incomplete antibodies. Addition of anti-human globulin antiserum leads to an agglutination of these cells, giving a positive result. This indicates both the presence of maternal iso-immunization and potential fetal haemolysis.

who abort spontaneously, have a therapeutic abortion or tubal pregnancy, or undergo amniocentesis (except for haemolytic disease due to Rh).

Anti-D globulin is about 98% effective in preventing Rh iso-immunization. However, its exact mechanism of action is uncertain.

Sensitized pregnancy

If antibodies are found during the antenatal course, this indicates that haemolytic disease is likely but it does not indicate the degree of severity. Amniocentesis is indicated to determine this.

The anti-D titre in the mother can be measured and provides some indication how seriously the baby will be affected.

Further management depends on the predicted severity of the anaemia as determined by the amount of bilirubin in the amniotic fluid. Repeated amniocentesis may be necessary to determine the optimal time for delivery (Fig. 5.5).

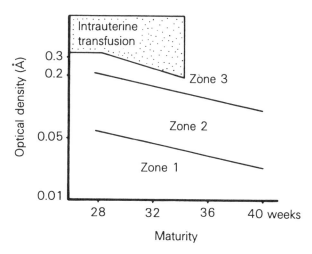

Figure 5.5 Chart for assessing fetal prognosis in Rh haemolytic disease. Amniocentesis results fall into one of the zones. In Zone 1, the baby is mildly affected and can safely be allowed to go to 38 weeks. In Zone 2, multiple amniocentesis may be required to determine in which direction the trend is developing. Early induction may be required. In Zone 3, after 34 weeks immediate delivery should be undertaken, while before 34 weeks, intrauterine transfusion will be necessary.

The mainstays of treatment are:

1. Premature induction of labour.
2. Exchange transfusion.
3. Phototherapy.

Occasionally, fetal intrauterine transfusion is indicated when the anaemia is severe enough to warrant treatment, but the pregnancy is not sufficiently advanced to allow indication of labour.

Other antibodies apart from Rh may cause haemolytic disease. It is important to remember that these may occur in Rh-positive as well as Rh-negative women. The antibodies include:

1. Kell (usually due to an incompatible blood transfusion).
2. Duffy.
3. MNS antibodies.

Remember, *all* pregnant women should be screened for antibodies, likely to cause haemolytic disease at their first antenatal visit.

5.13 GLYCOSURIA AND DIABETES MELLITUS

Glycosuria

During pregnancy the renal blood flow increases by 50% and the glomerular filtration rate by 45% above non-pregnant values. As a result, more glucose is presented to the renal tubules for reabsorption and often the T_m for glucose is exceeded and glycosuria occurs.

When 1% of glucose is found on two successive visits, a glucose tolerance test should be performed. Glucose tolerance tests should also be performed on potential diabetics when they are pregnant, such as women:

1. Who have an identical twin who is diabetic.
2. Whose parents are diabetic.
3. Who have one diabetic parent, and the other parent has diabetic siblings or parents.
4. Who have borne a live or stillborn child whose birth weight exceeded 4.5 kg.

5. Who have borne a stillborn child with islet cell hyperplasia not associated with Rh incompatibility.
6. Who weigh over 80 kg at conception.

There is a better likelihood of finding an abnormal response to a glucose tolerance test if the test is performed after 26–28 weeks of pregnancy.

Glucose tolerance test (GTT)

Following a 12-hour fast, a baseline fasting venous plasma glucose sample is taken and the patient is given a 75 g glucose load. Further samples are taken at 1 and 2 hours after the glucose. A normal fasting level should be less than 5.5 mmol/l while the 2-hour sample should be less than 8 mmol/l.

When the diagnosis of diabetes mellitus is made initially during a pregnancy, the patient is classified as gestational diabetic.

Effects of pregnancy on glucose metabolism

1. Glycosuria – previously described in the physiology of tubular reabsorption of glucose.
2. Human placental lactogen exerts an anti-insulin and lipolytic effect, which increases plasma glucose levels and makes more glucose available to the fetus.
3. Steroid hormones (oestrogens and progesterone) also have a mild anti-insulin effect.
4. Some insulin is probably destroyed by the placenta.

The net effect is a rise in maternal glucose levels throughout pregnancy, and in some women this is excessive and produces gestational diabetes.

Incidence of diabetes mellitus in pregnancy

Of the total population, 3% suffer from either juvenile or mature-onset diabetes mellitus. One-sixth of these people are women of child-bearing age, so that about one pregnancy in 400 is complicated by diabetes.

Effects of diabetes on pregnancy and vice versa

1. The infertility rate is slightly increased.
2. Hypoglycaemia is more common, due to nausea of pregnancy.
3. Ketoacidosis is more likely due to vomiting of early pregnancy.
4. Urinary tract infection is more common – 18% of pregnant women have asymptomatic bacteriuria (three times the usual rate).
5. Moniliasis is more common, and is often severe.
6. Pre-eclampsia is more common.
7. Polyhydramnios is more common.
8. Insulin requirements increase steadily during pregnancy, and it is easy to lose control of the diabetes.
9. Perinatal morbidity and mortality is increased.
   (a) There is a 6% incidence of major congenital malformations (three times the average rate).
   (b) Sudden intrauterine death may occur in late pregnancy.
   (c) Birth trauma may occur due to larger than average babies, predisposing to dystocia.

Management of insulin-dependent diabetes mellitus

1. A team approach ensures continuity of treatment by experienced people. The team includes obstetricians, physicians, paediatricians, dietitians, social workers, and pathology and nursing staff.
2. An early assessment of obstetrical and medical condition is necessary. In addition to usual investigations, renal function must be assessed.
3. Plasma glucose levels are used to regulate insulin dosage, rather than urinary glucose. The aim is to keep plasma glucose levels below 6 mmol/l. Fortnightly visits are indicated.
4. Fetal gestational age and morphology should be checked by ultrasound at 18–20 weeks.
5. Home glucose monitoring.
6. Twice-daily biphasic insulin should be given.
7. Admission may be required at any time for stabilization of diabetes or investigation of obstetric complications.

8. Admission at 32 weeks is indicated only in very severe cases.
    (a) Thrice weekly, 2-hour postprandial plasma glucose levels are determined.
    (b) Regular fetal movement charting is performed.
    (c) Serial ultrasound examinations every 2 weeks.
    (d) Daily weighing and girth measurements are made.
    (e) External cardiotocography is performed regularly.
    (f) Vaginal delivery at ± 38 weeks is preferable.

Delivery

1. If cervix favourable: amniotomy and oxytocin drip.
2. If cervix unfavourable: Caesarean section or PGE_2 to ripen the cervix before induction of labour.

Postnatal

1. Maternal insulin requirements drop suddenly to pre-pregnancy levels.
2. Urinary testing may be instituted soon after delivery.

Baby

The baby is prone to hypoglycaemia, so is fed at 1-hour intervals and regular plasma glucose levels are determined. Diabetic babies are also more prone to hyaline membrane disease, so should be monitored daily for this complaint.

With this routine, the perinatal loss can be reduced to 5–10%. With less strict regimes, the incidence of diabetic and obstetrical complications increases.

Gestational diabetes

Where the diagnosis of diabetes is made during pregnancy, initially control should be attempted through diet.

1. If diet is successful. Make fortnightly estimations of plasma glucose. Do not allow pregnancy to progress past term.
2. If diet not successful. Insulin (not oral hypoglycaemics) is needed. The routine for insulin-dependent diabetics should be followed.

5.14 AMNIOCENTESIS IN PREGNANCY

Amniocentesis is the withdrawal of fluid from the amniotic cavity. This involves passing a needle through the anterior walls of the mother's abdomen and uterus, always under ultrasound control. Amniocentesis may be performed:

1. Early in pregnancy for:
   (a) Therapeutic abortion.
   (b) Antenatal genetic diagnosis.
2. Late in pregnancy for:
   (a) Determining fetal lung maturity.
   (b) Management of Rh iso-immunization.

The ideal time for amniocentesis in early pregnancy is 14–15 weeks.

Antenatal diagnosis

It is possible to diagnose a variety of conditions, either directly from the amniotic fluid or as a result of cells cultured from the fluid. Such conditions include:

1. Chromosomal abnormalities. These occur either:
   (a) When the mother has previously had a baby with a chromosomal abnormality.
   (b) When the mother or the father is a mosaic carrier.
   Or may arise:
   (c) As the mother's age advances beyond 35 years.
2. Neural tube defects. Anencephaly, iniencaphaly, encephalo-coele, myelomeningocoele and spina bifida can be diagnosed when the fetal lesion is not skin covered. Approximately 90% of cases of spina bifida, can be detected by estimating the levels of alpha-fetoprotein (AFP) in amniotic fluid. AFP levels may also be raised when there is a large exomphalos or cystic hygroma, so it is not entirely specific for neural tube disorders. Hydrocephaly cannot be diagnosed by this procedure.
3. Biochemical disorders. A variety of such disorders are inherited as autosomal recessive genes. These may also be diagnosed. For example, adrenogenital syndrome, mucopolysaccharide disorders, some amino-acidurias.

4. X-linked disorders. Sexing of the fetus can be achieved by amniotic cell culture.
5. Haemoglobinopathies. These can be diagnosed by fetal blood sampling achieved by needling the umbilical cord under ultrasound at 18 weeks.

Tests of fetal lung maturity

The most common cause of respiratory distress syndrome in the newborn is hyaline membrane disease. Whether or not a baby develops this condition depends on the amount of surfactant in the lung alveoli. The appearance of surfactant in fetal lungs in sufficient amount to prevent hyaline membrane disease coincides with a sudden increase in the amount of lecithin in amniotic fluid.

Lecithin is a phospholipid, and its concentration and its relation to that of another phospholipid, sphingomyelin, is expressed as a ratio (L/S ratio). As a rule, the increase in lecithin occurs at 35–36 weeks (Fig. 5.6), but may occur earlier or later than this, depending on fetal maturation of adrenal tissue.

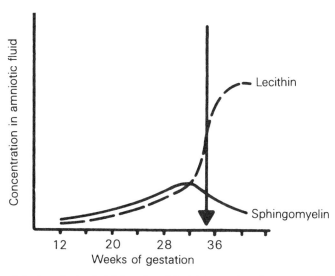

Figure 5.6 Amniotic fluid levels of lecithin and sphingomyelin indicate fetal lung maturity. After 36 weeks of gestation, there is usually a dramatic rise in lecithin levels compared with sphingomyelin, indicating that the fetal lung is mature and will probably easily sustain respiration after delivery.

Newer tests such as the TDX fetal lung maturity test use a fluorescent polarization immunoassay technique to estimate the quantity of lamella bodies which contain surfactant in the amniotic fluid.

Factors known to accelerate surfactant production in certain cases include:

1. Repeated small antepartum haemorrhage.
2. Maternal heroin addiction.
3. Prolonged premature rupture of the membranes.
4. Stress situations to the fetus, e.g. IUGR.

Factors that may delay lung maturation include:

1. Maternal diabetes mellitus.
2. Severe Rh iso-immunization.

Rhesus iso-immunization assessment

The severity of fetal haemolytic anaemia can be assessed by estimation of the amount of bilirubin in the amniotic fluid (see Rhesus iso-immunization, section 5.12).

Complications of amniocentesis

Fetal damage or death

A variety of types of fetal damage have been reported following amniocentesis, all of which are rare events. Death may be due to damage to a vessel in the fetus, placenta or umbilical cord.

Abortion or premature labour

The risk of abortion following an amniocentesis in early pregnancy is ±1% – only slightly higher than the normal incidence of midtrimester abortion (0.7%).

Pre-term labour may follow amniocentesis in late pregnancy in about 5% of cases, and is more likely to occur the closer the pregnancy is to term.

Infection

Amniocentesis is an invasive procedure and an aseptic technique is necessary to prevent the development of amnionitis.

Maternal morbidity

This is a rare occurrence, but complications due to maternal bleeding and formation of haematoma in the uterus have been recorded.

5.15 RADIOLOGY IN PREGNANCY

Because of the potential hazards of radiation and the emergence of diagnostic ultrasound, the role of radiology in obstetrics has diminished considerably. Attention to the possible teratogenic effects of radiology was first raised in the 1920s in relation to fetal microcephaly.

The effect of radiation to future generations because of irradiation of fetal gonads has not yet been evaluated. However, radiological examination is indicated in late pregnancy, in certain situations.

Radiology related to pregnancy

Pelvimetry: where cephalopelvic disproportion is suspected or there is a breech presentation during the last 3 weeks of pregnancy. The most useful view is a lateral radiograph of the pelvis with the mother standing erect. This will provide information about the following:

(a) Angle of inclination of the pelvic brim.
(b) Shape of the sacrum.
(c) Antero-posterior diameters of the pelvis.

In some instances (e.g. previous fractured pelvis), a Thom's view of the pelvic brim is indicated.

Where the uterus is larger than dates: multiple pregnancy may be diagnosed, as well as skeletal malformations that may be associated with polyhydramnios. Ultrasound has largely replaced X-radiography for this indication, except where more than three fetuses are present where X-radiography allows them to be counted.

Radiology incidental to pregnancy

When the pregnant woman develops an illness in which radiology would normally be used, radiology is indicated in special circumstances. These situations include:

1. Severe chest pain.
2. Pneumonia.
3. IVP for haematuria or suspected ureteric colic (single exposure only).
4. Suspected perforated viscus.
5. Suspected fractures.

With modern equipment and judicious use of X-rays, no deleterious fetal effects are believed to occur, and X-rays are no longer contraindicated in pregnancy.

5.16 ULTRASOUND IN PREGNANCY

Ultrasound is sound of a frequency greater than 2 mHz. It is a safe procedure for both mother and fetus. Two types of ultrasound are used during pregnancy:

1. Continuous ultrasound. Use is made of the Doppler effect to detect fetal heart movement. This is used in the portable fetal heart detectors, as well as by the external transducers found on fetal monitors.
2. Pulsed ultrasound. Impulses are released at several millisecond intervals and are reflected by the body tissues at differing speeds, depending on the density of the tissue. The reflected sound can be converted to dots of light and a picture is subsequently built up on a storage tube oscilloscope. Transverse and longitudinal tomograms are then used to build up a picture of the uterus and its contents.

Uses in early pregnancy

1. Diagnosis and prognosis of threatened abortion and diagnosis of missed abortion.

2. Diagnosis of hydatidiform mole.
3. Examination of the uterus that is apparently larger or smaller than dates.
4. Differential diagnosis of pelvic tumours.
5. Prior to amniocentesis.
6. Estimation of fetal age – between 14 and 24 weeks, fetal size and fetal age (duration of pregnancy) correlate with a great degree of accuracy (± 7 days). After this time the correlation between fetal size and age becomes less accurate using a single examination. However, serial examinations are helpful.

Uses in late pregnancy

1. Estimation of fetal age (see item 6 above).
2. Serial measurements of fetal size. These will give valuable information about the rate of fetal growth. If three readings are made at intervals of 10–14 days, the correlation with fetal size is accurate to 250 g in over 80% of cases.
3. Diagnosis of multiple pregnancy.
4. Investigation of polyhydramnios. Ultrasound can be very helpful in detecting both skeletal and non-skeletal conditions associated with polyhydramnios.
5. Diagnosis of fetal abnormalities.
6. Determination of abnormalities of fetal presentation, lie and position.
7. Placental localization. Ultrasound can accurately diagnose placental position in about 98% of cases. Any difficulties encountered are usually associated with posterior wall placentas. Because ultrasound is harmless and the method is accurate, it has superseded other methods of placental localization.

5.17 RADIOISOTOPES IN PREGNANCY

The principal use of radioisotopes was placentography, although the technique is now redundant. Radioisotope scanning is only used in pregnancy to confirm a diagnosis of pulmonary embolism.

5.18 INVESTIGATION OF SUSPECTED FETAL GROWTH RETARDATION

Fetal growth retardation is suspected when the size of the uterus is less than expected in relation to the period of amenorrhoea during the last trimester. To make this assumption, however, the date of the last menstrual period should be accurately known and corrections should have been made for:

1. Variations in menstrual cycle length.
2. Taking of oral contraceptives before conception.
3. Maternal height. Where a mother is taller than average, the fundus of the uterus will not reach the usual landmarks at the anticipated time. The uterus frequently appears smaller than dates would suggest. With a small woman, the uterine size may appear to be larger than dates.

Causes of fetal growth retardation

Fetal growth velocity can be expressed as a simple equation:

$$\text{Velocity of fetal growth} = \text{Intrinsic growth potential} \times \text{growth support}$$

Intrinsic growth potential is genetically determined. Thus two small parents will produce a small baby, while two large parents will produce a large baby. The growth potential can be altered in certain situations:

1. Chromosomal abnormalities. The total body cell number may be reduced.
2. Damage to the embryo during organogenesis. For example, the effect of rubella or cytotoxic drugs diminish the number of cells by damage or cell death.

Growth support is a measure of the amounts of nutrients and oxygen supplied to the fetus by the mother and placenta, and the amounts of waste products and carbon dioxide removed. Factors that interfere with these processes will diminish growth support. In the case of multiple pregnancy, the nutrients and oxygen supplied may be sufficient to maintain a single fetus in optimal conditions, but they may not be enough for more than one fetus.

Management

Initially this includes an adequate history to discover the likelihood of fetal abnormality by determining such factors as drug exposure and transplacental infection. In addition, the parent's own birthweight and her situation in her own family is important, as there is good correlation between fetal and parental birthweights.

Menstrual cycle length and exposure to oral contraceptives should be noted, and these factors taken into account when correlating uterine size with the duration of amenorrhoea at the first antenatal visit. If there is a discrepancy noted, an ultrasound examination before the uterine fundus reaches the umbilicus will help to ascertain fetal age accurately.

In instances other than these, growth retardation may be suspected from physical findings in the third trimester. When the uterus is smaller to palpation than expected:

1. Check available information with regard to such factors as duration of amenorrhoea and cycle length.
2. Assess maternal weight gain. Growth retardation is often associated with a low weight increase of the mother during pregnancy.
3. Check growth of the fundus by measuring the pubis to fundus distance serially.
4. Measure the mother's girth at the umbilicus and relate this to her weight, by using one of the available charts.
5. If these parameters are abnormal, repeat the assessments at subsequent visits.
6. Commence serial ultrasound measurements of the fetus.

Ultrasound growth patterns

These will show one of three types:

1. Normal.
2. Where growth has originally been satisfactory, but then proceeds slower than normal from early in the second trimester. These charts correlate with:
    (a) Genetically small, but normal children.
    (b) Fetuses whose growth potential has been altered by: chromosomal or genetic problems exposure to transpla-

cental infection, exposure to drugs including alcohol and nicotine, or malnutrition.

3. Where growth has proceeded normally until late pregnancy and has then slowed. This indicates failure of growth support, such as in:
   (a) Hypertension.
   (b) Repeated antepartum haemorrhage.

Where growth retardation is proven the mother should rest in bed to improve uterine blood flow. The optimal time of delivery is determined by:

1. Clinical information.
2. Ultrasound growth patterns.
3. Daily fetal movement charting.
4. Antenatal cardiotocography can be helpful in order to prolong a pregnancy where the fetus is retarded but immature.
5. An amniocentesis and estimation of either the L/S ratio or TDX test will help in trying to determine the optimal time to deliver the baby without the risk of hyaline membrane disease.

5.19 PRE-ECLAMPSIA AND ECLAMPSIA

Pre-eclampsia and eclampsia are diseases that are dependent on the presence of trophoblastic tissue. Their incidence is higher in conditions where the volume of trophoblast is greater than normal, such as diabetes mellitus, multiple pregnancy, Rh iso-immunization, and large hydatidiform moles.

Pre-eclampsia results in more admissions to hospital in the antenatal period than any other condition. In its more severe forms, it is a cause of both fetal and maternal morbidity and mortality.

Diagnosis

The diagnosis is made when any two of the following three signs are observed:

1. Hypertension.

2. Generalized oedema.
3. Proteinuria.

The first two signs almost invariably precede proteinuria. Additionally, generalized oedema may be accompanied by a sudden increase in maternal weight.

Elevation of the blood pressure above 140/90 mmHg, with the patient in the left lateral position, or a rise in the diastolic pressure of 15 mmHg or 25 mmHg systolic above pre-pregnancy or early pregnancy levels, should be regarded as significant.

Generalized oedema, which produces puffiness of the face and hands, is more significant than dependent oedema. However, dependent oedema will occur when oedema is generalized.

The detection of proteinuria on routine testing should be followed by testing a mid-stream specimen of urine and if still positive the sample should be sent for culture and sensitivity to exclude a urinary tract infection. A common cause of small amounts of proteinuria is the contamination of urine by vaginal secretions, or a urinary tract infection.

The presence of proteinuria during pregnancy has long been associated with a poor outcome for both the mother and the fetus. Women are encouraged to bring an early-morning sample of urine for testing in order to avoid false-positive results due to orthostatic proteinuria. About 50 years ago, the detection of proteinuria was an indication to take the mother's blood pressure. This practice continued until it was observed that with the exception of renal disease, hypertension occurring during pregnancy precedes proteinuria.

Incidence

In Australia about 6% of pregnancies are complicated by pre-eclampsia, but its occurrence is twice as common in primigravid and grand multiparous women.

Aetiology

The aetiology is unknown, but obviously is related to the presence of functioning trophoblast, and presumably placental hormones are responsible.

Pathology

The following conditions are known to be found in patients with pre-eclampsia.

1. Diminished plasma volume.
2. Increased extracellular fluid.
3. Vasospasm.
4. Disseminated intravascular coagulation in very severe cases.
5. Ischaemic changes in various organs, when the disease is severe.

Diminished plasma volume is probably associated with the increase in extravascular fluid. This results in increased vasopressin and aldosterone secretion, in an effort to maintain intravascular volume – and vasospasm occurs.

The resultant diminished renal blood flow causes increased renin secretion and glomerular damage, thus causing proteinuria. Diminished uterine blood flow will affect placental perfusion and fetal growth. Reduction in cerebral and hepatic perfusion can produce ischaemic change in these organs.

Disseminated intravascular coagulation will further diminish the calibre of small vessels, thus increasing blood pressure and further diminishing organ perfusion.

When left untreated, the following complications can arise:

1. Fitting (seizures) (eclampsia): related to cerebral hypoxia and oedema.
2. Cerebral haemorrhage: hypertension.
3. Left ventricular heart failure: hypertension and ischaemia.
4. Renal failure: ischaemia.
5. Liver failure: ischaemia.
6. HELLP syndrome. This is an uncommon severe form of pre-eclampsia which has a high morbidity associated with haemolysis, elevated liver enzymes and a low platelet count. Hypertension may be absent in 20% of cases.
7. Death: from any of the above causes, or due to failure of coagulation.

Fetal loss increases as the disease becomes more severe, and can be as high as 50% if the mother fits. The causes of perinatal death are hypoxia, placental separation and immaturity following premature delivery.

Classification

Pre-eclampsia can be classified according to blood pressure (BP) measurements:

- Mild: diastolic BP less than 100 mmHg
- Moderate: diastolic BP less than 110 mmHg
- Severe: diastolic BP more than 110 mmHg with proteinuria.

Management

Prophylaxis: a past history of pre-eclamptic toxaemia (PET), hypertension or renal disease, or a family history of the same conditions, may predispose to eclampsia.

Regular checks should be made of weight, blood pressure and urine during pregnancy, and greater vigilance is required for those mothers at risk, as determined from the history.

Early admission to hospital is indicated when there are abnormal findings.

Mild and moderate pre-eclamptic toxaemia

1. Bed rest. This will result in increased uterine and renal blood flow. A diuresis will almost always be achieved with bed rest.
2. Regular 4-hourly blood pressure recordings and urinalysis, together with daily weighing, are required.
3. Occasionally, sedation will benefit the patient. For example, diazepam (Valium) (5 mg 6-hourly) or temazepam 10–20 mg at night. Some have discouraged the use of diazepam-like products during pregnancy.

There is no indication for diuretics unless nerve compression syndromes (e.g. carpal tunnel) are present.

In mild cases, the blood pressure and oedema subside readily and after 3–4 days, the patient may be discharged from hospital after a period of mobilization. Usually further management is on an outpatient basis. If re-admission is required, the patient should remain in hospital.

In moderate cases, rest in hospital should continue if the blood pressure does not fall below 90 mmHg. Hypotensive agents are rarely, if ever, indicated unless the blood pressure remains above 100 mmHg. Besides the routine observations, the pregnancy should be monitored by fetal movement charts, cardiotocography and serial ultrasound. Induction of labour may be necessary between 37 and 40 weeks.

Severe pre-eclamptic toxaemia

Severe PET (or pregnancy-induced hypertension) is an obstetric emergency requiring intensive care both before and after delivery. Most patients recover quickly, usually after transient episodes of extreme hypertension or oliguria. If further complications arise, e.g. eclampsia, renal failure or intravascular coagulation, recovery may be delayed. Although PET is relatively common, most obstetricians will only see an occasional severe case.

Blood pressure recording

Before commencing management, it is important to standardize the recording of blood pressure. Due to hydrostatic pressure differences blood pressure should always be taken with the arm at the level of the heart. Thus patients in hospital should have their blood pressure taken as follows – the patient should lie on her back. If more than 26 weeks gestation, she should roll her lower abdomen and hips 45° to her left to prevent compression of the vena cava and aorta. The cuff is placed on the left arm with a pillow under the elbow. A pillow may also be placed under the abdomen.

Management of severe PET (BP higher than 110 mmHg diastolic, significant proteinuria) where delivery is indicated

1. Admit to labour ward.
2. Allocate *one* nurse to look after the patient.
3. Inform a physician and a paediatrician.
4. Deliver by the most expeditious means.
5. Fetal observation:
   Continuous CTG in labour.

6. Maternal observations:
    (a) Strict fluid balance chart.
    (b) Blood pressure – every 15 minutes.
    (c) Special nurse.
    (d) Urinalysis – 4-hourly.
    (e) Urine output – hourly measure with indwelling catheter.
    (f) Central venous pressure (CVP) – measure hourly. To be inserted by anaesthetist and checked with chest radiology.
    (g) Pathology: Full blood count and platelets.
                  Clotting time.
                  Fibrinogen, d dimers.
                  Urea, creatinine, electrolytes and uric acid.
                  Cross-match blood.
    Albumin, total protein, liver function tests may be performed later.
7. (a) Maternal treatment:
    Strict bed rest in a single, quiet, dark room.
    (b) Anticonvulsant therapy:
    Phenytoin infusion via IVAC infusion pump. Commence at 5 mg/h after initial statim dose. In the US, magnesium sulphate 4 g IV is much preferred.
    (c) Hypotensive therapy:
    If a patient is conscious, continue previous hypotensive agents.
    If unconscious, or blood pressure high, use:
    hydralazine (Apresoline), 20 mg parenteral or labetalol (Trandate), or magnesium sulphate IVI
      (i) Epidural block is sometimes used if patient is labouring
      (ii) Urine output maintain at more than 25 ml/h. If output less than 20 ml/h and CVP less than 12 mm use concentrated albumin.
      If output less than 25 ml/h and CVP more than 16 mm use frusemide (Lasix) 40 mg IV.
8. Remain in labour ward until blood pressure and urine output satisfactory – most patients become worse immediately postpartum, then eventually improve.

Patients in hospital requiring hypotensive therapy

1. Inform physicians and paediatricians.
2. Fetal observations:
   (a) Fetal movement chart and monitoring.
   (b) Serial CTGs.
   (c) Serial ultrasound every 2 weeks.
3. Maternal observations:
   (a) Fluid balance chart.
   (b) Weigh daily.
   (c) Blood pressure every 4 hours.
   (d) Pathology – as for severe PET, including uric acid and liver function tests.
   (e) 24-hour urine protein.
4. Maternal treatment:
   (a) Bed rest.
   (b) Hypotensive agents. Continue previous treatment. If blood pressure rises: hydralazine (Apresoline) or, labetalol (Trandate).
   (c) Sedation – preferably nil. Otherwise diazepam (Valium).
5. Deliver if there is:
   (a) Rising blood pressure.
   (b) Rising proteinuria.
   (c) Fetal compromise.
6. Continue treatment at least 48 hours postpartum.

Delivery

If the cervix is favourable, amniotomy should be performed and an oxytocin infusion commenced. If the cervix is unfavourable prostaglandin E_2 may be used to make it more favourable or Caesarean section can be considered.

Following delivery of the baby the maternal condition should be monitored until blood pressure returns to normal. This is frequently rapid, but may take several days. Remember that fitting (seizures) may recur at any time, but especially within the first 24 hours. In the long term, the mother should be observed for evidence of hypertension or renal disease.

Outcome

Eclampsia is still a cause of maternal mortality, usually associated with cerebral haemorrhage.

Fetal mortality is in excess of 50% when the mother has fitted either due to hypoxia *per se* or secondary to placental separation.

5.20 INTRAUTERINE FETAL DEATH

Fetal death may occur at any time during pregnancy due to a variety of causes, including:

1. Maternal hypertension (especially pre-eclamptic toxaemia).
2. Placental separation.
3. Transplacental infection.
4. Cord entanglement (rarely).
5. Rh iso-immunization.
6. Rarely maternal diseases, such as diabetes mellitus and chronic renal disease.

In a great number of instances, no obvious cause can be found.

Symptoms and signs

There may be a preceding history of one of the causes of fetal death. A loss of fetal movement is noted, which sometimes may be heralded by a period of unusual fetal activity. Fetal heart sounds are absent. After several days the uterus commences to shrink due to resorption of amniotic fluid.

Confirmation

1. Ultrasound. No heart movement will be detected either with a Doppler sensor or M-mode echography.
2. Radiology. Radiology is performed with 24–36 hours, gas may be seen in the fetal heart, great vessels and even the umbilical cord. Overlapping of the fetal cranial bones (Spalding's sign) takes about 3–10 days to develop, and is usually preceded by obvious separation of the cranial sutures.

Outcome

Labour usually commences within a few days or a week of the episode that kills the fetus. However, if labour has not commenced within 3 weeks of fetal death disseminated intravascular thrombosis may occur in the mother.

The mechanism for such coagulation is thought to be thromboplastin entering the maternal circulation from the degenerating placenta, causing widespread fibrin deposition. This is a chronic event that usually takes about 4 weeks to develop. As intravascular fibrin deposition occurs, there is a compensatory response from the plasma to convert plasminogen to plasmin. This in turn causes a further breakdown of fibrin and fibrinogen. The result of intravascular thrombosis and fibrinogen utilization is to produce hypofibrinogenaemia. Normal fibrinogen levels of 0.45 g/l fall slowly to under 0.1 g/l.

Management

If spontaneous labour does not ensue, it is natural for the parents to ask that labour be induced. Induction should not be embarked upon unless coagulation studies are normal.

The usual method of induction is by oxytocin infusion, but today prostaglandins are increasingly being used. The membranes are usually not ruptured due to the high risk of intrauterine infection.

After delivery, if there is no obvious cause, the mother should be investigated to exclude syphilis, iso-immunization or diabetes mellitus.

5.21 COAGULATION DEFECTS IN OBSTETRICS

These defects may be either chronic or acute.

1. Chronic, due to:
   (a) Fetal death *in utero.*
   (b) Missed abortion.
2. Acute, due to:
   (a) Severe placental abruption.
   (b) Severe pre-eclampsia and eclampsia.
   (c) Septic shock.
3. Amniotic fluid embolism.

The principle of management is the same, although the method is different. *Never* undertake a surgical procedure until the bleeding defect is corrected.

Investigations

1. Platelet count.
2. Fibrinogen and d dimer estimation.
3. Coagulation time and or bleeding time.
4. Prothrombin index.

Chronic coagulation disorders

The patient should be given heparin. This will inhibit fibrin deposition and allow fibrinogen and platelet levels, as well as other coagulation factors, to return to normal over a period of 48 hours.

Acute coagulation disorders

Transfusion with fresh whole blood under central venous pressure control. This will provide not only haemoglobin, but also all other coagulation factors including platelets (which are not present in stored blood).

Stored plasma protein substrate (SPPS) can be given while waiting for fresh blood.

If there is a fibrinolytic effect from plasmin production, then epsilon-aminocaproic acid (EACA) may be given to inhibit this reaction.

5.22 BREECH PRESENTATION (see Chapter 6)

The incidence of breech presentation falls as gestation advances with an incidence of 20% at the 30th week and 2–3% at term. The reasons for this are not known but two in particular are believed to play important roles: (i) the pear-shape of the uterus and the same shape of the head-down fetus at term; and (ii) the presence of the ala of the iliac bones of the maternal pelvis gives the kicking baby a solid purchase, resulting in its being able to kick itself round from a breech presentation, provided that the knees are flexed. Once in a cephalic presentation the fetus has only maternal soft tissues in the upper abdomen and is in effect unable to kick itself out of a head-down position.

In a small proportion of cases of breech presentation, there is either a structural or neurological abnormality in the fetus or a 'space-occupying' lesion preventing the fetus from turning. Examples of the latter are placenta praevia, large fibroids in the lower portion of the uterus, congenital uterine anomalies, contracted pelvis or a second fetus. The incidence of fetal anomalies in term breech presentations is at least twice that of term cephalic presentations and in pre-term breech presentations may be as much as four times higher, i.e. 17–20%.

Prognosis

In the absence of any other problems in pregnancy, pre-term breech births carry a perinatal mortality rate of up to 120 per 1000 and in term uncomplicated cases it has been reported as being 20–50 per 1000. The increased mortality, after excluding congenital abnormalities is due to:

1. Intracranial injury. The aftercoming head has less time for moulding and is in fact designed to mould in the opposite direction. Rapid compression and subsequent decompression are particularly likely to result in a tentorial tear and intracranial haemorrhage and this injury accounts for more than half the perinatal mortality of breech delivery.
2. Anoxia. Compression of the cord by the trunk and aftercoming head may interfere with placental circulation. Uterine retraction may initiate placental separation before delivery of the head. Cord prolapse in labour, rare with a frank breech but more likely with a flexed breech, may result in anoxia.

Management

Elective Caesarean section at term is presently performed in anything up to half the breech presentations. Where a breech presents at term in a patient with a normal or larger than normal gynaecoid pelvis and where the ultrasound assessment reveals a fetal weight of no more than 3.5 kg, vaginal delivery appears to carry no increased risk to the fetus. Where these criteria are not met or there is another complication of pregnancy such as hypertension, Caesarean section – despite its maternal morbidity – is advised.

External cephalic version (ECV) performed between the 36th and the 38th week will be successful in at least half the cases and reduce the incidence of a breech presentation in labour by at least 50%. ECV may require tocolysis using an intravenous bolus of a beta-adrenergic drug such as salbutamol or ritodrine to be successful. General anaesthesia was commonly used in the past, but it has now universally been abandoned.

Labour

The success of the vaginal delivery of a breech depends largely upon the skill and experience of the obstetrician. Diagnosis of a breech presentation may on occasion present the inexperienced with difficulty and it is only after rupture of the membranes that digital vaginal examination will reveal the true state of affairs. In the case of a flexed breech, the projecting heel will be readily distinguished from a hand. With a frank breech, although the rounded buttocks may superficially resemble a skull, the underlying bones and thus sutures are absent and with careful examination the sacrum and anus can be identified.

The denominator used to describe positions of the breech is the sacrum; thus the four positions conventionally used are sacroanterior and sacroposterior on both left and right sides.

In most cases, the bitrochanteric diameter (± 10 cm and similar to the BDP 9.5 cm) enters the pelvic brim in the transverse diameter with the back anterior (uppermost). As labour progresses the conical shape of the breech is a better dilator of the cervix than the rounded head and it descends into the pelvic cavity. When the buttocks reach the pelvic floor, the pelvic 'gutter' of the two levatores ani causes internal rotation, bringing the bitrochanteric diameter into the antero-posterior diameter of the pelvic outlet. The anterior buttock appears at the vulva and the breech is born by lateral flexion of the trunk. The rest of the trunk is born by further descent and external rotation of the buttocks occurs as the shoulders enter the pelvic brim in its transverse diameter. The arms normally remain flexed in front of the body unless injudicious traction on the legs has occurred resulting in the arm(s) becoming extended above the head. The shoulders then reach the pelvic floor and its shape encourages rotation such that the bis-acromial diameter comes to lie in the antero-posterior diameter of the pelvic outlet. The anterior shoulder emerges under the pubic arch, quickly followed by the posterior shoulder.

The flexed head enters the pelvis in its transverse diameter and forward rotation of the back is seen to occur as the head descends and undergoes internal rotation. The fetal neck comes to lie against the public symphysis and once the nape of the neck is seen, the lower limbs are swept in an arc describing a 'backward somersault', resulting in the chin and then face escaping over the perineum. With the appearance of the nose and mouth, these are sucked clear of mucus and the baby will often begin to breathe. Slow controlled delivery of the head, often with forceps, is now achieved and the baby placed on the maternal abdomen.

Occasionally the obstetrician will need to assist the fetus by flexing one or both extended legs. This is achieved by applying digital pressure in the popliteal fossa and abducting the leg. Similarly, delivery of the arms may require their flexion by pressure in the cubital fossa but the extent of obstetrical manipulation is best described as masterly inactivity.

Where a breech birth is going to occur, it is advised that the patient have an epidural block, since some form of manipulation may unexpectedly be required. A trial of labour may be conducted just as well with a breech presentation as with a cephalic presentation and for success in either, cervical dilatation should occur at a rate that exceeds 1 cm/hour in the active phase of labour.

Transverse and oblique lie (see Chapter 8)

When the fetus lies with its long axis transverse or oblique to the long axis of the uterus, the shoulder is usually the presenting point and this occurs in about 1 in 400 labours. This may occur in a multiparous patient with a lax abdominal wall and a lax uterus but may be associated with polyhydramnios, uterine malformation or placenta praevia.

When diagnosed after 36 weeks an ultrasound should be

obtained to seek a specific cause. In the absence of any cause, external version will often correct the lie, whereas Caesarean section should be used where a placenta praevia is present or if version fails.

Face presentation

Extreme extension of the head results in a face presentation and usually no specific cause is found. In some, however (1:7), the fetus is anencephalic or has a tumour of the front of the neck. Clinically the occiput is palpable on abdominal examination on the same side as the fetal back and at a higher level than the sinciput. On vaginal examination confusion with a breech may occur unless the supraorbital ridges and the chin are identified opposite each other.

In labour, the presenting diameter is the submento-vertical – 9.5 cm which is the same as a vertex; descent is slow and seldom occurs until late in the first stage. The denominator in this presentation is the chin, resulting in mentoposterior and mentoanterior positions. When internal rotation results in a direct mentoposterior position, spontaneous delivery is impossible and either rotation with Kielland's or a Caesarean section must be employed. With a mentoanterior position, delivery by flexion occurs.

Brow presentation

A rare presentation that generally develops as the head descends. The mentovertical diameter of 13.5 cm is generally too large to permit engagement so that once the head has entered the brim in a deflexed position further secondary extension in the pelvic cavity produces a brow presentation.

Where a brow presentation is present with the occiput lying posteriorly and the chin anteriorly, the cervix becomes fully dilated but the head becomes arrested. If the head can be rotated such that the occiput comes to lie anteriorly, flexion of the head usually occurs and vaginal delivery with forceps can be easily accomplished. Rotation is best performed with Kielland's forceps and the trial of forceps philosophy is the appropriate one with Caesarean section resorted to if any difficulty is experienced.

6

Normal labour and delivery

6.1 GENERAL INSTRUCTIONAL OBJECTIVE

The students should understand perinatal anatomy, physiology and psychology that occurs in both mother and baby so that he or she appreciates the principles of management of labour and knows how to supervise a spontaneous delivery.

6.2 SPECIFIC BEHAVIOURAL OBJECTIVES

1. Describe the anatomy of the female pelvis and the fetus relevant to labour and delivery.
2. Describe the uterine physiology and the mechanisms of labour.
3. Conduct a normal third stage of labour, examine the placenta, cord and membranes and describe the findings.
4. Discuss normal placental separation and the drugs affecting uterine muscle activity.
5. Provide emotional support to a woman in normal labour.
6. Recognize the onset of labour and the normal progress of labour by history, abdominal and vaginal examination and record the findings.
7. Assist with the conduct of a normal delivery.
8. Discuss the nutritional and fluid requirements of the mother during labour and be aware of how to assess them clinically.
9. Assess and discuss the condition of the fetus during labour.
10. Demonstrate a knowledge of pain relief with drugs and other measures during labour and discuss the possible effects on the fetus and mother.
11. Describe the management of an assisted breech delivery.
12. Discuss the indications for and the technique of episiotomy, and the principles of repair of episiotomy or lacerations.

6.3 REASONS FOR UNDERSTANDING NORMAL LABOUR AND DELIVERY, AND RESUSCITATION OF THE NEWBORN

The basis of obstetrics is to care for a woman during her pregnancy, to assist with the delivery of an infant who is born in an optimal condition, and to prevent any complications occurring to either mother or baby during this process. To achieve this skill in practice requires an understanding of the physiological processes and the mechanisms of labour, as well as the techniques of management of labour, delivery, resuscitation of the newborn and the management of the puerperium. This chapter will provide the basic information necessary for students to understand these processes.

6.4 ANATOMY OF THE FEMALE PELVIS

The obstetric anatomy of the female pelvis is divided into the bony structure of the pelvis and the soft tissues therein, including the uterus, cervix, vagina, pelvic fascia, ligaments, bladder, rectum, muscles and perineum.

The bony pelvis is made up by four bones: the sacrum, coccyx and the two innominates (consisting of the ilium,

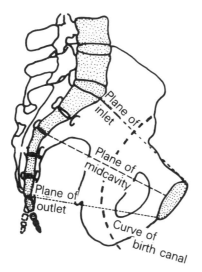

Figure 6.1 Showing the three planes of the pelvis – brim, midcavity and outlet – and illustrating that the coccyx will bend backwards to accommodate a large fetal head.

ischium and pubic bones). These bones are divided into three obstetrically significant sections (Fig. 6.1).

1. Inlet or brim: this is bounded in front by the symphysis pubis, at the sides by the pubic crest, pectineal eminence, ilio-pectineal line, sacro-iliac joint and posteriorly by the sacrum itself.
2. Mid cavity: this is the true pelvis, and is that area lying between the pelvic brim or inlet and the pelvic outlet. It is bounded in front by the lower border of the back of the symphysis pubis, by the ischial spines laterally, and by the lower border of the last sacral vertebrae posteriorly.
3. Outlet: this is bounded by the lower border of the symphysis pubis, the ischial tuberosities and the coccyx.

Diameters of the obstetric pelvis

1. The true or direct conjugate diameter of the brim extends from the centre of the back of the symphysis pubis to the sacral promontory. In a normal gynaecoid pelvis, this measures about 11.5 cm. The sacral promontory is the most protuberant point on the sacrum.
2. The oblique diameters of the pelvic brim extend from the sacro-iliac joint to the diagonally opposite pectineal eminence. Normally, in a gynaecoid pelvis, this distance is about 12.5 cm.
3. The transverse diameter of the pelvic brim extends across the pelvis at its widest point. It normally measures about 13.5 cm.

In the gynaecoid pelvis (see below), the average diameters of the mid-cavity measure about 12 cm, whereas at the outlet, the diameters are the reverse of the brim – with the antero-posterior diameter being 13.5 cm and the transverse or bi-ischial diameter being about 11.5 cm.

The plane of the brim is an imaginary line at the obstetric inlet which, in the erect female with a gynaecoid pelvis, makes an inclination of 55° to the horizontal (Fig. 6.2).

The axis of the pelvis is a line drawn through the mid-cavity of the pelvis from the brim to the outlet. Normally it curves forward through 90° in the mid-pelvis (Fig. 6.1).

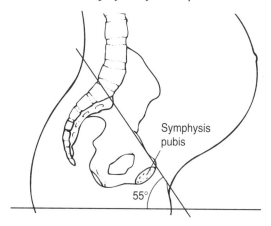

Figure 6.2 Illustrating that in the erect position the plane of the pelvic brim makes an angle of 55° with the horizontal.

Pelvic brim shapes

Caldwell and Moloy in 1934 performed anatomical studies on female pelves and were able to describe four major categories of pelvic shapes. Although there are many variations on these basic brim shapes, most women will have a pelvis that is described by one of these major subdivisions. The shape and size of the obstetric inlet dictates the mechanisms of labour and influences the progress in labour. It is important to understand these variations in pelvic shapes (Fig. 6.3).

1. Gynaecoid pelvis
This is the most common type (50%) of the pelvic brim shape among Caucasian females. This has a basically rounded brim and a well-rounded sacral curve, an adequate pelvic cavity, a well-rounded subpubic arch and an adequate obstetric outlet. The sidewalls of this pelvis are parallel.

2. Anthropoid pelvis
The anthropoid pelvis is also common (30%) and is character-ized by a long antero-posterior diameter, a normal transverse diameter and a deep pelvic cavity. The obstetric diameters are generally large and the subpubic angle is well-rounded. The sidewalls are parallel.

3. Android pelvis

The android pelvis occurs in about 20% of women and is associated with a generally triangular brim shape, with the maximum transverse diameter close to the posterior portion of the obstetric inlet. There is usually a flattened sacrum, convergent pelvic walls and a narrow subpubic arch.

4. Platypelloid pelvis

The platypelloid pelvis (5%) is relatively uncommon and is characterized by a shortened antero-posterior diameter and

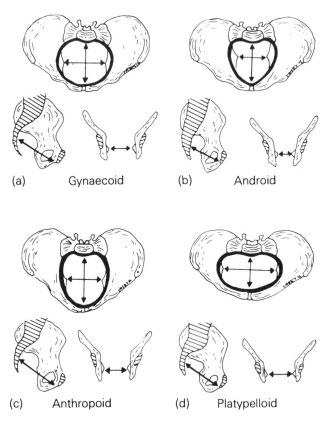

(a)   Gynaecoid   (b)   Android

(c)   Anthropoid   (d)   Platypelloid

Figure 6.3 Common types of pelvic brim shapes. (a) Well-rounded brim. Rounded sacral curve, parallel pelvic side walls; (b) Triangular-shaped brim. Flattened sacrum, narrow sacro-sciatic notch. Convergent pelvic side walls; (c) Large pelvic brim with long anteroposterior diameter. Wide but deep sacrum. Parallel side walls; (d) Flattened pelvic brim with small anteroposterior diameter. Short but good pelvic curve. Parallel side walls.

wide transverse diameter of the brim, with a shallow pelvic cavity having divergent walls and a wide subpubic arch. Obstetric problems usually are encountered at the brim only.

Soft tissues of birth canal

The pelvic floor comprises those muscles, ligaments and fascia that fill in the pelvic outlet and support the intrapelvic viscera. During the process of labour, these soft tissues stretch and dilate to allow the fetus to pass through the bony pelvis. The uterus and cervix form a muscular sac in which the muscle bundles are arranged to produce an efficient expulsive unit, which forces the fetus through the pelvis, stretching the soft tissue in the pelvic floor during the process.

The main anatomical structures of the pelvic floor (pelvic diaphragm) are:

1. The levator ani muscles and their investing fascia, which slope forwards, downwards and inwards. By this inclination, they exert an important influence on the movement and rotation of the fetal head as it passes down the pelvis (Fig. 6.4). The levator ani muscle arises from a broad expanse over the sides of the pelvis, extending from the ala of the sacrum, the ileo-pectineal line and around to the front of the pelvis behind the symphysis pubis. The muscle fibres pass round the vagina, urethra and rectum to insert

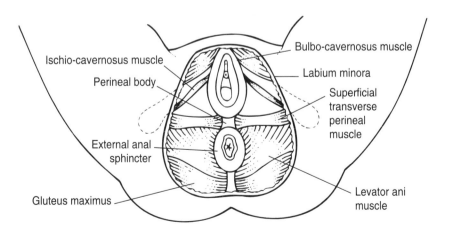

Figure 6.4 Soft structures of the pelvic floor.

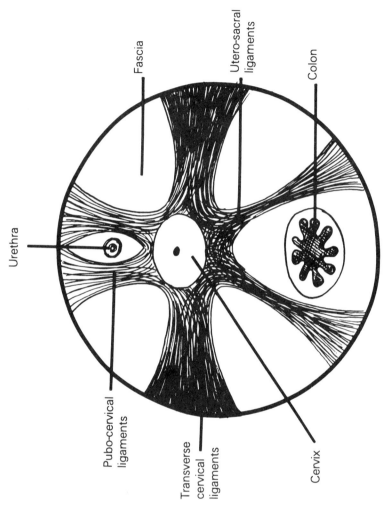

Figure 6.5 Ligamentous supports of the cervix and uterus.

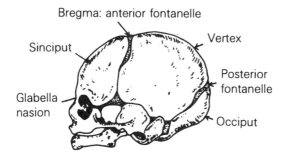

Bregma: anterior fontanelle

Sinciput

Vertex

Posterior fontanelle

Glabella nasion

Occiput

Figure 6.6 Lateral view of the fetal skull.

into the lateral borders of the coccyx and the sacrum.

2. The endopelvic fascia and its condensations which form the transverse cervical ligaments, the utero-sacral ligaments and the pubo-cervical ligaments. With the surrounding fascia, these support the uterus, cervix and upper third of the vagina (Fig. 6.5).

3. Perineal muscles consisting of the bulbo-cavernosus and ischio-cavernosus muscles, as well as the superficial and deep transverse perineii muscles, and the external anal sphincter which together with the fascia investing these muscles make up the remainder of the support for the vagina and introitus (Fig. 6.4).

Normally, all those soft structures which form the pelvic diaphragm and provide support for the pelvic floor are softened, stretched and dilated during labour. However, during difficult deliveries (such as prolonged labour, disproportion and forceps delivery) tears, overstretching or cuts may occur to produce an anatomical weakness or deficiency. If these are not properly managed, a permanent deficiency may occur, predisposing to prolapse.

6.5 THE FETUS

Normally the fetus presents by the head (97%), so the anatomical arrangement of the fetal skull is important in understanding the process and mechanisms of labour.

The fetal head is generally oval in shape and will pass

through the pelvis relatively easily when in an ideal attitude and position.

The attitude of the fetal skull is usually one of flexion, so that the suboccipito-bregmatic diameter (9.5 cm) will enter the pelvic brim. This is the presenting diameter when the head rotates into an occipito-anterior position so that the fetal head may pass through the pelvis and extend from under the symphysis pubis. If the head is deflexed and presents in an occipito-posterior position, then the presenting diameter may be either suboccipito-frontal (10.5 cm) or occipito frontal (11.5 cm). In a face presentation as the result of extension of the fetal head, the diameter is the submento-vertical (9.5 cm) whereas in a brow presentation, it is mento-vertical (13.5 cm) (Figs 6.6 and 6.7).

The skull is composed of the bones forming the base, the face and the vault. Those bones at the base and in the face are firm and incompressible, whereas the skull bones of the vault are soft cartilaginous plates joined at their edges by fibrous tissue. These fibrous joints are called *sutures*. This arrangement of the vault bones allows for considerable moulding or overlapping of these bony plates during labour. The sutures easily identified on a fetal skull are the sagittal, frontal, coronal and the lambdoid sutures (Fig. 6.7).

The anterior fontanelle is diamond-shaped and is formed by the junction of the sagittal, frontal and coronal sutures. The

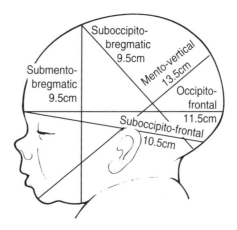

Figure 6.7 Landmarks and diameters of the fetal skull.

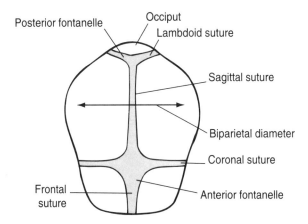

Figure 6.8 Sutures and fontanelles of the fetal skull.

posterior fontanelle is much smaller and triangular-shaped and the junction of the sagittal and lambdoid sutures (Fig. 6.8).

The vertex is the area bounded by the anterior and the posterior fontanelles and laterally by the parietal eminences. It is usually the presenting part of the well-flexed head as it passes down through the pelvis (Fig. 6.7).

The occiput (the posterior vault bone) extends from the lambdoid sutures to the foramen magnum. Because of its size and the occipital ridge, it is easily identified and is used as a point of reference (denominator) when identifying the position of a fetus in relationship to the maternal pelvis.

Sinciput is the opposite of occiput and is the area between the anterior fontanelle and the glabella (Fig. 6.6).

Definitions of importance regarding the fetus in its relationship to the mother before and during labour

Fetal attitude. This is the term applied to fetal parts in their relationship to each other. Normally a fetus is universally flexed with the head flexed on the trunk, the back flexed and all the limbs flexed. In this position of universal flexion, the fetus presents (vertex presentation) the smallest possible diameters to the pelvic brim (suboccipito-bregmatic and biparietal diameters of skull – 9.5 cm).

Fetal lie. This is the term given to the relationship of the long axis of the fetus to the long axis of the mother. Mostly, the fetus takes up a longitudinal lie, but may have a transverse or oblique lie.

Fetal presentation. This is the term given to the part of the fetus that is lowest in the pelvis. This is usually the head (cephalic) but may be the breech, shoulder, abdomen or even cord, etc., depending on the lie of the fetus.

Fetal position. This is defined as the relationship of the denominator of the presenting part of the fetus to the maternal pelvis. When the head is presenting, there are two possible denominators (occiput or mentum). Because the mentum or chin is only used as the denominator in relation to the fully extended head (face presentation), most reference will be to the occiput. Normally at the onset of labour, the fetus presents with the head in the occipito-lateral position (OL, 65%), right or left; occipito-anterior (OA, 25%), right or left; occipito-posterior (OP, 8%) right or left; and direct occipito-anterior (OA) or occipito-posterior position (OP, 2%).

Engagement of the fetal head. This is said to occur when the widest transverse diameter of the head (biparietal diameter,

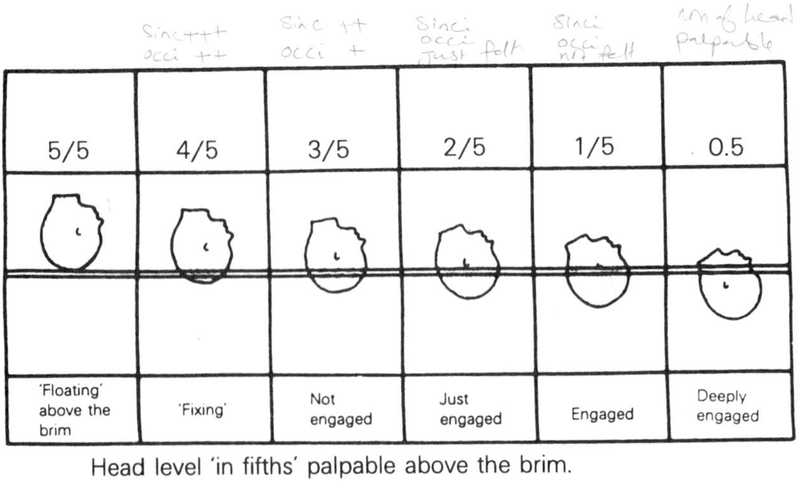

Sinc+++ occi ++	Sinc ++ occi +	Sinci occi just felt	Sinci occi nit felt	on of head palpable	
5/5	4/5	3/5	2/5	1/5	0.5
'Floating' above the brim	'Fixing'	Not engaged	Just engaged	Engaged	Deeply engaged

Head level 'in fifths' palpable above the brim.

Figure 6.9 Showing the assessment of descent of the fetal head into the pelvis, measured in fifths.

9.5 cm) has passed through the pelvic brim. On vaginal examination, the vertex will be at the level of the ischial spines.
Descent of the fetal head is usually assessed abdominally. The
head is divided into fifths below the pelvic inlet (see Fig. 6.9).
Descent of the presenting part is probably the result of
increased uterine activity as well as formation of the lower
uterine segment, which develops from the anatomical isthmus
of the uterus. The fetal head engages by 38 weeks in primigravid patients but may not engage in multiparous patients
until they are in labour.

Asynclitism. This occurs when there is asymmetrical presentation of the parietal bones. On examination, the sagittal suture
of the fetal skull does not lie midway between the sacral promontory and the symphysis pubis. When the sagittal suture is
posterior near the sacrum and the anterior parietal bone is
lower in the pelvis than the posterior parietal bone, it is called
anterior asynclitism (Fig. 6.10). When the reverse occurs and
the posterior parietal bone is lower, it is called posterior asyn-

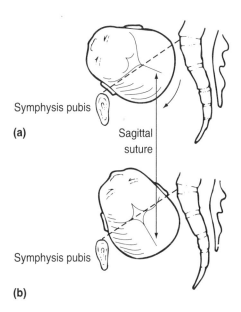

Symphysis pubis

(a)

Sagittal
suture

Symphysis pubis

(b)

Figure 6.10 Demonstrating how a head may enter the pelvic brim by
asynclitism, with (a) first one parietal bone presenting and then, (b)
following pressure and moulding, the other parietal bone sliding
through the pelvic brim.

clitism. The head usually engages by lateral flexion. This phenomenon occurs in association with occipito-lateral positions,
cephalopelvic disproportion and with a platypelloid pelvis.

6.6 PHYSIOLOGICAL PROCESS IN LABOUR
(THE POWERS)

Physiology of labour

1. Effective labour contractions are initiated by a complex
   process beginning in the fetus. It appears that maturation
   of fetal adrenal tissue produces cortisone, which acts on the
   placenta to produce a change in the oestrogen/progester-
   one ratio, and which also appears to initiate the production
   of increased amounts of prostaglandin. The prostaglandins
   produce not only increased amplitude in the uterine contractions, but also an increase in the rate of contractions.
   Eventually, as well as softening the cervix with partial effacement, contractions force the presenting part onto the
   lower uterine segment and as this is thinned out and stretched, a reflex (Ferguson's reflex) initiates the production of
   oxytocin from the posterior pituitary gland. Stretching of
   the cervix in turn also leads to prostaglandin production.
   These hormones enhance uterine contractions by increasing
   the rate, tone and amplitude of contractions, and so labour
   becomes established.
2. Painful contractions. The pain of labour contractions is
   almost entirely cervical in origin and is associated with the
   resistance of the cervix to the dilating forces. As labour
   progresses, pain is felt as soon as the intrauterine pressure
   rises above 25 mmHg (Fig. 6.11).

In well-established labour, a uterine contraction lasts for
about 50–60 seconds and occurs every 2–4 minutes. During
contractions, the intrauterine pressure varies from 50–70 mmHg
in the late first stage. Thus the pain lasts for the entire duration
of the contraction, whereas in early labour the pain may be
only mild and occur near the peak of the uterine contraction.

As labour progresses, the spiral muscles of the fundus of the
uterus become more dominant, pulling up and thinning the
cervix and lower segment. Normally, in primipara, the cervix is

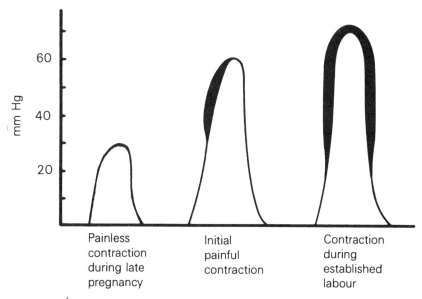

Figure 6.11 Showing pain in relation to amplitude of contraction. The duration of 'pain' is shown by the thickened line.

effaced before dilation begins whereas in multigravida, the cervix begins to dilate as the lower segment and cervix are pulled up.

As the cervix dilates in early labour, the mucous plug blocking the endocervical canal is dislodged. This, together with some bleeding that occurs as the chorionic membrane 'shears' off the lower segment, forms a blood-stained 'show'.

The uterus and cervix are an active unit of muscular power providing the force by which the fetus (passenger) is pushed through the pelvis (passage).

Secondary powers in labour

When the presenting part reaches the pelvic floor (usually after full dilatation), the distension of the vagina and pressure on the rectum produces a sensation that results in the expulsive 'bearing down' exertion. During this process the diaphragm is fixed, and the thoracic and abdominal muscles are contracted to assist expelling the fetus. The pressure on the fetal skull during this stage may reach 100–120 mmHg.

6.7 MECHANISMS OF LABOUR

The mechanism of labour is the mechanical changes that take place throughout the process of labour and delivery. These are physiological processes and occur spontaneously. The following steps normally occur in a fetus with a cephalic presentation:

1. **Flexion.** Most fetuses present in the occipito-lateral position at the onset of labour. Uterine contractions exert pressure on the upper pole of the fetus to produce flexion of the head on the neck and so reduce the presenting diameter (Fig. 6.12).
2. **Descent.** The next stage in the mechanism is descent through the pelvic brim. When the head is well flexed, the presenting diameters (biparietal 9.5 cm, sub-occipito breg-matic 9.5 cm) pass easily through the brim and descent is rapid. Delay may occur when extension of the head persists (occipito-posterior position), the head is abnormally large, the pelvis is of an abnormal shape (android brim) or the pelvis is small in size.
3. **Internal rotation.** The underlining principle in rotation is that whichever part of the fetus hits the pelvic floor first,

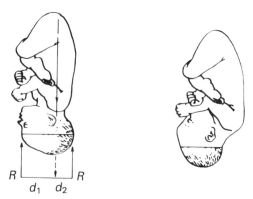

Figure 6.12 Flexion: resistance at the pelvic brim and the asymmetry of the fetal head encourages flexion of the neck. d_1 and d_2 – distances to foramen magnum. R = resistance of pelvic brim. $R \times d_1$ is greater than $R \times d_2$, thus resulting in flexion.

will usually rotate *anteriorly*. If the fetal head is well flexed, the occiput hits the pelvic floor first and then rotates anteriorly. This is called 'internal rotation' and varies from 45–90–135 degrees depending upon whether the head was in an occipito-anterior or occipito-lateral or occipito-posterior position. The shoulders always rotate 45° less than the head. If the head rotates through 45° then the shoulders at this stage remain unchanged in their position. Should the head rotate through 90°, then the shoulders will rotate to 45°.

4. **Descent.** Further descent of the presenting part now occurs.

5. **Extension.** The head, as it passes out of the birth canal, extends with the symphysis pubis acting as a fulcrum. This process is called crowning and leads to delivery of the fetal head (Figs 6.13–6.15).

6. **Restitution.** As the head is no longer flexed inside the birth canal, it rotates through 45° to return to the position that it held prior to internal rotation. At this stage, the head is once again at right angles to the shoulders.

7. **External rotation.** There is now further descent until the leading shoulder reaches the pelvic floor where it rotates anteriorly, followed by rotation of the head by 45°. This is called *external rotation* as it occurs outside the pelvis and is visible to the observer. The sagittal suture is now in the transverse position.

8. **Birth of the shoulders.** The anterior shoulder comes into view under the symphysis pubis where it remains while

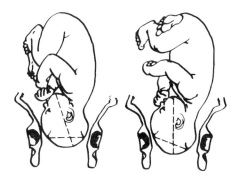
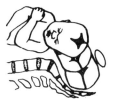

Figure 6.13 Showing that descent occurs as the head flexes. It usually enters the pelvic brim in the occipito-lateral position and then undergoes internal rotation deep in the pelvic cavity.

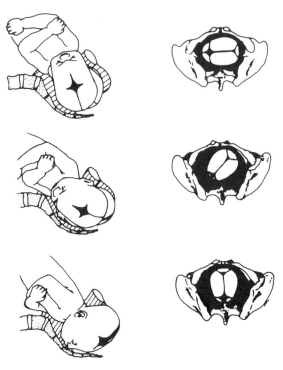

Figure 6.14 Demonstrating how internal rotation occurs deep in the pelvic cavity, so that the occiput normally comes to lie in an anterior position.

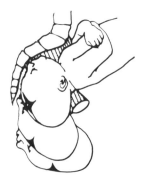

Figure 6.15 Demonstrating how the head extends as it descends and is born from under the symphysis pubis.

the posterior shoulder is born following lateral flexion of the fetal spine.

9. **Birth of the trunk.** The remainder of the trunk is also born by lateral flexion.

Occipito-posterior position

Long rotation
In 90% of these cases, the fetal head flexes and the occiput will undergo *internal rotation* through 135° into the occipito-anterior position. The shoulders rotate through 90°. The remainder of the delivery is identical to the mechanisms outlined above.

Short rotation
In 10% of occipito-posterior positions, the head extends with descent allowing the sinciput to hit the pelvic floor first; this rotates anteriorly. *Internal rotation* through 45° occurs resulting in the head being in the direct occipito-posterior position.

Delivery of the head (face to pubis). As the head is already extended, this occurs by a combination of flexion to allow the head to deliver and extension to allow the face to be born. The presenting diameter is the larger suboccipito-frontal (10.5 cm). The remainder of the mechanism of delivery is similar to all the other positions.

Deep transverse arrest

In less than 1% of births, the head neither fully flexes nor extends. The head rotates 45° to the occipito-lateral position and then stops. This occurs at the level of the ischial spines. It may also be due to the fact that the transverse diameter of that pelvis may be inadequate to allow full rotation to occur. This is a deep transverse arrest. For delivery to occur, the head needs to be rotated either by:

1. Manual rotation.
2. Vacuum extraction.
3. Kielland's forceps rotation and delivery.

If attempts at rotation fail, a Caesarean section is indicated.

Moulding

As labour progresses, the shape of the fetal head alters to better fit the maternal pelvis. This leads to overlapping skull bones and assists in producing a smaller head diameter.

Caput succedaneum

If the fetal scalp is compressed against the cervix or the pelvic soft tissue, it interferes with venous return. This in turn leads to oedema of a small portion of the scalp which is known as caput succedaneum.

Mechanism of placental separation and delivery

Separation of the placenta is accomplished by marked uterine contractions. This leads to a reduction of the internal surface area of the uterus by over 50%. The placenta, however, which has been firmly adherent by the trophoblastic invasion of the decidua has a fixed mass. It is unable to reduce its surface area and so begins to separate from the uterus (Fig. 6.16). The site for separation occurs in the decidua with many small cleavage sites. Blood collects in these small cleavage sites, forming small

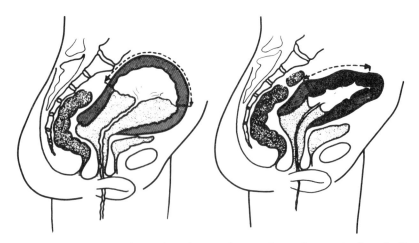

Figure 6.16 Showing how the placental site of attachment is drastically reduced following the end of the second stage, thus aiding separation of the placenta from the uterus.

pools behind the placenta. In some instances this retroplacental bleeding will also help to shear the placenta from the uterine wall. Some of this bleeding tracks behind the chorionic membranes and appears in the vagina as a 'show'.

Placental expulsion

Uterine contractions expel the placenta into the vagina 5–20 minutes after delivery of the infant. This is usually indicated by a gush of blood from the vagina and lengthening of the cord as the placenta descends into the upper vagina. The now empty and firmly contracted uterus rises up on the full vagina to form a 'large ball' at the level of the umbilicus. Removal of the placenta can then be completed either by bearing down by the mother or by applying traction to the umbilical cord and lifting the uterus off the placenta (Brandt–Andrews technique).

Control of haemorrhage

This is effected by contraction and retraction of the myometrium after the placenta has been expelled. Although contraction of the muscle compresses the vessels and stops it bleeding at the time of placental separation, the permanent arrest of haemorrhage is due to myometrial retraction which causes a permanent shortening of the muscle fasciculi. This compresses the vessels which pass between the muscle bundles and effectively stops bleeding in the long term.

6.8 NORMAL LABOUR

Throughout pregnancy, the uterus contracts in a rhythmic fashion but these are impalpable and undetected by the mother. After the 32nd week of pregnancy, these contractions become more dominant and are felt by the mother and are known as Braxton Hicks' contractions. They are usually not painful and do not lead to any permanent shortening of muscle fibres (retraction) and therefore there is no cervical dilatation. These contractions usually lead to formation of the lower uterine segment and can be distinguished from labour contractions which are usually painful.

Labour is said to begin when the uterine contractions are

regular, strong enough to cause pain (more than 25 mmHg) and lead to cervical dilatation.

Admission

Women are advised to present to the hospital for admission when the uterine contractions are painful and occurring regularly at intervals of less than 10 minutes, when the 'waters break', or if there is any fresh bleeding. In 10% of patients, rupture of the membranes precedes the onset of labour.

Each woman admitted to the labour ward will:

1. Have a relevant obstetric history taken.
2. Be examined to determine the state of pregnancy and labour.
3. Be given a suppository or enema only if the bowel is very full.

History

The history on admission will include previous pregnancies, the relevant information regarding the present pregnancy, when the labour commenced and whether the membranes are ruptured or not.

Examination

Examination will include palpation of the fetus for size, lie, presentation, position and engagement. The strength, duration and interval of contractions are also determined. The maternal blood pressure is recorded and urine is tested for sugar, protein and ketones. The fetal heart rate is also recorded before, during and after contractions. A vaginal examination is usually performed.

Management of labour

Although the entire labour should be regarded as a continuum, for convenience it is divided into the following stages:

First stage of labour

The first stage of labour commences when uterine contractions are sufficiently efficient to lead to cervical dilatation and ends when the cervix is fully dilated. Established labour is considered to have occurred when uterine contractions are painful and last more than one-third of a 10-minute period. Contractions should be regular, last more than 45 seconds in duration and occur every 2–3 minutes with good relaxation in between. The patient usually experiences pain only when intrauterine pressure rises more than 25 mmHg. Once the pressure reaches 40 mmHg, the uterus is no longer indentible on palpation. This is the maximum pressure that can be palpated or determined using external tocodynomometry. For labour to progress in the first stage, intrauterine pressures of 50–70 mmHg are required. In between contractions, the intrauterine pressure should not exceed 10 mmHg as this is the pressure above which choriodecidual blood flow ceases.

The first stage of labour is divided into two phases:

1. **Latent phase.** This commences at the onset of contractions and is completed when the cervix reaches 3 cm of dilatation. In a primigravid patient this takes approximately 8 hours, while in a multigravid patient, it lasts an average of 6 hours.
2. **Active phase.** This commences when the patient reaches 3 cm of dilatation, and is completed when the patient is fully dilated. The average total duration of labour in a primigravid patient is 12 hours, while in a multigravid patient, it is 7 hours. Primigravid patients will progress at approximately 1.5 cm/hour during the active phase, while multigravid patients progress at $\geqslant$ 2 cm/hour during the active phase of labour.

During this stage the mother should be encouraged to keep herself occupied by reading or watching television and where the father is present, he should be involved in activities to provide support and encouragement. Once admitted to the labour ward, the patient's observations are charted on a partogram (Fig. 6.17). This is a graphical recording of all the patients observations which include:

1. Fetal heart rate observations before, during and after each contraction and recorded every 15 minutes during the first stage of labour.
2. Strength, duration and frequency of uterine contractions recorded over a 10-minute period.

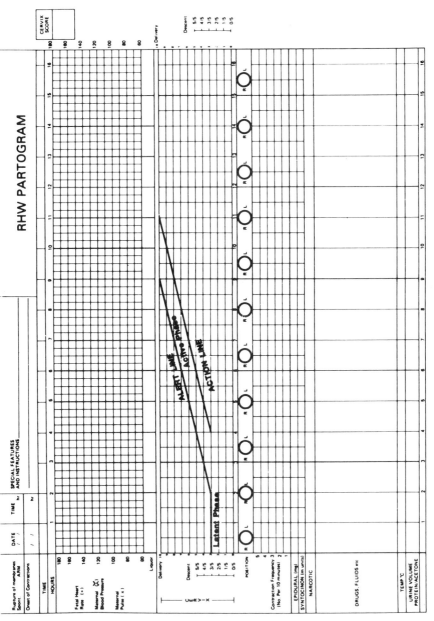

Figure 6.17 A partogram demonstrating the rate of progress in labour and use of alert and action lines. If the rate of progress in labour crosses the alert line then closer review must be undertaken. If the rate of progress is even slower and crosses the action line then some positive steps must be taken to expedite delivery.

3. Observation of the presenting part with regard to its descent and engagement as well as its position.
4. Maternal pulse rate and blood pressure are recorded every hour, but temperature is taken every 4 hours.
5. Observations of maternal fluid intake are recorded as well as the urinary output and its chemical analysis.
6. Any drugs given to the mother are recorded on the partogram.

A vaginal examination is done every 4 hours unless there is an indication to do so more frequently (Table 6.1).

Table 6.1 Observations to be made during each vaginal examination

Vulva and vagina	Bleeding
	Draining amniotic fluid (clear or meconium-stained)
	Vulval ulceration (herpes simplex)
	Vulval varicosities or warts
	Vaginal cysts or septum
Cervix	Dilatation
	Effacement
	Application to the presenting part
	Position
	Texture
Presenting part	What is it? (head or breech)
	Station (relative to ischial spines)
	e.g. −2 cm = 2 cm above the spines
	Position, e.g. LOA or ROP
	Degree of flexion
	Degree of caput or moulding
Membranes	Intact or ruptured
Amniotic fluid	Clear
	Meconium: Grade 1 Lightly stained amniotic fluid
	Grade 2 Equal parts meconium to amniotic fluid
	Grade 3 Thick meconium staining

Use of the partogram (see Fig. 6.17)

Once the patient's cervix reaches 3 cm of dilatation (the active phase), the minimum rate of dilatation should be >1 cm/hour and a line is drawn to mark this rate. This is known as the *alert line*. Studies have shown that active intervention is rarely required in patients whose rate of dilatation exceeds this. A parallel line may be drawn 2 hours later than the alert line and this is called the *action line*. Once the rate of dilatation, as recorded on the partogram, crosses the alert line, a vaginal examination should be done after a further 2 hours. If at this stage, progress has been satisfactory, no intervention is required. If the labour has not progressed at the second examination, then a critical review of the patient, her labour and her fetus are needed. It needs to be established by means of a vaginal examination as to whether there is obvious cephalo-pelvic disproportion, relative cephalo-pelvic disproportion due to a malposition or the slow rate of progress has been due to inadequate uterine activity.

1. The vaginal examination should determine the degree of cervical dilatation, descent and position of the presenting part, whether there is caput or moulding and to ensure that the membranes have ruptured.
2. An intravenous Syntocinon infusion may be required if uterine contractions are inadequate. Uterine contractions can be measured by means of external tocodynomonetry or, if this presents difficulty, by direct intrauterine pressure recording.
3. The fetal heart rate should be monitored continuously using a cardiotocograph.
4. Intravenous dextrose/saline to rehydrate and provide adequate nutrition for the mother.
5. Adequate analgesia should be provided, preferably by means of epidural anaesthesia, but if this is not possible parenteral analgesics will suffice.
6. Blood should be taken for cross-matching.
7. Should an abnormal fetal heart rate pattern be present, then a fetal scalp blood sample analysis may be necessary to determine fetal pH, PCO_2 and base deficit levels.

Cervical dilatation

Normally, the cervix dilates slowly up to about 5 cm, after which the progress is more rapid. When the cervix reaches full dilatation (10 cm) the cervix and lower segment of the uterus are usually thinned out and thus easily drawn out round the presenting part of the fetus. Once the cervix is fully dilated, the first stage is said to have been completed. During the late first stage of labour pain and discomfort increases as the head passes through the cervix into the vagina. This causes increased rectal pressure and a sensation of 'bearing down' or the desire to push.

Analgesia

During the first stage analgesics such as nitrous oxide may be administered via a face mask, or the patient may require intramuscular analgesics such as pethidine or morphine to provide pain relief. If, however, the pain becomes more severe later in labour, epidural anaesthesia may be the only way of providing adequate relief.

Local anaesthesia

Local anaesthesia, such as perineal infiltration or a pudendal block provides adequate analgesia for delivery but does not provide relief in late first stage. The longer labour lasts, particularly in late first stage, the more anxiety and tension are created in the mother. Pain, low backache and the feeling of helplessness, may cause the mother to become hysterically anxious and distressed. If this distressful situation continues, the obstetrician may also be under severe pressure to bring about completion of the labour, perhaps performing otherwise unnecessary procedures. This situation can be avoided by the judicious use of epidural anaesthesia to provide adequate pain relief and the administration of Syntocinon by intravenous infusion to enhance uterine contractions if required.

It is most important to reassure the mother that all is under control, even though the labour may be proceeding slowly. Knowledge, empathy, understanding and sympathy will probably do more to protect a mother from a poor obstetric outcome than the most sophisticated technical aids.

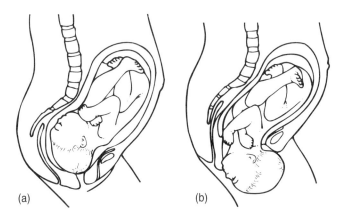

Figure 6.18 (a) Descent; (b) Extension.

Second stage of labour

The second stage of labour lasts from full dilatation of the cervix to delivery of the infant. In primigravid women, this normally takes about 1 hour, while in a multigravid patient the time is usually halved. Once the cervix is fully dilated, the fetus will proceed through the pelvis with the aid of uterine contractions and maternal expulsive efforts. The head flexes, descends, moulds and undergoes internal rotation so that the occiput comes to lie anteriorly under the symphysis pubis. From this position, expulsive efforts assist the fetal head undergoing extension and delivery from under the symphysis pubis (Fig. 6.18).

Normal uterine contractions in association with bearing down by the mother may increase the intrauterine pressure to 100–120 mmHg and assist delivery of the infant.

As the head delivers, the perineal tissue will stretch and may tear. If this seems likely, it is wise to perform an episiotomy under local anaesthesia.

Episiotomy

An episiotomy is a cut in the perineum that enlarges the vaginal introitus. It aids delivery by removing the resistance of the perineum. It is usually used for primigravid women in whom the perineum is less elastic and less dilated than that of a multigravid woman. It also may be indicated in a patient who has delay in the second stage of labour or where there is any complication associated with delivery. There are two types of episiotomy:

1. **Medio-lateral.** This is the most common type and is usually 'J'- or 'L'-shaped. It begins in the midline of the fourchette and extends along a line that would run just lateral to the external anal sphincter. This divides the vaginal and perineal epithelium, the transverse perineii muscle, the posterior fibres of the bulbo-cavernous muscles and the decussating fibres of the levator ani muscle.
2. **Median.** This incision starts in the centre of the fourchette and extends posteriorly towards the anus for about 2–3 cm.

The advantages of an episiotomy are:

1. It avoids tears and rupture of the anal sphincter or tears into the rectum.
2. It hastens delivery when the head is arrested on the pelvic floor.
3. It may assist in preventing future prolapse by avoiding over-distension and tearing of vaginal tissue.
4. It avoids undue pressure on the fetal tissue, particularly in pre-term infants.
5. It makes vaginal manipulations (such as rotation and forceps delivery) easier to perform.

Indications for an episiotomy are:

1. To prevent perineal tears.
2. To avoid arrest of the presenting part at the perineum.
3. When delivering small premature infants.
4. When delivering large babies who are at risk of shoulder dystocia.
5. When performing obstetric manipulations such as rotations or forceps delivery.
6. When fetal distress necessitates a rapid delivery.

The repair of an episiotomy (Fig. 6.19) should be performed with care, as an inadequate repair may lead to haemorrhage, infection, haematomas, painful scars, a tight vagina or to severe dyspareunia. The incision is sutured in layers, using minimal amounts of tension with the thinnest possible suture material.

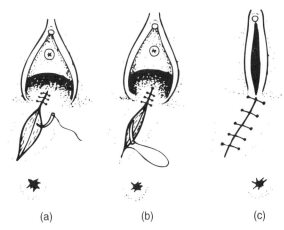

(a)   (b)   (c)

Figure 6.19 Episiotomy repair. Demonstrating the technique of: (a) Sewing the vaginal epithelium from apex of cut to introitus of vagina. Then uniting transverse perinei muscle; (b) Uniting fascia of perineal body; (c) Suturing skin of episiotomy.

Initially, the vaginal cut should be completely visualized and care taken to place the first suture high in the vagina, at the apex of the incision. A continuous chromic catgut or synthetic absorbable suture can be used to unite the vaginal epithelium as far as the introitus, making sure that the hymeneal remnants are opposed at the introitus. When the vagina is intact, the levator ani, transverse perineii and bulbo cavernosus muscles are united in that order, together with their investing fascia by means of interrupted sutures. Finally, the skin is sutured using a sub-cuticular absorbable suture or with interrupted sutures.

A rectal examination is always done afterwards to ensure that no sutures have inadvertently penetrated the rectal epithelium.

Delivery of the baby

The natural method for delivery is for the mother to squat on her haunches. This allows the maximum intra-abdominal pressure to be generated by the mother and also the alteration of the angle of inclination of the pelvis leads to an increased surface area being available to the advancing presenting part. However, it is usually more convenient for the accoucheur to assist or manipulate during delivery if the mother is in the dorsal or lateral position. In most developed countries as a result of adequate maternal nutrition, the relationship between the fetal skull and brim area is such, that alteration of the angle of inclination is not critical for a normal delivery. The mother is usually propped up on pillows, her legs and abdomen are draped with sterile towels and the midwife/obstetrician stands at the side.

In this position, one hand can be used to guide the vertex as it 'crowns' and is born from under the symphysis pubis, while the other hand feels deep between the anus and the coccyx for the fetal chin. Once the chin has been 'caught', the patient is asked to stop bearing down while delivery of the head occurs by extension. To relieve pain at this stage, the woman may be given nitrous oxide to inhale unless an injection of local anaesthetic into the perineum or a pudendal block has been given before this stage (Fig. 6.20).

Once the head has been delivered by extension, the nasopharynx may be sucked free of mucous and fluid. The neck is gently palpated to ensure that the cord is not wrapped around it. If it is, it is freed by slipping it over the head or shoulders. If, however, it is tight or encircles the neck two or more times it should be clamped and cut. By this stage restitution will

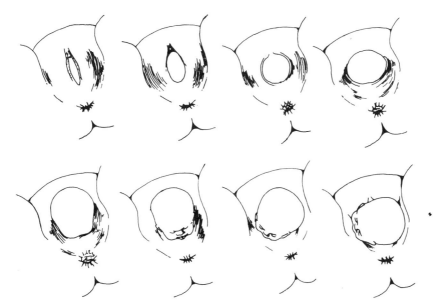

Figure 6.20 Crowning, extension and delivery of the fetal head.

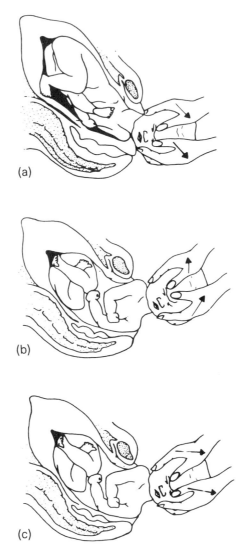

Figure 6.21 (a) Demonstrating the technique of delivering the anterior shoulder. Stand on the side to which the occiput is pointing and with a hand pressing firmly over either parietal bone, pull the head out and down to deliver the anterior shoulder; (b) Demonstrating the technique to deliver the posterior shoulder. With the hands grasping the head on either side of the parietal bones, the head is lifted upwards until the posterior shoulder slides out of the vagina; (c) Once the shoulders have delivered, the body of the baby is delivered in a downward and outward motion.

have occurred and with further descent, external rotation will take place. Both hands are then placed on either side of the fetal skull, over the ears and parietal bones, ensuring that no pressure is placed on the infant's carotid arteries (see Fig. 6.21). Firm pressure is then exerted in a posterior direction to aid the delivery of the shoulder. By pulling out and downwards, the anterior should slide under the symphysis pubis. By lifting the head upwards as the baby is delivered, the posterior shoulder will also slide out. Once the shoulders are free, the baby is easily delivered. The baby is then placed on the mother's abdomen and the cord is clamped and cut. The mother is encouraged to touch and hold her baby. After a short while the baby is wrapped in a warm blanket and given to the mother to hold.

Routine following delivery of the baby

1. The baby is checked immediately for gross abnormalities and identification tags are tied around the baby's wrist and ankle.
2. If the mother's blood group is Rhesus-negative, then cord blood is obtained to assess the infant's blood group, anti-bodies and haemoglobin. After the third stage, venous blood is taken from the mother to ensure that she has not developed Rhesus antibodies and to do a Kleihauer test to measure the volume of infusion of fetal cells that may have occurred during the delivery. This enables the volume of anti-D globulin given to the mother to be adjusted appro-priately.
3. The fundus of the uterus is checked to ascertain whether signs of placental separation have occurred.

Third stage of labour

This is the shortest and the most hazardous stage of labour for the mother. It commences with the delivery of the infant and is completed with the delivery of the placenta. It is concerned with separation and expulsion of the placenta and control of haemorrhage from the placental site and normally lasts 5–20 minutes. Separation of the placenta normally occurs when the uterus contracts and the muscle retracts following the delivery of the fetus.

Steps in management

1. When the anterior shoulder of the fetus is born from under the symphysis pubis, Syntocinon (10 units) is usually given by intramuscular injection. This results in uterine contractions after 3–4 minutes.
2. The vaginal introitus is observed so that the 'show' of blood and lengthening of the cord (which indicates separation and expulsion of the placenta into the upper vagina) can be noted.
3. The uterus is gently palpated so that when the placenta separates and is expelled from the upper vagina, the firmly contracted small uterus can be identified just above the level of the umbilicus.
4. When the placenta has been identified to have separated and passed from the uterus into the upper vagina, the cord is grasped firmly in one hand while the uterus is steadied by the other hand and lifted off the placenta. This technique of delivery is known as the Brandt–Andrews technique.
5. Following delivery of the placenta, the patient's blood pressure is checked and if not elevated, ergometrine (0.25–0.5 mg) may be given by intramuscular injection if there is persistent bleeding.

Action of oxytocics

1. Oxytocin is absorbed rapidly from an intramuscular injection site and will produce a uterine contraction within 3–4 minutes. It is rapidly broken down by the enzyme oxytocinase. When given by intramuscular injection, ergometrine will only produce uterine contractions after 5–6 minutes and its action lasts a number of hours.
2. Oxytocin produces contractions of higher amplitude than ergometrine.
3. Oxytocin produces contractions with an intervening relaxation phase, thus simulating physiological contractions.
4. Ergometrine produces contractions of high tone and frequency, but of small amplitude. Because of the longer duration of action, ergometrine provides more reliable contractions and aids in preventing postpartum haemorrhage.

These differing properties of oxytocin and ergometrine are used to advantage in the third stage of labour. By giving oxytocin on delivery of the anterior shoulder, physiological contractions occur that aid in separation and expulsion of the placenta. Following expulsion of the placenta, ergometrine then provides prolonged tetanic contractions that help to prevent postpartum haemorrhage. Syntometrine which is a combination of 5 units of oxytocinon and 0.5 mg of ergometrine is also widely used with the delivery of the anterior shoulder. The action of ergometrine if given by intramuscular injection commences after 4–6 minutes and lasts 6–8 hours. The main danger of using the combination is the presence of undiagnosed twins which may then result in the second twin being trapped in the uterus. Ergometrine should not be used in the presence of cardiac disease or hypertension.

If the patient is at risk from postpartum haemorrhage (e.g. from multiple pregnancy, grandmultiparity, antepartum haemorrhage, etc.), then an intravenous infusion should be commenced during labour. The oxytocin or ergometrine can be given directly intravenously. If postpartum bleeding occurs due to uterine atony (e.g. from retained placenta, prolonged labour, APH, etc.), then ergometrine (0.25–0.5 mg) can be given directly intravenously or an oxytocin infusion (40 units in 1 litre Hartman's solution) can be commenced.

6.9 BREECH DELIVERY

Breech presentation in labour occurs in 4–5% of all deliveries. It should be managed as for a woman with a cephalic presentation. However, because of the greater risks associated with complications of a breech delivery, it should take place in a well-equipped hospital with an experienced obstetrician in attendance. Before labour is allowed to proceed, care should be taken to ensure that the maternal pelvis is adequate. Ideally the patient should be multiparous with a large, well-formed pelvis whose dimensions are known (by the use of a standing lateral radiograph). The fetus should have extended legs and the ideal weight for a breech delivery is between 2500–3500 g. If there are any doubts as to the adequacy of the pelvic dimension, then an elective Caesarean section should be performed at between 38 and 40 weeks.

Care should be taken to maintain intact membranes, as premature rupture of the membranes is associated with a high incidence of cord prolapse.

Most breech presentations will progress to a normal vaginal delivery, so the management includes the following principles:

1. Do not interfere, unless some obstetric situation (such as fetal distress) indicates that this is necessary.
2. The fetus should be monitored continuously throughout labour using external cardiotocography or, if the membranes are ruptured, a scalp electrode may be placed on the buttocks.
3. Keep the patient in bed throughout the labour.
4. Do not rupture the membranes in the early stage of labour.
5. Maintain an intravenous drip and only use Syntocinon if the contractions are inadequate.
6. Judicious use of adequate analgesia, in particular epidural anaesthesia, prevents the mother from bearing down before the cervix is fully dilated leading to entrapment of the fetal head.
7. Perform a vaginal examination regularly throughout labour or when the membranes rupture so as to exclude cord prolapse or other complications.
8. Ascertain that the nursing staff, medical staff and anaesthetist are notified of the presence of a breech in labour so that they may be readily summoned if needed.
9. Use of local anaesthesia (pudendal nerve block) and an episiotomy is necessary to permit easy delivery of the trunk and after-coming head.

Delivery technique

During each contraction the patient is encouraged to bear down so that the buttocks distend the perineum (Fig. 6.22). By this stage, if the patient has not had an epidural anaesthetic, then local anaesthesia is injected into the perineum prior to performing an episiotomy. Bearing down is encouraged with contractions, until the buttocks are delivered to the trunk and the umbilicus is seen. At this stage, a loop of cord is pulled down and the legs are freed from inside the vagina. As the umbilical cord is now compressed, it is important to deliver the baby

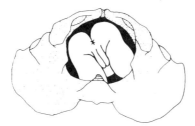

Figure 6.22 Right sacro-anterior position in a breech with extended legs.

within 5 minutes to avoid the risk of hypoxia. A towel is wrapped around the limbs of the fetus to support it, and the mother is encouraged to bear down. Unnecessary traction on the fetal trunk may lead to extension of the fetal arms and their entrapment above the pelvic brim. If this occurs, then it may require rotation of the lower trunk in the reverse direction to allow the delivery of the shoulders from under the symphysis pubis (Lovset manoeuvre) (Fig. 6.23).

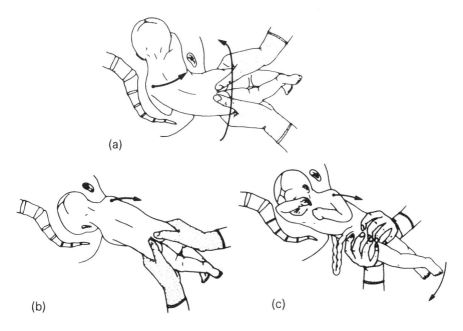

(a)

(b)

(c)

Figure 6.23 The Lovset manoeuvre. (a) Hands grasp buttocks with thumbs over the sacrum. By pulling down and rotating the lower part of the body through 180°, the anterior shoulder slides from under the symphysis pubis.

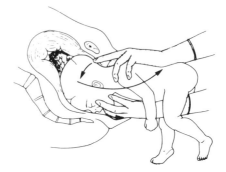

Figure 6.24 The after-coming head of the breech delivered by the Mauriceau–Smellie–Viet manoeuvre.

Delivery of the fetal head

This can be the most difficult part of the delivery.

Burns–Marshall method: once the shoulders have delivered, the baby is allowed to hang, using its own weight to allow the head to engage. When the nape of the neck is visible, the legs are grasped by the ankles with a finger between the legs to maintain steady traction. The trunk is swung upward and forward in a wide arc. The other hand controls the perineum allowing the mouth and face to deliver. The mouth is suctioned immediately to allow the infant to breathe.

Mauriceau–Smeilie–Veit manoeuvre (Fig. 6.24): once the head has engaged as described above, a hand is passed into the vagina until the face and mouth are felt. The index and ring fingers are placed on the fetal maxilla and the middle finger is placed in the fetal mouth to assist in maintaining flexion. The fingers of the other hand exert traction on the fetal shoulders as well as using the middle finger of that hand to push on the occiput to help flex the head. The major expulsive force in this manoeuvre should be from an assistant applying supra-pubic pressure.

Forceps to the after-coming head: more commonly, forceps are applied to control the delivery of the fetal head as this technique is probably safer. An assistant holds the infant's legs in the air while the blades are applied. Care should be taken not to

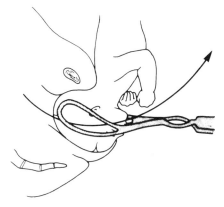

Figure 6.25 The after-coming head of a breech delivered by forceps.

hyperextend the fetal neck. Slow and steady traction is applied to deliver the fetal head. It is important that the head should be delivered slowly as it is the compression and sudden decompression that leads to tentorial tears and intracerebral haemorrhage (Fig. 6.25).

The newborn infant

7.1 GENERAL INSTRUCTIONAL OBJECTIVE

The students will develop competence in examining a normal newborn infant and recognize abnormalities which require investigation and treatment.

7.2 SPECIFIC BEHAVIOURAL OBJECTIVES

1. Take a perinatal history.
2. Examine and follow-up normal newborn babies (including feeding).
3. Recognize minor abnormalities (in newborn infants) that require no treatment.
4. Examine and manage low birthweight babies.
5. Plan investigations and management of a jaundiced infant.
6. Plan investigations and treatment of an infant with infection.
7. Plan investigations and treatment of an infant with neurological problems.

7.3 EXAMINATION OF THE NEWBORN

It is the duty of the attendant at delivery to record the Apgar score (Table 7.1) at 1 and 5 minutes (and subsequently if the baby has problems with establishing regular respiration), and note the presence of major malformations (e.g. meningomyelocoele) which might cause difficulty to the baby in adapting to extrauterine life. All well babies must be examined (in the presence of the mother) as soon after birth as possible and again before discharge from hospital. The aim of the first examination is to detect abnormalities, to establish a baseline for subsequent

Table 7.1 Apgar scoring chart

Sign	0	1	2
Heart rate	Absent	Slow (below 100)	Over 100
Respiratory effort	Absent	Weak cry, hypoventilation	Good strong cry
Muscle tone	Limp	Some flexion of extremities	Well flexed
Reflex response			
(i) Response to catheter in nostril (tested after oropharynx is clear)	No response	Grimace	Cough or sneeze
(ii) Tangential foot slap	No response	Grimace	Cry and withdrawal of foot
Colour	Blue, pale	Body pink, Extremities blue	Completely pink

examination and to reassure the mother that the baby is normal. The second examination aims to determine the progress of the infant and to detect any minor problems that may have surfaced or been overlooked at the first examination.

History

Before examining the baby it is important to check the mother's notes to determine the history of pregnancy, labour and the state of the infant at birth. Nursing notes also give essential information regarding the birthweight of the infant, the changes in weight since birth, feeding pattern of the infant and observations such as colour, respiratory rate, heart rate, passage of meconium and urine. It is best to examine the baby in the mother's presence, as this will allow the examiner to demonstrate to her some of the normal findings in the newborn and also to answer any questions.

The examination of the baby is described systematically here,

Table 7.2 Assessment of gestational age

Characteristic	Gestational age in weeks			
	28–30	32–34	36–38	40+
Breast nodule development	Absent	Absent	3–5 mm	7 mm+
Sole creases	Absent	Single anterior creases	2–3 creases	Many creases
Ear lobe	No cartilage	No cartilage	Pliable, some cartilage present	Stiff
Male genitalia	Testis unpalpable: small, smooth scrotum	Testis in inguinal canal; small, smooth scrotum	Testis often descended: some scrotal rugae	Testis descended: scrotum fully rugose
Female genitalia	Prominent labia minora, labia majora flat	Prominent labia minora, labia majora flat	Labia majora almost cover labia minora, few rugae	Labia majora completely cover labia minora, marked rugae
Posture	Hypotonia	Some flexor tone at hips and knees	Some flexor tone at hips knees and elbows	Marked flexor tone all joints
Scarf sign	Elbow past midline	Elbow past midline	Elbow reaches midline	Elbow does not reach midline
Toe to ear	Usual	Usual	Difficult	Impossible

but this is usually not possible in the newborn. However, the same procedure should be used each time so as to avoid omissions, and a check list should be kept to ensure that no abnormalities are overlooked.

General observations

Much information is obtained by general observations which include posture, activity, peripheral perfusion, colour, type and rate of respiration, shape and size of the skull, the presence of abdominal distension and features which indicate the maturity of the infant (Table 7.2).

Skull

Most full-term newborn infants examined in the first 24–48 hours will show some evidence of moulding of the skull. A caput succedaneum or a cephalhaematoma may be present in some cases. The occipito-frontal head circumference is measured routinely, but it may be difficult to interpret if severe moulding is present. The fontanelles are examined for size and tension and the sutures felt for overlapping, synostosis or separation.

Facies

Most newborn infants show some facial asymmetry. In facial nerve palsy there is evidence of flattening of the nasolabial folds in addition to facial asymmetry. If the appearance of the infant suggests dysmorphic features, a more detailed examination is indicated. This includes the palpebral slant, size of the orbits, the distance between the inner canthi (hypo- or hypertelorism), the position of the ears in relation to the outer canthi of the eyes (low-set ears), the appearance of the bridge of the nose, the size of the philtrum, mouth and chin. Unless measurements are carried out (e.g. distance between the inner canthi) and compared with normal standards it is very easy to draw wrong conclusions. If a specific condition is suspected (e.g. Down's syndrome), one should look for other stigmas of the condition.

The eyes are usually closed but will open if the baby is held upright and gently rocked forward and backward. There may be evidence of subconjunctival haemorrhage or infection (sticky eye). Unless the eyes are examined carefully it is very easy to miss abnormalities such as congenital cataracts and glaucoma, coloboma of iris and abnormalities of pupillary reflex. The presence of bilateral red reflexes suggests the absence of cataracts or of intra-ocular pathology.

The external ears should be examined carefully as minor abnormalities of the ears (periauricular skin tags, pits and shape of pinnae) are not uncommon.

The oral cavity is examined for the presence of abnormalities (especially posterior cleft palate) and infection (thrush). A bifid uvula should alert the physician to the possibility of a submucous cleft palate. The hard palate usually has some small white nodules (Epstein's pearls) which consist of an accumulation of epithelial cells and should not be confused with monilial infection. Retention cysts of similar appearance may also be seen on the gums. The tongue is relatively large and the frenulum may be short but does not require cutting.

The neck is relatively short. Abnormalities include lumps (goitre, cystic hygroma, sterno-mastoid tumour) and redundant skin seen in Turner's syndrome. Both clavicles should be palpated for fractures and abnormalities.

Chest

The chest of the newborn is symmetrical in shape and moves equally on respiration. Abnormalities of the respiratory system would be suspected from the general observations (respiratory rate, chest recession, grunting). Normal respiration (rate 25–40/minute) in the newborn is usually diaphragmatic. Percussion and auscultation of the chest in infants who are breathing normally are unlikely to reveal any abnormalities and are best omitted.

The mammary glands are hypertrophied and may produce secretions.

Cardiovascular system

The normal heart rate is 100–140 per minute and sinus arrhythmia is usually very marked. The praecordium should be palpated to localize the position of the heart. The apex beat is difficult to palpate and usually does not reflect the size of the heart, but the cardiac impulse may help in identifying ventricular hypertrophy. The sounds over the pulmonary area are louder than the aortic sounds. Systolic murmurs are not uncommon and vary from day to day but do not necessarily indicate the presence of congenital heart disease. Conversely, the absence of murmurs does not exclude congenital heart disease. Femoral pulses should be examined to exclude coarctation of the aorta. Blood pressure should be measured in both upper and lower limbs in infants with abnormal femoral pulses.

Abdomen

The abdomen usually appears distended and a scaphoid abdomen may be the only sign of a diaphragmatic hernia. The abdomen should be palpated for the presence of masses and in particular for enlargement of kidneys, liver or spleen. The liver is palpable 1–2 cm below the right costal margin in the mid-clavicular line. The spleen can be tipped in most cases. The umbilicus should be examined for infection and number of blood vessels. The male genitalia should be examined for hernias, hydrocoeles, undescended testis and the position of the urinary meatus. In the female infant hymenal skin tags are common and there is mucoid or bloody vaginal discharge. Though labial adhesion may be seen in normal infants, labial fusion with an enlarged clitoris with or without hypospadius suggest adrenogenital syndrome.

Skeletal system

The skin of the newborn manifests signs indicative of vasomotor instability. These include mottling, acrocyanosis and harlequin colour change. Most newborn infants have capillary nevi. These include salmon patches (nevus simplex) that occur most commonly on the glabella and eyelids, nevus flammens (usually seen on the nape of the neck), cavernous haemangioma (strawberry nevus) and portwine stain. Other minor abnormalities of the skin include milia, sucking blisters, cutis marmorata, transient neonatal pustular melanosis, erythema toxicum and café-au-lait spots. Children of Asiatic, Mediterranean and Negroid descent may have a blue spot (Mongolian spot) over the back, which has no medical significance.

Skeletal anomalies such as polydactyly may be obvious. However, careful examination will be required to note the presence of sternomastoid tumour, fractured clavicle, paronychia, Sydney line or a Simian crease. The spine should be examined carefully to exclude skin defects, small closed menningocoele dermoids and sinuses. Particular attention should be paid to the examination of the hips by the method described by Ortolini and telescoping to exclude the presence of congenital dislocation of the hip. Other abnormalities to observe in the lower limbs include torsion of the femur or tibia and the presence of congenital talipes.

Nervous system

Well newborn infants will demonstrate the presence of primitive reflexes such as grasping, rooting, sucking, glabella tap, Gallant and Moro. Abnormalities of these reflexes do not necessarily indicate brain damage, but a more detailed neurological examination should be performed. The Moro reflex is probably the most useful guide to the infant's neurological status.

7.4 DEFINITIONS

- *Gestation* is regarded as being the time from the first day of the last menstrual period.
- The *low birthweight* baby has a birth weight of 2500 g or less, irrespective of the gestation period.
- The *pre-term* baby has a gestation period less than 37 weeks (i.e. 36 weeks 6 days, or less).
- The *full-term* baby has a gestation period of 37 weeks to 41 weeks 6 days.
- The *post-mature* baby has a gestation period of 42 weeks or more.
- The *small-for-dates* baby has a birth weight below the 10th percentile for the gestation period.
- The *large-for-dates* baby has a birth weight above the 90th percentile for the gestation period.

- The *appropriate-for-gestation* baby has a birth weight between the 10th and 90th percentile for the gestation period.

Any of these combinations may be present in a particular infant. Unless the gestation period can be determined accurately, it is not possible to place an infant in a definite category. The gestational age of the infant may be determined from maternal history (last menstrual period), and checked by ultrasound examination. After birth, gestational age can be estimated within an accuracy of 2 weeks by careful physical and neurological examination of the newborn. However, the neurological examination cannot be performed on a sick, depressed infant. The physical and neurological characteristics that are most useful in diagnosing gestational age are shown in Table 7.1.

7.5 PRE-TERM BABIES

Most pre-term (premature) infants also have a low birthweight (i.e. birthweight of 2500 g or less), but a premature infant may weigh more than 2500 g. A premature infant may also be small-for-dates if the birthweight is below the 10th percentile for the gestation period.

In the majority of cases, the cause of premature birth is not clear. Until the exact mechanism that causes the onset of labour is known it is unlikely that the cause of prematurity will be understood. However, it is well recognized that prematurity is associated with antepartum haemorrhage, multiple pregnancy, incompetent cervix, amnionitis, toxaemia of pregnancy, urinary tract infection of the mother and possibly malnutrition of the mother. Some of the features of prematurity are described in Table 7.1. Others include reddish skin due to lack of subcutaneous fat, presence of lanugo hair, oedema of the feet, large fontanelles with widely separated sutures, and poorly developed primitive reflexes.

Clinical problems

These are due to immaturity of organ function. The most serious of these is immaturity of the respiratory function, which results in difficulties in establishing regular respiration at birth, idiopathic respiratory distress syndrome (hyaline membrane disease), apnoeic attacks and periodic respiration. Respiratory problems may also result from aspiration of liquor amnii or meconium, retained lung fluid or infection.

Hepatic immaturity results in increased and prolonged jaundice, and immaturity of the nervous system predisposes the premature infant to kernicterus at a lower level of bilirubin than a full-term infant. Premature infants also have low protein levels, which further increases the hazard of bilirubin toxicity and also restricts the use of drugs that are bound to protein (such as sulphonamides and cloxacillin). As renal function is immature, drugs such as streptomycin, kanamycin or gentamicin must be used with caution.

The cardiopulmonary circulation is transitional between fetal and adult, which results in increased shunting of blood through the ductus arteriosus and foramen ovale in response to stress and hypoxia. This may cause circulatory insufficiency or under perfusion of vital organs, leading to renal failure, necrotizing enterocolitis, periventricular leucomalacia and intraventricular haemorrhage. The patent ductus arteriosus may lead to congestive cardiac failure or pulmonary hypertension.

Premature infants have very little subcutaneous tissue and brown fat, which limits their ability to control their body temperature. They are also liable to increased risk of infection as a result of low serum immunoglobulins and the need for invasive procedures. Problems in feeding result from poorly developed sucking and swallowing reflexes, poor gastrointestinal motility and increased incidence of necrotizing enterocolitis. Hypoglycaemia may result because of difficulties in feeding and because of the presence of low energy stores in the form of fat and glycogen. Premature infants have a greater tendency to develop cerebral birth trauma (during delivery) and intraventricular haemorrhage. Anaemia results from frequent blood sampling, low iron stores and hyoplasia of the bone marrow.

Long-term problems include oxygen dependency, bronchopulmonary dysplasia, retinopathy of prematurity, refractive errors of vision, cerebral palsy and developmental delay.

Management

As premature infants are more liable to infection, appropriate precautions should be taken by rigorous attention to the problem of cross-infection.

To help maintain body temperature, the pre-term infant should be nursed at a temperature much greater than that for the average nursery; even healthy babies may need to be nursed in an incubator. The smaller the baby, the higher the environmental temperature it will require to maintain normal body temperature. The temperature of the incubator is adjusted to the needs of the baby, and this is best achieved by the use of a thermostat attached to the abdomen of the infant. One pitfall in recording temperature of newborn premature infants is that their body temperature may be below 35°C. Unless a low-reading thermometer is used, it may not be apparent that the baby's body temperature is very low.

The management of other problems of premature infants is discussed later.

7.6 SMALL-FOR-DATES INFANTS

Small-for-dates babies may result as a consequence of inadequate potential for growth (intrinsic growth retardation) resulting in similar growth reduction of weight, length and head. Such infants have a decreased number of cells, as well as decreased cell size, and do not have the potential for normal growth. These infants are small before the second trimester. Recognized causes include chromosomal abnormalities, congenital viral infections, drugs, irradiation in the first trimester, growth-retarding dysmorphic syndromes, e.g. Russell–Silver syndrome and constitutional growth retardation related to parental stature, racial and ethnic factors.

Other small-for-dates infants result from abnormalities of the placenta or are due to maternal factors which prevent the fetus from achieving its full potential of growth caused by impaired delivery of oxygen and nutrients from the placenta. The magnitude of the growth retardation will depend on the duration of the adverse factors. In these infants, weight gain is more affected than length, which is more affected than the brain (head). Placental factors include pregnancy-induced hypertension, multiple pregnancy, small placenta (due to antepartum haemorrhage or infarcts) and twin-to-twin transfusion. Recognized maternal factors include smoking, alcohol and narcotic abuse, hypertension, hypoxia (e.g. cardiac or pulmonary disease, living at high altitude and diabetes mellitus with vascular complications).

Clinical problems

All small-for-dates babies should be examined carefully for the presence of congenital malformations and congenital viral infections. The other problems include perinatal asphyxia, meconium aspiration, respiratory problems due to meconium aspiration, polycythaemia with or without increased viscosity of the blood which may also cause respiratory problems and a tendency to bleeding (particularly massive pulmonary haemorrhage). Metabolic problems include hypoglycaemia due to inadequate stores of fat and glycogen and hypocalcaemia.

These infants lose little weight, feed well and gain weight rapidly after birth. Full-term growth-retarded infants usually catch up with their peers, particularly if the growth retardation is due to maternal factors. Catch-up growth rarely occurs if it has not done so by the age of 6 months. Follow-up studies have shown that small-for-dates infants are more likely to show developmental, behavioural and learning problems than full-term normal infants and those born mildly premature. The risk of serious neurological abnormality is greatest in a premature small-for-dates infant.

7.7 LARGE-FOR-DATES INFANTS

Some large babies (usually born to tall parents) are constitutionally large. Such infants do not have any problems other than complications of delivery. The most common pathological cause of a large-for-dates infant is maternal diabetes mellitus, which may be gestational or permanent. The large size of the infant is thought to be due to increased production of insulin by the fetus in response to intermittent hyperglycaemia in the mother. Other known causes of large-for-dates infants include cyanotic congenital heart disease in the infant, haemolytic disease of the newborn, and Beckwith's syndrome.

7.8 INFANT OF THE DIABETIC MOTHER

Diabetes mellitus in the mother is associated with subfertility, increased fetal and neonatal wastage, polyhydramnios and increased incidence of congenital malformations (particularly of the central nervous system) in the infant. Characteristically the infant is large (due to increase in fat and generalized organomegaly), appears overfed, is plethoric and has a Cushingoid appearance. Though large in size, these infants may be born prematurely and have all the problems related to prematurity.

More than 50% of infants of diabetic mothers develop hypoglycaemia but only a small percentage of these infants become symptomatic. The risk of hypoglycaemia increases if cord blood glucose or maternal fasting blood glucose levels are high.

Infants of diabetic mothers have an increased incidence of aline membrane disease which is ably related to an .tagonistic effect between cortisone a sulin on surfactant synthesis, transient tachypnoea of the wborn, hyperbilirubinemia, polycythemia, cardiac failure ue to hypertrophic subaortic stenosis, congenital anomalie or hyperviscosity), lumbo-sacral agenesis and abdominal distension due to the transient delay in the development of the left side of the colon (the small left colon syndrome). The hyperviscosity predisposes to renal vein thrombosis which should be suspected in the presence of a flank mass, haematuria and thrombocytopenia.

Management

All infants of diabetics mothers should be admitted to the special-care nursery for observation. Blood sugars should be monitored by 'Dextrostix' and readings below 2 mmol/l should be confirmed by formal blood sugar measurements. The infants should be fed early (within 1 hour of birth). An intravenous 10% dextrose infusion should be set up for emergency treatment of hypoglycaemia. These infants can be successfully treated with glucagon in an emergency. The detailed management of hypoglycaemia is discussed below.

7.9 HYPOGLYCAEMIA IN THE NEWBORN

Newborn infants have low blood sugar levels compared with those of an adult. As the condition may be asymptomatic there is no consensus regarding normal glucose levels, though a plasma glucose level of less than 2 mmol/l (35 mg/100 ml) in the first 72 hours and less than 3.5 mmol/l (65 mg/100 ml) thereafter would be regarded as hypoglycaemic by most investigators. Neonatal hypoglycaemia is associated with low birthweight or small-for-dates infants, infants of diabetic mothers, infants with haemolytic disease of the newborn, hypoxia, respiratory distress syndrome, cerebral haemorrhage and difficult delivery. The diagnosis is usually made by routine monitoring of blood sugar levels by 'Dextrostix' examination at frequent intervals in the babies at risk. The diagnosis should be confirmed by formal blood sugar measurements.

Reported signs and symptoms of neonatal hypoglycaemia are vague and may occur in infants who do not have hypoglycaemia. They are as follows:

- Respiratory   cyanosis, irregular respirations, apnoea.
- Neurological   tremors, jitteriness, convulsions, apathy, limpness, eye-rolling and a high pitched or weak cry.
- Cardiac   hypotension, bradycardia, tachycardia, heart failure, cardiac stand-still.
- Miscellaneous   pallor, refusal to feed.

Management

Infants at risk should be fed early and their blood glucose monitored closely by 3-hourly Dextrostix examination before feeds. If asymptomatic hypoglycaemia is detected in this way, true plasma glucose levels should be determined by the glucose oxidase method. In the event of absence of facilities for measuring true plasma glucose, blood specimens for glucose should be collected and the infants should be treated as for hypoglycaemia.

If true plasma glucose is low or if symptoms develop, a single dose of intravenous dextrose of 0.5 g/kg as a 10% solution over 2–3 minutes should be followed by a 10% intravenous glucose drip at 6–8 mg/kg per minute. Oral feeding is introduced as soon as possible, but the intravenous infusion should be continued until such time as feeding is established fully. If hypoglycaemia persists or recurs in spite of the above measures, investigations should be undertaken to exclude hyperinsulinaemia and other rare causes of neonatal hypoglycaemia (Table 7.3).

Table 7.3 Causes of neonatal hypoglycaemia

1. Depleted stores of glycogen: low birthweight or small-for-dates infants, hypoxia, respiratory distress syndrome, difficult delivery, hypothermia

2. Endocrine disorders
   (a) hyperinsulinism: maternal diabetes, erythroblastosis, Beckwith–Wiedmann syndrome, pancreatic β-cell abnormalities (islet cell tumour, functional β-cell hyperplasia, nesidioblastosis)
   (b) Panhypopituitarism
   (c) Isolated growth hormone deficiency
   (d) Adrenal insufficiency: cortisol deficiency, maternal steroid therapy, adrenal haemorrhage, adrenogenital syndrome, corticosteroid unresponsiveness
   (e) Hypothyroidism
   (f) Glucagon deficiency

3. Inborn errors of metabolism
   (a) Carbohydrate metabolism: galactocaemia, glycogen storage disease and fructosaemia
   (b) Amino acid metabolism: maple syrup urine disease, methylmalonic acidaemia, tyrosinosis
   (c) Fatty acid metabolism: acyl CoA dehydrogenase deficiency

4. Iatrogenic
   (a) Abrupt cessation of hypertonic glucose infusion
   (b) Following exchange transfusion

5. Miscellaneous
   (a) CNS abnormalities
   (b) Chronic diarrhoea
   (c) Sepsis
   (d) Liver disease
   (e) Hyperviscosity
   (f) Maternal drugs, e.g. propranol, tolbutamide, tocolytic agents

7.10 JAUNDICE IN THE NEWBORN

About one-half of the infants in a postnatal nursery will show visible jaundice. It is therefore not surprising that its occurrence may be taken for granted by the medical attendants. However, it may be the only symptom that occurs in many serious illnesses in the newborn. The jaundice may be due to enzyme deficiencies in the liver, haemolysis, infection, metabolic disturbances and obstruction to the bile passage. High levels of indirect reacting bilirubin can cause brain damage, which may be so mild as to cause only disturbance of cognitive function or so serious as to cause kernicterus and deafness. Although 340 mmol/l is quoted as the level at which bilirubin toxicity may occur, factors such as the maturity of the infant, hypoxia, acidosis, rate of rise of bilirubin, and the presence of substances that compete with bilirubin for albumin-binding sites must also be taken into consideration when planning treatment for an infant with raised indirect bilirubin.

Physiological jaundice

This condition occurs in newborn infants and requires no treatment. It is mainly due to relative deficiency of the enzyme glucuronyl transferase, though red cell destruction and the enterohepatic circulation may be partially responsible. The infant is usually well, and the jaundice does not appear before the age of 24 hours and begins to wane by the seventh day in the full-term and by the 10th day in the pre-term infant. Usually it is maximum on the third or fourth day in full-term infants and on the fifth or sixth day in pre-term infants. The serum level of unconjugated (indirect) bilirubin remains below 250 μmol/l, and the conjugated (direct) bilirubin level does not exceed 16–25 μmol/l.

Haemolytic jaundice

This may be due to blood group incompatibility (Rh, ABO and other rare blood groups), abnormalities of the shape of the red blood cells (e.g. hereditary spherocytosis) red blood cell enzyme deficiency (e.g. glucose-6-phosphate-dehydrogenase deficiency), or abnormal haemoglobins (e.g. Bart's). The haemolysis may also be secondary to the administration of drugs. It may occur in extravascular sites secondary to bleeding in the tissues, as in ecchymosis and caphalhaematoma.

Bacterial and viral infections

These may cause jaundice in the neonatal period, and the infection may be congenital or acquired. Bacterial infections (particularly septicaemia due to Gram-negative organisms) should be considered in all cases of neonatal jaundice. In jaundice due to infection there is usually a rise in both direct and indirect bilirubin.

Metabolic conditions

Those that tend to cause hyperbilirubinaemia include hypoxia, hypoglycaemia, hypothyroidism, galactosaemia, alpha-1-antitrypsin deficiency, cystic fibrosis and many disturbances of amino acid metabolism. The mechanism of jaundice in these conditions is complex, and the type of bilirubin will depend on the underlying disease process. Other symptoms will sometimes aid in the diagnosis.

Bile-duct atresia

This type of jaundice is rarely recognized in the first week of life, and is difficult to distinguish from neonatal hepatitis. In both these conditions there are signs of obstructive jaundice (raised direct bilirubin, clay-coloured stools, bile in urine). Bile-duct atresia and neonatal hepatitis must be distinguished from other conditions causing a raised direct bilirubin (e.g. galactosaemia and cystic fibrosis).

Enzyme deficiencies

Certain congenital liver cell enzyme deficiencies cause neonatal hyperbilirubinaemia, but these conditions are rare. Crigler–Najjar syndrome is an example of unconjugated hyperbilirubinaemia due to glucuronyl transferase deficiency, and Dubin–Johnson syndrome is an example of direct hyperbilirubinaemia due to a defect of hepatic excretory function.

Bilirubin competitors

Many substances compete with bilirubin for conjugation by the liver and will tend to cause hyperbilirubinaemia in the neonatal period. Examples of some commonly used drugs in the perinatal period that compete are salicylates, water-soluble analogues of vitamin K, diazepam by injection which contains benzoate, certain sulphonamides and steroids.

Other drugs that have been implicated in the causation of neonatal jaundice include phenothiazines and oxytocin given to the mother.

Breast milk jaundice

The exact mechanism of breast milk jaundice is not clear, though pregnanetriol and unsaturated fatty acids (which are bilirubin competitors) in the milk have been implicated in its causation. More recently, it has been shown that bilirubin reductase in breast milk breaks down conjugated bilirubin in the gut, which increases bilirubin load via the enterohepatic circulation.

Management of hyperbilirubinaemia

There are many causes of hyperbilirubinaemia, so the investigations and treatment will depend on individual cases. Investigations aim to exclude haemolysis (blood group of infant and mother, direct Coombs' test, peripheral blood smear and enzymes), infection (urine and blood cultures) and metabolic conditions (reducing substances in urine).

Exchange transfusion is the most reliable and quick method for reducing bilirubin concentration, whatever the cause of hyperbilirubinaemia. However, phototherapy has greatly reduced the need for exchange transfusion in neonatal nurseries. The exact mechanism by which phototherapy reduces bilirubin is not clear, but so far two types of reaction have been demonstrated: photo-oxidation, in which the bilirubin molecule is broken down into monopyrroles and dipyrroles, and photo-isomerization, in which the molecule remains intact and can be excreted without hepatic glucuronization in the bile. *In vitro* studies suggest that photo-isomerization is the more important reaction. Although phototherapy has been known to cause retinal damage, growth retardation and the early onset of puberty in experimental animals, no such problems have been reported in infants. It appears that these effects are mediated through the retina and it has been recommended that the eyes of newborn babies be shielded during phototherapy.

It has been observed that phenobarbitone given to the

mother or the newborn infant activates the enzyme glucuronyl transferase over a period of approximately 48–96 hours. It is not a useful drug for reducing bilirubin levels, but in selected cases it may be given prophylactically to the mother prior to delivery.

7.11 INFECTIONS IN THE NEWBORN

Infections in the newborn may be acquired transplacentally from the mother. The baby may be born with the TORCH (Toxoplasma, Other, Rubella, Cytomegolovirus, Herpes simplex) syndrome: hepatosplenomegaly, jaundice, nervous system abnormalities, chorioretinitis and rashes. The diagnosis may be suspected from the maternal history, and routine examination of cord blood for immunoglobulin M (IgM). Viral studies and examination of cord blood for specific IgM will further help to elucidate the diagnosis.

Congenital syphilis can be acquired in the second and the third trimesters. Bacterial infections including septicaemia, pneumonia, pyelonephritis, meningitis and tuberculosis may also be acquired *in utero*, though they usually occur during parturition or postnatally.

Factors that predispose the newborn to infection include prolonged labour, prolonged rupture of membranes and manipulative and resuscitative procedures on the infant. Other conditions that may predispose to infection are immaturity, respiratory distress and invasive procedures such as intermittent positive-pressure ventilation, arterial and venous lines.

Newborn babies are susceptible to infection by most microorganisms, but the local and systemic response to infection is poor: most infections become generalized and have non-specific symptoms. Clinical features that should arouse suspicion of infection include changes in behaviour (e.g. irritability, lethargy, poor feeding, and vomiting), or simply that the baby does not 'look well'. Other symptoms include failure in temperature control (hypothermia or hyperthermia), prolonged or unexpected jaundice (particularly in urinary tract infections and septicaemia), disturbances in respiration, abdominal distension due to ileus, and the presence of purpura and pustules on the skin. In the presence of specific signs, investigations are directed towards the appropriate organ system. However, in most cases it is necessary to do a 'septic work up' which includes swabs for culture of the ear and umbilical cord, full blood count (including differential and band count), blood, urine and cerebrospinal fluid cultures. Infants with infection develop secondary problems, and in severe cases it is necessary to measure blood glucose, serum bilirubin, acid–base balance and electrolytes.

The management of the newborn with suspected infection includes anticipating problems in 'at risk' situations, carrying out appropriate investigations and instituting treatment on clinical grounds (rather than relying on prophylaxis or bacteriological investigation). Antimicrobial therapy is indicated if the infection is thought to be bacterial. The choice of antibiotics will depend on the sensitivity of the organisms in a particular nursery, until bacteriological results are available. The usual practice is to use a combination of two drugs, such as a penicillin and an aminoglycoside. Supportive measures include nursing in a neutral thermal environment, adequate fluid and nutrition, and the management of the complications that occur in severe cases, such as anaemia, shock, hypoglycaemia and disseminated intravascular coagulation.

7.12 RESPIRATORY PROBLEMS OF THE NEWBORN

Respiratory failure causes more than 50% of the deaths of normally formed live-born infants during the first 48 hours of life. The respiratory failure may be central or peripheral.

Central respiratory failure. This is characterized by apnoea and slow, irregular, gasping respiratory movements. Table 7.4

Table 7.4 Causes of central respiratory failure

---

1. CNS: drugs, haemorrhage, congenital malformation, immaturity (prematurity), seizures
2. Respiratory: laryngeal reflex, intrapulmonary disease
3. Infections: sepsis, meningitis
4. Metabolic: hypoglycaemia, hypocalcaemia, high environmental temperature
5. Miscellaneous: anaemia, circulatory failure, gastro-oesophageal reflux

---

Table 7.5 Causes of peripheral respiratory failure

Condition	Salient clinical features	Specific therapy
Respiratory		
Transient tachypnoea of newborn	Is due to failure to absorb lung fluid. Predisposing factors are caesarean section, rapid delivery. Chest X-ray is non-specific, may show streakiness starting from the hila, prominent intralobar fissure, slight hyperinflation	Nil
Hyaline membrane disease	Predisposing factors are prematurity, infant of diabetic mother, hypoxia, acidosis and Caesarean section. Chest X-ray shows generalized reticular-granular (ground glass, snow storm) pattern with air bronchogram	Surfactant
Pneumonia	Prolonged rupture of membranes, maternal infection (fever, vaginal discharge). Low white cell count suggests infection. Blood cultures positive	Broad-spectrum antibiotics
Meconium aspiration	Fetal distress, meconium-stained liquor. Term infants. Chest is hyperinflated. Chest X-ray shows hyperinflation with diffuse patchy opacities. Pneumothorax, pneumomediastinum and interstial emphysema may be present	Suction of mouth and pharynx prior to delivery of thorax of infant

Table 7.5 Causes of peripheral respiratory failure

Condition	Salient clinical features	Specific therapy
Pulmonary air leaks	Seen as a complication of hyaline membrane disease, meconium aspiration, hypoplastic lungs. Present as sudden deterioration of babies with respiratory distress. Diagnosis can be made by chest transillumination and confirmed by chest X-ray	Chest drain for pneumothorax. Cardiac drain for pneumo-pericardium
Congenital abnormalities		
Choanal atresia	These babies are blue while quiet and pink while crying	Train baby to breathe through the mouth by placing a large oral gastric tube
Pierre–Robin syndrome	These babies have a large tongue, receded chin and cleft palate	May respond to nursing in the prone position, failing which the tongue is stiched to the floor of the mouth to prevent it falling back and causing obstruction
Tracheo-oesophageal fistula	Maternal hydramnios, mucousy after birth, aspiration following a feed, failure to pass nasogastric tube	Frequent sucking of saliva, surgical repair
Diaphragmatic hernia	Difficulty in resuscitation, respiratory distress, displacement of apex beat, scaphoid abdomen, bowel sounds in the	If resuscitation is needed, it should be via an endotracheal

Condition	Features	Treatment
	chest, chest X-ray shows loops of bowel. May develop persistent pulmonary hypertension	tube and never by bag and mask, surgical repair, NO and ECMO for persistent pulmonary hypertension
Pulmonary hypoplasia	Seen in association with neuromuscular disorders, space-occupying lesions in the thorax and oligohydramnios. May have characteristic facies (beaked nose, low-set abnormal ears, prominent epicanthic folds and antimongolian slant to the eyes) seen in renal ageneses	Nil
Bronchopulmonary dysplasia	Seen in infants requiring pulmonary support and high concentrations of oxygen. Chest X-ray in advanced cases shows irregular honeycomb appearance, over-inflation, extensive fibrosis and multiple cysts of irregular size	Dexamethasone, diuretics
Wilson–Mikity syndrome	Seen in pre-term infants in the second or third week without previous history of respiratory distress. Chest X-ray initially shows bilateral coarse, streaky infiltrates which progress to a small cyst. The latter enlarge and the lungs become over inflated	Nil
Extrapulmonary causes		
Persistent pulmonary hypertension of newborn	Predisposing factors are hypothermia, underlying congenital heart disease, hypoxia, acidosis, polycythaemia with hyperviscosity and lung diseases such as diaphragmatic	Correct aetiological factors if possible, e.g. polycythaemia. Hyperventilation

Table 7.5 Causes of peripheral respiratory failure

Condition	Salient clinical features	Specific therapy
	hernia, pneumonia and meconium aspiration. Diagnostic criteria include raised pulmonary artery pressure, hypoxemia with or without acidosis and evidence of right-to-left shunting of blood and normal cardiac anatomy	and alkalinization (maintain pH 7.45–7.50). Pulmonary vasodilators including nitric oxide. ECMO
Congenital heart disease	Signs and symptoms of congenital heart disease: cyanosis, congestive cardiac failure, heart murmurs, arrhythmias	Make exact diagnosis, treat congestive cardiac failure, offer palliative or curative surgical treatment

lists some of the recognized causes of central respiratory failure. Besides specific therapy, general measures include careful monitoring of heart rate and respiration, tactile stimulation and oral or intravenous theophylline. Infants who fail to respond to these measures require constant positive airway pressure or intermittent positive-pressure ventilation.

Peripheral respiratory failure. This is characterized by tachypnoea (respiratory rate more than 60/minute), intercostal and/or subcostal recession and an expiratory grunt. The persistent of two or more of these signs for 4 hours or more is required for the diagnosis of respiratory distress syndrome. As there are many causes of respiratory distress syndrome (Table 7.5), an aetiological diagnosis should be attempted in all cases in order to carry out specific therapy. As a general rule, all patients with respiratory distress syndrome are given broad-spectrum antibiotics (e.g. amoxicillin and gentamicin) until such time that it is clear that the infant has no infection as clinical, haematological and X-ray findings may not indicate infection. General measures include:

1. Oxygen: amount will depend on blood gases or haemoglobin saturation. The aim is to maintain a PO_2 between 60–80 mmHg or a haemoglobin saturation of 92–95%.
2. Monitor blood gases in order to plan oxygen therapy as well as to diagnose respiratory failure. If the PO_2 is less than 60 mmHg in 60% oxygen or the PCO_2 is more than 60 mmHg, the patient will need respiratory support in most cases.
3. Correction of acid–base disturbance: alkali administration is rarely indicated. Plasma expanders (e.g. SPPS) will be useful in patients showing low blood pressure or other evidence of circulatory failure.
4. Nurse infant in neutral thermal environment to minimize oxygen and glucose needs.
5. Provide adequate fluids and calories.

7.13 NEONATAL CONVULSIONS

Convulsions in the neonatal period most frequently are subtle (when they are easily overlooked) or obvious (multifocal clonic movements, focal clonic movements and tonic or myoclonic movements). Generalized convulsions are rare. Subtle manifestations include eye movements (horizontal deviation, jerking, blinking or fluttering), drooling, sucking, unusual limb movements ('rowing' or 'swimming') and apnoea. Jitteriness (rhythmic limb movements) which is fairly common in the newborn may be confused with convulsions. However, unlike convulsions, jitteriness is rhythmic, stimulus sensitive and is not accompanied by abnormalities of eye movements. Furthermore, jitteriness can be stopped by flexion of the affected limb.

Common causes of neonatal convulsions

Hypoxic ischaemic encephalopathy

Hypoxic ischaemic encephalopathy, including oedema, haemorrhage and perinatal anoxia.

Metabolic conditions

Hypoglycaemia (usually in the first 48 hours in low birthweight infants and within the first 24 hours in infants of diabetic or pre-diabetic mothers), hypocalcaemia (first or second day usually in association with maternal complications of pregnancy and delivery or fifth day in bottle-fed babies), disturbances of amino acid metabolism (usually 24–48 hours after commencement of feeding) and miscellaneous conditions such as hypomagnesaemia, electrolyte imbalance, hyperbilirubinaemia and pyridoxine dependency.

Drug withdrawal

Heroin, methadone, barbiturates (usually present within 48–72 hours of birth, though may present a week later).

Infections

Central nervous system (e.g. meningitis) or systemic.

Intracranial malformations

Intraventricular haemorrhage

In premature infants.

8

Abnormal labour

8.1 GENERAL INSTRUCTIONAL OBJECTIVES

The students should recognize deviations from normal labour and understand their effect on mother and fetus so that in an emergency they can initiate management.

8.2 SPECIFIC BEHAVIOURAL OBJECTIVES

1. Identify failure of progress in labour.
2. Identify the symptoms and signs that are suggestive of disproportion.
3. Describe the clinical features of a patient with obstructed labour.
4. Identify the signs that may indicate fetal distress, and discuss their causes and the implications to the fetus.
5. Distinguish between normal and abnormal uterine action.
6. Identify the effects of prolonged labour on mother and fetus.
7. Assist in the management of a patient with a prolonged labour, and discuss the problems that are identifiable.
8. Discuss the use of continuous fetal heart rate monitoring.
9. Discuss the initial management of a transverse lie, cord prolapse, shoulder dystocia and unsuspected second twin.
10. List the common indications for and the complications of Caesarean section.
11. List the criteria necessary for the safe application of forceps.
12. Discuss the causes of postpartum haemorrhage.
13. Examine a patient with a postpartum haemorrhage, diagnose the cause and initiate the appropriate emergency management.
14. List the causes of shock during labour and early puerper-

ium, and indicate the emergency management of these
patients.
15. Discuss the causes of intrapartum haemorrhage.
16. Discuss the causes and management of women who have a
    pre-term labour.

8.3 REASONS FOR STUDYING ABNORMAL LABOUR

Almost every labour progresses to delivery with some minor
deviations from normal which do not produce any marked problems to the mother or fetus or which require minimal interference to correct. However, some labours become so abnormal
that continuation may produce increased morbidity or death of
the mother or fetus. It is important that the competent student
will have the ability to recognize these deviations and to assess
their significance and then to initiate the appropriate steps in
management. Every student should spend as much time as
possible in the labour ward, learning to recognize abnormalities
in women during the first and second stages of labour. The
student should recognize these minor deviations and be prepared to discuss their observations with the staff in charge of
the patient. Because of the earlier recognition, major deviations
become easier to define and appropriate management instituted
at a much earlier stage.

8.4 DELAY IN LABOUR

Although there is wide variation in the duration of labour,
most multiparous patients will deliver in about 8 hours while
primiparas patients take 12–14 hours. It is now recognized that
the fetal skull is probably the best pelvimeter (indicator of
pelvic adequacy). Unless labour is contraindicated, all primi-
gravidas should be allowed to have a trial of labour.

Once patients are in established labour, their progress is
recorded on a partogram and regular vaginal and clinical
examinations should be performed every 4 hours.

Indication of delay in labour

1. Should the rate of cervical dilatation fail to exceed 1 cm/
   hour in a primiparous patient or 1.5 cm/hour in a multi-

parous patient, once the patient is in the active phase of labour (more than 3 cm dilated), then the staff should be alerted that a problem may exist.

2. Where there is failure of descent of the presenting part. Like cervical dilatation, the presenting part of the fetus descends into the pelvis at a gradually increasing rate. Disproportion or poor uterine contractions may delay the descent of the presenting part.

Once the 'alert line' (see Fig. 6.17) has been crossed, a further vaginal examination is done after another 2 hours. If the rate of progress has now been satisfactory, no further intervention is necessary. If however, no further progress has occurred (i.e. the cervix has not dilated any further) then the action line will be crossed. At this point it is necessary to establish a diagnosis as to why the labour has not progressed and a critical vaginal examination and pelvic assessment should be made by an experienced observer to exclude obvious cephalo-pelvic disproportion.

Delay may be due to cephalo-pelvic disproportion (absolute or relative) or abnormal uterine activity.

Cephalo-pelvic disproportion

This is one of the most common causes of obstructed labour and the underlying condition may be due to one of the following:

Absolute disproportion

1. Large baby
   (a) Hereditary factors. Most babies have a birthweight similar to that of their mother/father. Big babies have large heads. Large mothers tend to have large babies.
   (b) Post-maturity. When the placenta functions normally, the fetus continues to grow at a regular rate. If the pregnancy continues beyond 40 weeks then the fetus will be larger than average.
   (c) Diabetes. The increased maternal levels of glucose pass to the fetus, so stimulating insulin production, deposi-

tion of glucose in tissue and initiation of growth hormone-like activity.

(d) Multiparity. Up to the fifth baby, each succeeding baby tends to be heavier and larger than the preceding infant.

2. Small pelvis

Normal women who are 160 cm tall have a true conjugate diameter of the pelvis of about 11.5 cm. Taller women tend to have larger pelvic diameters while shorter women have smaller diameters. The risks of absolute cephalo-pelvic disproportion increase if the woman is less than 150 cm in height. Approximately 25% of mothers who are 155 cm or smaller have some form of surgical interference (forceps, Caesarean section) to their labour, whereas mothers of 163 cm and taller have only a 5% chance of surgical interference.

3. Abnormal shape to pelvic brim

Most women will have either a **gynaecoid** (45%) or an **anthropoid** (40%) shape to their pelvic brim and the brim, cavity and outlet will be adequate for most fetuses to pass through the pelvis. However, about 15% of women have an android shape to the brim, a flattened sacrum, narrow subpubic angle and prominent ischial spines. In these women, the sidewalls of the pelvis tends to be convergent (funnel-shaped) and the fetus, which often presents in the occipito-lateral or occipito-posterior position may become jammed in the mid-pelvis, unable to undergo or complete internal rotation and unable to descend further. This arrest of internal rotation occurs at the level of the ischial spines and is called **deep transverse arrest** of the fetal head. This may be managed by rotating the head to an occipito-anterior position, either manually, with Kielland's forceps – or by means of a vacuum extractor. If this is not possible it may be necessary to perform a Caesarean section.

Another abnormal pelvic shape is associated with a **platypelloid** pelvic brim, where there is general flattening of the brim in an antero-posterior diameter. The true conjugate diameter is about 10.5 cm with a wider (12.5 cm) transverse diameter. Because the pelvic cavity is usually divergent, the fetus will deliver easily, once it has negotiated the brim (usually by the process of asynclitism).

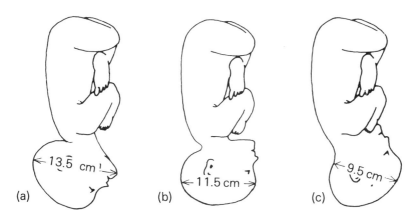

Figure 8.1 Fetal attitude. (a) Extension to a brow presentation with a mentovertical diameter (13.5 cm); (b) Extension in the military attitude with an occipito-frontal diameter (11.5 cm); (c) A normal flexed head with an suboccipito-bregmatic diameter (9.5 cm).

Relative disproportion

4. Abnormal positions
    Normally a fetus delivers in the occipito-anterior position with the head well flexed so that the suboccipito-bregmatic (9.5 cm) and the biparietal (9.5 cm) diameters will easily pass through a normal pelvis.

    If however, the fetus is in an occipito-posterior position then the presenting diameter may be either suboccipito-frontal (10.5 cm) or occipito-frontal (11.5 cm).

    If there is a brow presentation (mento-vertical, 13.5 cm) then cephalo-pelvic disproportion will occur. With the onset of contractions forcing the extended head against the pelvic brim, flexion of the head normally occurs (or in brow presentation, further extension to a face presentation) until a smaller diameter presents. When this occurs, the fetal head descends, and with moulding and long internal rotation, the baby will eventually deliver in the occipito-anterior position. Because of the added mechanisms of flexion and long internal rotation, fetuses in the occipito-posterior and occipito-lateral position have a longer labour (Fig. 8.1).

5. Abnormality of the genital tract
    Vagina: can be due to congenital abnormalities such as septa.
    Cervix: obstruction can be due to post-surgical scarring or congenital rigidity.
    Pelvic tumours very rarely cause obstruction to labour. Ovarian cysts or uterine fibroids only obstruct labour if they are large and situated posteriorly in the Pouch of Douglas.

Abnormal uterine action

If the labour fails to progress then careful observation should be made of the uterine contractions. The contractions can be monitored by means of external tocodynamometry or by means of an intrauterine catheter to measure the intrauterine pressure directly. Note should be taken of the pressure, the frequency and the duration of each contraction. Care should also be taken to ensure that the uterus is relaxed between contractions.

An accurate diagnosis should be made as to the precise type of abnormal uterine action present and appropriate steps taken to deal with it. It is most important to exclude cephalo-pelvic disproportion.

8.5 TYPES OF ABNORMAL UTERINE ACTIVITY

Overactive hypertonic

Hypertonic incoordinate uterine activity

This generally occurs in anxious primigravid patients and may be associated with a malposition such as an occipito-posterior position. The contractions are incoordinate, irregular and ineffectual. There is an absence of fundal dominance and an increased uterine tone in between contractions. Because of the elevated resting tone, patients experience pain between contractions (Fig. 8.2).

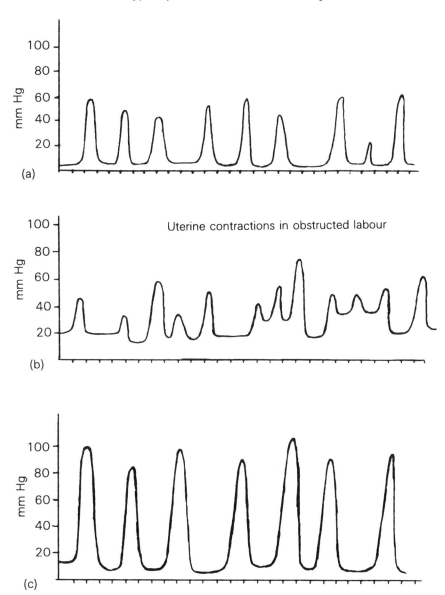

Figure 8.2 Uterine contractions. (a) Uterine contractions during the first stage of a normal labour. Low resting tone, good amplitude, lasting for 50–70 seconds every 3–5 minutes; (b) Uterine contractions in a primigravid in the first stage of labour, who is responding poorly to obstruction. High resting tone, poor amplitude, irregular time and amplitude. A non-productive uterine action; (c) Obstructed labour in a multigravid. Regular contractions with high amplitude. May cause ruptured uterus.

Management
1. Adequate analgesia: usually in the form of epidural anaesthesia. If this is not available, then adequate dosage of intramuscular pethidine will suffice.
2. Reassurance: it is important to reassure the patient and husband that the problem can be dealt with as maternal anxiety may play a role in the aetiology of this condition.
3. Beta-adrenergic agents: provided there is no contraindication, a small intravenous bolus dose (i.e. salbutamol, 100–300 µg or Ritodrine) can be used to inhibit uterine activity. When contractions restart 15–20 minutes later, they are often more regular. This treatment is indicated if epidural analgesia fails or is contraindicated.

Constriction ring

In this form of abnormal activity there is localized spastic contraction of a ring of circular muscle, usually at the junction of the upper and lower uterine segment around the fetal neck in cephalic presentations. They are normally associated with the injudicious use of oxytocics, premature rupture of membranes or premature attempts at instrumental delivery under inadequate local anaesthesia. Diagnosis is difficult and should be suspected if there is failure of the presenting part to descend in spite of what appears to be adequate uterine contractions and an adequate pelvis. It is sometimes revealed during a Caesarean section in the first stage or during a manual removal for a retained placenta (hour-glass uterus). The ring cannot be felt per abdomen.

Retraction ring

This condition occurs late in obstructed labour after the membranes have ruptured. As a consequence of the progressive permanent shortening (retraction) of the muscle fibres with each contraction, the upper segment becomes thickened and the lower segment progressively thinner. This ring and thickening rises progressively up the uterus as the lower segment becomes thinner. When it rises to an abnormally high level, it is termed a *Bandl's ring* and is an indication of impending uterine rupture.

Management
This is by Caesarean section.

Precipitate labour

This is said to have occurred when the duration of both the first and second stage of labour is less than 2 hours. The major risk to the mother are those of trauma to the cervix and lower genital tract. Dangers to the infant are mainly trauma and includes intracranial haemorrhage as a result of sudden compression and expansion of the fetal skull during the rapid delivery.

Treatment
Little can be done in the present pregnancy but in future pregnancies, patients should be admitted and induced near term so that delivery of the head can be controlled.

Underactive or hypotonic uterine activity

The uterine contractions are weak and infrequent and the intrauterine pressure will be below 30 mmHg.

Primary hypotonic inertia

Causes

- Overdistention of the uterus, due to multiple pregnancies, polyhydramnios or fibromyomata.
- Multiple pregnancies.
- Congenital uterine abnormalities such as bicornuate uterus.
- In association with antepartum haemorrhage and marked anaemia.
- As a result of cephalo-pelvic disproportion.

Secondary hypotonic inertia

This is where the uterus has been contracting adequately and then the contractions become inefficient later in labour.

Causes

- Cephalo-pelvic disproportion, particularly in multiparous patients.
- Overdistention of the uterus in association with multiple pregnancy or polyhydramnios.
- A rigid cervix or perineum.
- Malpresentations.
- Oversedation.

Management

1. Exclude cephalo-pelvic disproportion, obstruction.
2. Syntocinon stimulation.
3. Adequate analgesia.
4. Prevent postpartum haemorrhage by the use of oxytocic drugs.

8.6 PROLONGED LABOUR

Definition

The definition of prolonged labour has changed over the years and it is believed now that any labour which lasts more than 18 hours is prolonged. However, there is a good reason to believe that no patient should be in the active phase of labour (commences at 3 cm of dilatation) for more than 12 hours. This is because of the trend towards practising preventative obstetrics and the consequences of prolonged labour.

Prolonged latent phase

It is abnormal for the latent phase to exceed 20 hours in a primigravida or 14 hours in a multigravida. The causes include:

- Unripe cervix.
- Malposition or malpresentation.
- Cephalo-pelvic disproportion.
- Premature administration of sedation.

Management
If vaginal delivery is not contraindicated, then this is by oxytocin stimulation.

Consequences of prolonged labour

Maternal

- Maternal metabolic abnormalities.
- Potential infection.
- Psychological disappointment.
- Anxiety.
- Mechanical complications such as a rupture of the uterus and fistulae.
- Exhaustion.

Fetal

- Fetal distress.
- Fetal infection.
- Fetal brain damage.
- Intrauterine death – stillbirth.
- Neonatal death.

Management of prolonged labour

The most important part of the management of prolonged labour is prevention and the recognition of potential causes. If patients are correctly managed using a partogram and appropriate attention is paid to the alert and action lines, prolonged labour should not occur. The possible causes may be:

1. Abnormalities of the passenger
   (a) Malpresentation.
   (b) Malposition.
   (c) Fetal malformation.
   (d) Large fetus (Fig. 8.3).
2. Abnormalities in the passage:
   (a) Contracted pelvis.
   (b) Abnormalities of the uterus and lower genital tract as well as pelvic tumours.
3. Abnormalities in the power:
   (a) Abnormal uterine contractions (see previous section).

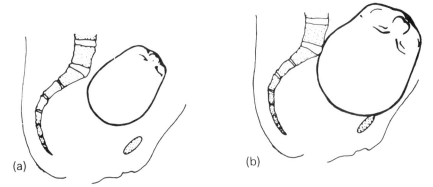

Figure 8.3 (a) Non-engaged head without disproportion. The skull does not overlap the symphysis pubis; (b) Non-engaged head. The skull overlaps the symphysis pubis.

Procedure

1. Establish an intravenous line, adequate fluids and nutrients.
2. Reassure the mother that you are aware of the problem and of her needs and anxiety, and that you are taking appropriate steps to manage the problem.
3. Judicious use of Syntocinon if the contractions are inadequate.
4. Use of epidural anaesthesia for pain relief.
5. Monitoring of fetal well-being by the use of a cardiotocography.
6. Ensuring that the membranes are ruptured.
7. Chemoprophylaxis by using the appropriate antibiotics should the patient be pyrexial or there be any suspicion of intrauterine infection.
8. Instrumental delivery to manipulate the fetus when indicated.
9. Perform a Caesarean section if no progress is made.

8.7 FETAL DISTRESS

During any labour, but particularly during the labour of an 'at risk' pregnant mother, the signs of fetal distress may develop. These signs imply metabolic abnormalities and may reflect fetal hypoxia and acidosis. These abnormalities can arise as acute events (prolapsed cord, placental abruption), subacute, (hypertonic uterine activity) or be chronic (as a result of placental insufficiency).

Fetal distress is a term applied to a set of signs indicating that if the fetus is not delivered, it will be born dead, or will suffer some brain damage as a result of the hypoxia. Fetal distress needs to be separated from signs of fetal 'stress' which do not have such ominous implications.

Signs of fetal stress

1. Meconium staining of the amniotic fluid. Meconium staining of infants who are term or post-term in gestational age is less sinister in its incidence in pre-term infants. The major danger of meconium-stained amniotic fluid is aspiration at the time of delivery.
2. Intrauterine growth retardation.

Signs of fetal distress

1. Rapid fetal heart rate (tachycardia), greater than 160 beats/minute.
2. Slow fetal heart rate (bradycardia), less than 100 beats/minute.
3. Heart rate deceleration (particularly late decelerations).
4. Loss of fetal heart reactivity (beat-to-beat variability).
5. Low fetal scalp pH and increased base deficit.
6. Fetal gasping or absence of fetal respiratory movements *in utero* as seen on ultrasound.

Although many of these signs often indicate fetal distress, all of these may be found in a fetus that is born healthy and active with an excellent chance of normal growth after delivery. The art in obstetric management is to decide what is abnormal, when to interfere and how to interfere with the normal processes of labour.

Fetal heart rate patterns

For a normal fetal heart rate to be maintained, the fetus requires an adequate supply of nutriment (glucose and glycogen) and oxygen. Placental inadequacy or reduced placental blood flow (occurring in conditions such as maternal hypertension, excessive maternal smoking or poor maternal nutrition) reduce the amount of glucose that can be actively or passively transferred to the fetus, so that it is born small-for-gestational age and with poor glycogen reserves. If such a fetus has a labour which is prolonged or overstimulated, there is superadded hypoxia, and the fetus will become acidotic. All fetuses that are at risk should be observed in labour by continuous fetal heart rate monitoring. The significance of any abnormality in heart rate pattern depends on their severity as well as the number of abnormalities present.

Fetal heart rate variability

Short-term (beat-to-beat) variability

When measured directly from a scalp electrode it gives a measure of the R–R wave interval and true beat-to-beat variability. They are measured over seconds. Beat-to-beat variability is thought to provide a measure of the balance between the sympathetic and parasympathetic nervous systems. This in turn is thought to provide some measure of central nervous system integrity.

Long-term variability

These fluctuations occur over minutes and are associated with fetal movements or uterine contractions. Reduced beat-to-beat variability may indicate alterations in the fetal sleep state which either occur spontaneously or as a result of maternal sedation or it may indicate fetal hypoxia.

Fetal heart rate changes

Non-periodic changes

The normal fetal heart rate varies between 110–160 beats per minute. Should the fetal heart rate rise above 160 beats/minute and be sustained for more than 10 minutes, this is regarded as tachycardia. If the fetal heart rate slows to less than 100 beats/minute for the same duration, this is regarded as bradycardia.

The most common cause of a fetal tachycardia is maternal pyrexia. One of the earliest signs of fetal compromise is a fetal tachycardia and can easily be missed.

Periodic changes

These are changes in the fetal heart rate that last less than 10 minutes and are associated with uterine contractions or fetal movements. These are classified as:

1. **Accelerations**
An increase in heart rate associated with either uterine contractions or fetal activity and usually indicate a healthy active fetus.

2. **Decelerations**
   (a) Early decelerations (Type 1). This slowing of the fetal heart rate usually occurs in association with contractions and is probably due to vagal nerve stimulation due to head or trunk compression. The lowest point of the deceleration (nadir) occurs in association with the apex of the contraction.
   (b) Late decelerations (Type 2). Here the slowing of the fetal heart rate starts after the apex of the contraction and the nadir of the deceleration occurs well after it. This may be a sign of fetal hypoxia.
   (c) Variable decelerations (Type 3). These are a combination of early and late decelerations and usually are associated with cord compression.

Relative risks of fetal distress:

1. Approximately 5% of patients who have a normal intra-partum cardiotocograph will be born with low Apgar scores.
2. Meconium-stained amniotic fluid alone carries a risk of about 5% that the fetus will have a low Apgar score.

The greater the number of abnormal features present in the cardiotocographic tracing, the greater the chances are of the fetus being compromised. The risk depends upon the underlying baseline heart rate, the degree of beat to beat variability plus the extent of the decelerations (if any are present).

To help differentiate true fetal distress in labour from any abnormal heart rate pattern due to other reasons, fetal scalp blood analysis can be undertaken. A small sample is taken from the fetal scalp and analysed for pH, $P\text{CO}_2$ and base deficit. A normal fetal pH level in the first stage of labour is usually greater than 7.25. A level of <7.20 indicates the need for urgent delivery. During the second stage the normal fetal scalp pH may drop to 7.15. It may be necessary to assess the maternal acid–base status as alterations in the maternal acid base balance can affect the fetal base status.

Management of an abnormal heart rate pattern

When any abnormal pattern is present, a cause for it should be sought (Fig. 8.4). The patient is turned to the lateral position (to avoid the supine hypotensive syndrome) and also to try to exclude cord compression. If a Syntocinon drip is running, this should be stopped in case the abnormal heart rate pattern is a result of hyperstimulation. A vaginal examination should be

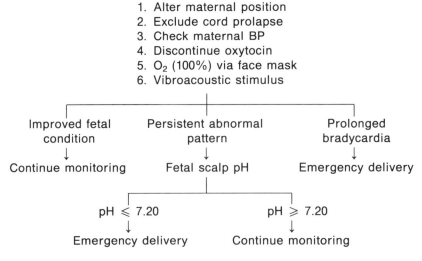

Figure 8.4 Management of an abnormal heart rate pattern.

done if cord prolapse is suspected. The mother should be given 100% O_2 via a facemask.

If the fetal heart rate abnormality persists, then a fetal scalp blood sample should be taken. Preliminary evidence with vibroacoustic stimulation suggests that if the fetus is stimulated in labour and responds with a heart rate increase of more than 15 beats/minute then the risks of the scalp pH being less than 7.25 is small. If the fetal scalp sample is abnormal or the facilities are not available to do this test and the fetal heart rate abnormality persists, then delivery should be expedited by whichever means is safest to both mother and fetus. If the cervix is fully dilated and the head already engaged if may be delivered by forceps delivery or if this is not possible an emergency Caesarean section should be performed.

Intrauterine resuscitation

In the presence of a severely abnormal fetal heart rate, while preparations for Caesarean section are being made a small bolus dose of a beta-adrenergic drug (salbutamol, ritodrine) or magnesium sulphate can be given to inhibit uterine activity and improve placental perfusion in the interim period.

8.8 TRANSVERSE AND OBLIQUE LIE

An unstable lie is one in which the presenting part alters from week to week. It may be either a transverse (long axis of the fetus at right angles to the maternal spine) or oblique lie (long axis of the fetus oblique to the maternal spine) or possibly a breech presentation. These are relatively uncommon events but are found in association with the following conditions:

1. Grand multiparity. This is by far the most common factor, due to the lax uterine and abdominal walls, which prevent the 'splinting' effect found in women with lesser parity.
2. Polyhydramnios. The volume of fluid distends the uterus and allows the fetus to 'swim like a goldfish in a bowl' – often taking up an oblique or transverse lie.
3. Prematurity. Here there is a relative excess of fluid to fetus. If pre-term labour occurs, the fetus may be found to have a transverse lie.

4. Subseptate uterus. The septum prevents the fetus from turning *in utero*.
5. Pelvic tumours such as fibroids and ovarian cysts may not only prevent the lower pole from engaging, but cause it to take up a transverse lie.
6. Placenta praevia. This usually prevents engagements of the presenting part. Because of this it may present with the fetus in an oblique or transverse lie.
7. Multiple pregnancies may present with a transverse lie. If this does occur, it is more common in the second twin.

Management of oblique and transverse lie

It is not uncommon for the fetus to have a transverse lie until about the 32nd week of pregnancy. If the transverse lie persists after this time, a **cause** should be determined. An ultrasound examination should be done to exclude placenta praevia, ovarian tumour or fibroid and if either of these conditions are present an elective Caesarean section should be performed at 38–39 weeks of gestation. The ultrasound is also used for identifying twins and a subseptate uterus, while a vaginal examination will confirm a pelvic tumour.

The main risk of a transverse or oblique lie is in association with pre-term rupture of the membranes and cord prolapse. When diagnosed, the state of the cervix should be checked. If the cervix is dilated, the patient should be admitted to hospital. If, however, the cervix is closed and the membranes are intact, the patient may be reviewed on a regular basis. If no easily identifiable cause is found, attempted external cephalic version can be made after 37 weeks. In grand multiparous patients, the fetus will usually turn easily but will often swing back to an abnormal lie. If the abnormal lie persists or constantly reoccurs, the woman should be admitted to hospital by the 38th week. If external version is successful at this stage and the patient's cervix is favourable then artificial rupture of the membranes can be performed with the head held over the pelvic brim and a Syntocinon drip commenced to augment uterine activity. If the cephalic presentation is maintained, labour may be allowed to continue. If the transverse or oblique lie re-occurs in labour then a Caesarean section must be performed.

Complications of a transverse lie

If a mother goes into labour with a transverse or oblique lie, several catastrophes may occur. Because this occurs more commonly in multiparous women and their uterine activity is often much stronger the rupture of the uterus is more likely. When the membranes rupture, there is a greatly increased danger of cord prolapse.

8.9 CORD PROLAPSE

Cord prolapse is that condition when the membranes rupture, allowing a loop of cord to prolapse through the cervical os. The cord is found either in the vagina or protruding outside the labia. This complication has a high fetal mortality rate because the cord is compressed either by the presenting part or the vessels go into spasm due to a change in temperature and drying effects of the air (Fig. 8.5).

Factors associated with cord prolapse

1. Transverse and oblique lie.
2. Breech presentation.
3. Disproportion.
4. Multiple pregnancy.
5. Polyhydramnios.
6. Pre-term rupture of the membranes.

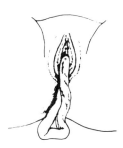

Figure 8.5 Cord prolapse leads to drying and cooling of the cord causing spasm of vessels or the cord may be compressed at the pelvic brim by the fetal presenting part.

7. Pelvic tumours.
8. Placenta praevia (not Type 4).

Management of cord prolapse

A cord prolapse is an acute obstetrical emergency, and is often first seen by those people who are least experienced to cope with it. Steps in the acute management:

1. Determine if the cord is still pulsating.
2. If pulsating, push any exposed loop of cord back into the vagina to keep it warm and moist.
3. Determine the dilatation of the cervix. If fully dilated the patient can be encouraged to bear down or an emergency forceps delivery can be performed.
4. If not possible to deliver the patient safety vaginally then the patient is placed in the knee–chest position to allow gravity to keep the presenting part from compressing the cord at the pelvic brim (Fig. 8.6).
5. The operator's hand is inserted into the vagina with the fingers apart so that the cord is kept in the vagina and the presenting part can be pushed up from the pelvic brim.
6. An alternative to this is to insert a number 16 Foley catheter into the patient's bladder which in turn is inflated with 500–700 ml of normal saline. This will distend the bladder and elevate the presenting part off the cord, thereby reducing the need for the operator to elevate the presenting

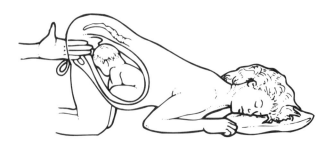

Figure 8.6 Prolapsed cord. Demonstrating the maternal position and a hand in the vagina in an attempt to replace the cord into the vagina and to keep the presenting part away from the pelvic brim.

part. This makes the anaesthetic management of the patient less complicated as she can then be anaesthetized on her back without great jeopardy to the fetus. Inserting a catheter and filling the bladder takes time and this technique is best suited if the patient needs to be transported to hospital or if there is a delay in being able to perform a Caesarean section.

7. Arrange an emergency Caesarean section. When the patient is anaesthetized and the obstetrician is ready to carry out this procedure then the bladder can be deflated and/or the operator can remove his hand from the patient's vagina.

8.10 SHOULDER DYSTOCIA

This can be defined as the arrest of the delivery of the body after the successful delivery of the head. This is one of the most urgent problems that the attendant at delivery will need to be able to manage. Most commonly the anterior shoulder is lodged behind the symphysis pubis at or above the inlet of the pelvis with the shoulders in the antero-posterior diameter. Occasionally, the shoulders may be in the transverse after failure of restitution of the head.

Predisposing factors

1. Large fetus. If >4.5 kg risk is 15–30%; if <4.5 kg risk is 3–5%.
2. Maternal obesity.
3. Insulin-dependent diabetes.
4. Post-maturity.
5. Previous shoulder dystocia.
6. Delay in the second stage.
7. Abnormal fetus: i.e. sacral tumour.

Fetal risk

1. Death or severe neurological damage from asphyxia as a result of cord compression.
2. Brachial plexus injuries.
3. Fractures to the humerus or clavicle.

Management

1. Place in lithotomy position.
2. Large episiotomy.
3. Posterior lateral traction plus suprapubic pressure.
4. Check that posterior fetal arm and hand not in sacral bay holding up delivery.
5. McRobert's manoeuvre – the maternal thighs are flexed against the maternal abdomen to alter the angle of inclination between the sacrum and spine making it easier to deliver the shoulders.
6. Check the fetal heart – if no bradycardia, reduced urgency for delivery.
7. Try and deliver the posterior arm.
8. Disimpact shoulders and try and rotate shoulders into the transverse with an assistant helping to rotate the shoulders per abdomen – bigger pelvic diameter.
9. Deliver posterior arm by placing a hand up the posterior vaginal wall and grasp the posterior arm and pull it across the chest and downwards. This will allow the posterior shoulder to deliver. It may result in a greenstick fracture of the humerus and once present allows the arm to bend at the fracture site. Such a fracture is usually minor and heals after 10 days of splinting and is preferable to a brachial plexus injury or asphyxia.
10. When shoulder dystocia follows a forceps delivery for delay in the second stage and all of the above fails then the Zavanelli manoeuvre may be tried. The head is flexed and pushed back into the vagina and an emergency Caesarean section is performed.

Prevention

1. Anticipate patients at risk with large babies. Do not allow them to go post-term.
2. Experienced attendant present at delivery.
3. Do elective Caesarean section if baby thought to be >4.5 kg.

8.11 TWIN PREGNANCY AND UNSUSPECTED SECOND TWIN

Occasionally, a woman will deliver an apparently normal small infant but before giving ergometrine, the attendant may notice that the uterus is still sufficiently enlarged to contain a second fetus. The first twin will be managed as for all normal pregnancies but special care must be taken for the second twin. Under ideal circumstances unless the patient has an epidural anaesthetic *in situ*, twin deliveries should take place in an operating theatre. However, this may not be possible when the second twin is undiagnosed.

1. Make sure that ergometrine is not given.
2. Palpate the lie of the fetus. If it is transverse or oblique, an external cephalic version is attempted.
3. Insert an intravenous line, with a side drip containing Syntocinon, if this is not already running.
4. Arrange for an anaesthetist and a paediatrician to be available. Ideally a mother delivering a twin pregnancy should have an epidural anaesthetic in labour.
5. If the lie is longitudinal, wait 5–10 minutes for uterine contractions to return so that the intrauterine pressure will push the presenting part into the pelvis.
6. The fetal heart rate should be continuously monitored. A clamp should be put on the umbilical cord of the first twin and blood should not be allowed to run out from the cord.
7. If there are no contractions start an oxytocic drip.
8. When the contractions are sufficiently strong to push the presenting part into the pelvis, the membranes are ruptured and a normal spontaneous delivery will follow.
9. If the fetus persists in an oblique or transverse lie after the return of uterine contractions, then should it prove impossible to do an external cephalic version, a Caesarean section should be performed.
10. Following delivery of the second twin and the placenta, ergometrine or Syntocinon should be given by intravenous injection.

8.12 INDICATIONS FOR CAESAREAN SECTION

In the absence of complications, it is safer to allow a normal vaginal delivery than to perform a Caesarean section. However, in those circumstances where difficulty may occur in labour, the risks attached to a Caesarean section may be less than those of a complicated instrumental delivery. The indications for Caesarean section are variable and may include:

1. Absolute disproportion.
2. Relative disproportion.
3. Fetal distress, where the continuation of a vaginal delivery increases the risk of fetal mortality or morbidity.
4. Maternal disease (such as pre-eclampsia) that increases the risk to the fetus and mother.
5. Prolonged labour.
6. Previous Caesarean section.
7. Breech presentation.
8. Unstable fetal lie at the onset of labour.
9. Placenta praevia.
10. Prolapsed cord.
11. Obstructed labour.

8.13 VAGINAL BIRTH AFTER CAESAREAN SECTION (VBAC)

It used to be believed that once a woman had a Caesarean section for cephalo-pelvic disproportion then she should have repeat elective Caesarean section with her next pregnancy. Many studies have shown that when a previous Caesarean section wound has healed without evidence of infection, i.e. where the integrity of the scar is not in doubt, all women can safely be allowed a trial of scar in a subsequent pregnancy. The risk of uterine rupture is less than 0.1%. The chances of a successful vaginal birth are in the order of 60–70%. There are studies demonstrating that a greater than 50% VBAC rate can be achieved, even after two Caesarean sections.

There are, however, provisos that must be met before attempting a VBAC, the most important of which is that it should occur in a well-equipped hospital with appropriately experienced staff and not in a Birth Centre setting. The labour should proceed steadily without any delay. An intravenous cannula should be inserted to allow venous access should it be required. Blood should be taken for group and hold/crossmatch. The fetal heart rate should be monitored continuously as one of the earliest signs of uterine rupture is the development of an abnormal fetal heart rate pattern. Scar tenderness is a very unreliable indicator of impending uterine rupture. An epidural can be used if required. Antenatal X-ray pelvimetry does not help in determining who will have a successful vaginal delivery.

If there is any delay in the second stage, the delivery should be assisted with forceps to reduce the pressure on the intrauterine scar and reduce the risk of uterine rupture.

After the delivery of the placenta, if possible, a gentle attempt should be made to palpate the lower uterine segment to ensure that it is intact.

8.14 APPLICATION OF OBSTETRIC FORCEPS

Forceps fall into two major groups:

1. **Traction**
   Neville–Barnes, Simpson and Wrigley forceps, which are used to deliver the fetus when sagittal suture is in the occipito-anterior position and the fetus presents in either an occipito-anterior or as a direct occipito-posterior position.
2. **Rotational forceps**
   Kielland's forceps, which are used to rotate the occiput either from an occipito-transverse or an occipito-posterior position.

Indications for forceps

1. When the delivery process needs to be expedited for maternal reasons (hypertension, maternal distress, previous Caesarean section, cardiac disease, delay in the second stage, epidural anaesthesia, maternal exhaustion).
2. When the delivery needs to be expedited for fetal reasons (fetal distress, prolonged delivery, prolonged labour or failure to progress to the second stage).
3. When the fetus has an abnormal position (occipito-posterior/occipito-transverse) which is delaying the progress of labour. (This is the major use for Kielland's forceps.)

Conditions that must exist before application of forceps

1. The cervix must be fully dilated.
2. The fetal head must present (except for forceps to the after-coming head of breech).
3. The internal suture should be in the occipito-anterior position (except when applying Kielland's forceps).
4. The fetal head must be engaged in the pelvis.
5. The bladder and rectum must be empty.
6. The membranes must be ruptured.
7. The operator should be sufficiently experienced.

Before applying forceps, it must be ascertained that there is a reasonable chance of a normal vaginal delivery. Should there be any doubt in the mind of the operator as to the likelihood of success of the forceps delivery, then the patient should be taken to the operating theatre, preparations made for a Caesarean section and a trial of forceps may be undertaken in the theatre with all facilities available for an immediate Caesarean section should any complications arise.

8.15 POSTPARTUM HAEMORRHAGE

Postpartum haemorrhage is the loss of more than 500 ml of blood following the delivery of the infant. If this occurs within the first 24 hours, it is called primary postpartum haemorrhage. The causes of primary postpartum haemorrhage are:

1. Atonic uterus, which may follow:
    (a) Retained placental tissue.
    (b) Full bladder.
    (c) Prolonged labour.
    (d) Forceps or other traumatic delivery.
    (e) Grand multiparity.
    (f) Twins and polyhydramnios (causing over distension of the uterus).
    (g) Antepartum haemorrhage.
    (h) Anaesthesia.
    (i) Relaxant drugs.
2. Trauma. Bleeding may occur from:
    (a) Episiotomy.

    (b) Perineal, vaginal or cervical tears.
    (c) Ruptured uterus.
3. Coagulation failure may follow:
    (a) Accidental haemorrhage.
    (b) Amniotic fluid embolus.
    (c) Intrauterine death.

Management of primary postpartum haemorrhage

1. Give ergometrine (0.25 mg) by intramuscular or intravenous injection, except in cases of hypertension.
2. Set up an intravenous line and add 40 units Syntocinon or Pitocin to 1 litre Hartman's or Ringer's lactate solution.
3. Arrange for blood to be cross-matched.
4. Examine the patient for signs of uterine atony (bulky, soft uterus). If present, massage the fundus of the uterus (rubbing up the uterus) as this will decrease the bleeding by physically stimulating the uterus to contract.
5. Inspect the perineum and vagina for tears and lacerations that may be bleeding.
6. Determine whether the placenta has been removed, and if it has then inspect it for completeness – looking particularly for missing cotyledons, succenturiate lobes and possible fragmented membranes.
7. Ensure that the bladder is empty. A full bladder may inhibit uterine contractions.
8. If it is suspected that some or all of the placenta is retained *in utero*, arrange for an anaesthetic. Once the patient has been fully resuscitated a manual exploration and removal of the placenta is done. If no placental tissue is retained, the bladder is empty and the uterus is well contracted but the bleeding persists then a local cause for the bleeding should be determined.
9. If no apparent cause is found, then blood clotting should be checked.
10. If the uterus does not contract adequately, uterine rupture or retained products of conception should be suspected.
11. Finally, make sure that the vaginal and perineal lacerations are re-sutured. Care should be taken to reach the apex of any vaginal laceration when suturing, as it is a common site for continuing postpartum haemorrhage.

Secondary postpartum haemorrhage

This is dealt with in Chapter 10.

8.16 INTRAPARTUM HAEMORRHAGE

Intrapartum haemorrhage may be due to:

1. Placenta praevia.
2. A heavy 'show' caused by the chorionic membrane shearing off from the decidua.
3. Tears and lacerations to the uterus, cervix and vagina.
4. Vasa praevia. This occurs in 1 in 5000 pregnancies. In all placenta praevias, the trophoblast contains poor attachment to the lower segment decidua – the placenta is therefore often membranous in type, with fetal vessels coursing over the chorionic membrane. Because these vessels may run across the cervical os, they may tear open when the membranes rupture, producing antepartum haemorrhage of fetal origin.

Management

Should bleeding occur during labour, a sample of the blood should be tested to ensure that it is maternal and not fetal blood. Blood taken is tested by means of the Kleihauer test or its resistance to denaturing in the presence of an alkali solution (Apt test).

8.17 SHOCK IN LABOUR

Any woman who has spent some hours in labour may become shocked, collapse or die. It is important to recognize that certain conditions and problems predispose to these catastrophes. However, a woman in prolonged labour who is poorly managed, becomes dehydrated, ketoacidotic and infected will also be a prime target for some hypotensive condition to occur. The causes of shock may be:

1. Blood loss.
2. Rupture of the uterus.
3. Endotoxic shock from Gram-negative organisms.

4. Amniotic fluid embolus.
5. Intracranial haemorrhage (severe hypertension, rupture of a Berry aneurism during straining in the second stage).
6. Uterine inversion.
7. Cardiac failure (valvular heart disease and severe anaemia).
8. Pulmonary embolism.
9. Myocardial infarction.
10. Adrenal crises.
11. Hypoglycaemia.

Management

This is related to avoiding the cause and making certain that the mother enters labour in a physically fit condition. By preventing the complications of labour, most of the causes can be prevented.

8.18 PRE-TERM LABOUR (see Chapter 5, section 5.8)

Any labour that occurs before 37 weeks is regarded as pre-term. Approximately 7–10% of women will begin their labour between the 20th and 37th week of pregnancy and the perinatal loss in these labours is proportionate to the degree of prematurity. The survival rate for pre-term infants at 28 weeks (1000 g) is 80%, 90% for infants born between 29 and 32 weeks (1200–1500 g), 95% for infants born between 32 and 34 weeks (1500–2000 g) and 99.5% over 34 weeks (2 kg).

Women may go into pre-term labour for many reasons:

1. Cervical incompetence.
2. Premature rupture of the membranes.
3. Amnionitis (beta-haemolytic streptococcus).
4. Uterine overdistension – multiple pregnancy, poly-hydramnios.
5. Placental abruption.
6. Any severe infection.
7. Pyelonephritis.
8. Congenital uterine abnormalities.

General management of patients

If the fetus is more than 34 weeks, the labour is allowed to continue. Should the patient be less pregnant than this, an attempt should be made to stop the labour to allow the fetus to gain a few vital weeks of maturity. Patients are:

1. Admitted to hospital for bed rest.
2. They may be given a mild sedative such as diazepam.
3. If experiencing painful contractions, they can be given Omnopon 15 mg by intramuscular injection.
4. Set up an intravenous drip.
5. A vaginal swab should be taken to exclude infection (beta-haemolytic streptococcus) as a cause of the preterm labour.
6. A gentle vaginal examination should be done to assess cervical dilatation, but care must be taken not to stimulate further release of prostaglandin from the cervix. A digital examination is never done in the presence of ruptured membranes unless delivery is planned.
7. If the membranes are ruptured a cervical swab should be taken after passing a sterile bivalve speculum under aseptic conditions.
8. After hydration, magnesium sulphate may be administered: 4–6 g as a bolus over several minutes followed by an infusion of 2 g/hour. A tocolytic such as salbutamol (Ventolin) or ritodrine may also be given. This has a specific stimulant effect on the beta-adrenergic receptors and thus relaxes smooth muscle.
9. Alert the paediatric staff that a pre-term infant may require special nursery care.
10. If the fetus has a gestational age of less than 34 weeks it may be advisable to give steroids intramuscularly to the mother to try and accelerate fetal lung maturity and thus prevent hyaline membrane disease.
11. Should the patient still persist with uterine contractions, consideration can be given to the judicious use of anti-prostaglandin agents such as Indocid. This can be given as a suppository but care should be taken as there is a danger that prolonged use may lead to closure of the ductus arteriosus *in uterus* and thus pulmonary hypertension.
12. More recently, nitroglycerine transdermal patches have also been used to arrest pre-term labour.

There is also some evidence that beta-adrenergic agents themselves play some role in developing fetal lung maturity. Oral beta-adrenergic agents suffer from the problem of tachyphylaxis and this leads to down-regulation of the receptors and the drug, which becomes less effective.

Some recent studies have suggested that prophylactic antibiotics given in the absence of obvious infection may prolong the pregnancy. This area is still controversial and it is unresolved whether antibiotics should be given routinely. In the presence of ruptured membranes regular checks should be made to exclude infection and to monitor fetal well-being.

9

Analgesia and anaesthesia in obstetrics

9.1 GENERAL INSTRUCTIONAL OBJECTIVES

In order to enable them to choose the optimal technique for the management of pain in labour, students should have a comprehensive understanding of the options of analgesia available to mothers in labour. While students will not be expected to describe or administer major regional blocks, they must be able to understand the indications for, success rate, degree of acceptance, and complications of these techniques. Students should have a simple blueprint for the administration of general anaesthesia at term. They should understand the importance of supine hypotensive (vena cava compression) syndrome, aspiration pneumonitis and preoxygenation in relation to general anaesthesia for obstetrics. They should know the major differences in the management of a cardiac arrest in a pregnant woman as compared with the non-pregnant adult patient.

9.2 SPECIFIC BEHAVIOURAL OBJECTIVES

1. Describe the pain of labouring women and understand the physical and psychological factors that may influence the perception of this pain.
2. Describe the sensory nerve supply to the uterus and birth canal and the anatomy of the lumbar and caudal epidural spaces and the pudendal nerve.
3. Know the basic pharmacology and maximum allowable dosages of lignocaine and bupivacaine.

4. Know the dangers and limitations of pudendal, lumbar epidural and caudal regional blocks.
5. Appreciate the clinical pharmacology, dosage regimens, limitations and hazards to mother and fetus of parenteral and oral narcotic, sedative and analgesic medications as well as analgesic gases and inhalational agents used in labour and delivery.
6. Describe the hazards of and indications for general anaesthesia for obstetric patients.
7. Understand the important differences between pregnant and non-pregnant women when dealing with a cardiac arrest.

9.3 THE PAIN OF PARTURITION

Preamble

The only constant feature of the parturition pain suffered by women is its extreme variability. Though truly painless labour is a rarity, in any group of 100 labouring women, about 10 of them will have a rapid normal delivery with relatively little discomfort. Most of this group will have had previous confinements. Another 20 or 30 will be less fortunate. They will have a much longer labour and will suffer severe pain for many hours. Unless they are helped effectively, they will always remember their labour as a dreadful ordeal. The remaining 60 or 70 patients will experience something between these two extremes. Their contractions will be most uncomfortable and painful at certain stages and they will have a lot of pain during the actual delivery. In general, labour pain is one of the most severe a woman will ever experience and compares in intensity with severe cancer pain or the pain of renal colic. However, with competent medical and nursing care, their degree of discomfort can be reduced to a tolerable level.

As in any other field of pain relief, an assessment of the severity of pain being experienced by a patient depends on observation of the patient's reaction and on her own description of the pain. Any complaint of pain must be given sympathetic consideration and related to both the clinical situation and the patient's personality.

The pattern of labour pain

In an average normal labour, contractions usually become painful when the cervix is dilated 3–4 cm, and the intensity of the pain increases as cervical dilatation proceeds. The last quarter of the first stage may be accompanied by severe pain.

When full dilatation of the cervix is reached, the pain will change in character. As the presenting part descends onto the pelvic floor, the distention and stretching of the perineal tissue causes sensations of pressure and pain and an intense urge to bear down with the contractions. The patient feels the pain of intense contractions not in the uterus but as a colicky pain across the lower abdomen. It is also frequently referred to the back and sometimes radiates down the thighs. It starts soon after each contraction begins, rises to a peak as the intrauterine pressure increases and dies away completely between contractions.

Factors that influence severity of pain of childbirth:

1. Physical factors
    (a) The intensity and duration of uterine contractions.
    (b) The resistance of the cervix to dilatation.
    (c) The resistance to distention of perineal tissues.
    (d) The presence of any degree of cephalopelvic disproportion.
    (e) Other obstetric conditions prolonging labour, especially occipito-posterior position of the fetal head, which can produce a most distressing backache.
    (f) Fatigue, anaemia, general debility and malnutrition influence the patient's tolerance to the painful experience.
2. Psychological factors
    (a) Cultural patterns and customs. A noisy patient is not necessarily having more pain than a silent one.
    (b) Antenatal education and emotional preparedness for labour. Fear, apprehension, ignorance and loneliness lower the tolerance to discomfort.
    (c) The attitude of the patient's attendants, both medical and nursing. Cheerful, sympathetic and competent management will do a great deal to make pain more tolerable.

Nerve pathways

Pain from the isometric contractions of the first stage of labour originate mostly in mechanoreceptors in the uterus and cervix and is carried along fine unmyelinated C and myelinated A fibres which gather together at the base of the broad ligaments. Nociceptive afferents pass via various plexuses to reach the lumbar and lower thoracic sympathetic chains, and then via white rami communicantes to the dorsal nerve roots of the T10 to T12 and L1 nerves. They converge on wide dynamic range neurons in the dorsal horn grey matter producing referred deep-seated 'visceral' pain.

In the late first stage, as the fetal presenting part starts to descend, pressure on the lumbosacral plexus may produce pain referred to the dermatomes of L2 to L5 and S1. As the second stage is approached, the deep, intense, diffuse 'visceral' pain of uterine contraction is replaced by a sharper, more localized 'somatic' pain.

This pain of second stage labour and delivery results from high threshold mechanoreceptors (via A fibre afferents) and nociceptors (via polymodal C afferents) responding to pressure, distention, stretching and tearing of the lower birth canal and perineum. Sensory nerve supply is provided by the pudendal nerve, which is a somatic nerve made up from the 2nd, 3rd and 4th sacral roots. This somatic pain reaches its zenith during crowning of the baby's head.

9.4 PAIN RELIEF IN LABOUR

As far as the patient is concerned, the desire for a healthy infant and adequate relief of pain are the most important aspects of her labour. The aim of any pain relief programme should be to reduce pain and distress to a degree that is tolerable and to ensure that the patient's recollection of her labour is pleasant. At the same time, there should be no added risk to mother or child. Indeed, most mothers are happy to accept some discomfort to ensure the safety to their baby. For example, if an additional opiate will reduce the motor weakness and potential local anaesthetic toxicity of a standard epidural bloc, many women will be content to put up with minor abdominal and rectal pain.

Pain relief is not easily accomplished in all patients. It depends on a combination of many factors which include:

1. Ethnic and cultural differences.
2. Education (antenatal classes).
3. The mother's personality.
4. Compassionate, sympathetic and competent nursing and partner support.
5. The severity and duration of pain and its associated hormonal stress response.
6. Degree of fatigue, dehydration and nausea imposed by a protracted labour.
7. Type and quality of analgesia provided by the intelligent use of drugs and other techniques.

Local anaesthesia

Local anaesthesia occurs when a drug produces a reversible blockade of conduction in nerves. Conduction in all types of axons is blocked, but fibres of small diameter are usually (though not always) more susceptible to local anaesthetics and are slower to recover than fibres of larger diameter.

Action: local anaesthetics inhibit the transient increase in permeability of excitable membranes to sodium ions, thereby producing a temporary inability of the nerve fibre to transmit the nerve impulse.

Metabolism: the amide local anaesthetics (lignocaine, bupivacaine, mepivacaine, ropivacaine) are metabolized by hepatic cyclooxygenase microsomal enzymes while the esters (chloroprocaine, procaine), which are used far less commonly, are hydrolysed by pseudocholinesterase. The by-products then undergo biotransformation in the liver.

The local anaesthetics can be used in a large variety of locations:

First-stage pain. This can be managed with a lumbar or low thoracic epidural (with or without continuous epidural infusion) or a continuous intrathecal (spinal) blockade.

Second-stage pain. This can be controlled with a lumbosacral epidural, a caudal, a subarachnoid 'spinal', a pudendal nerve block or local infiltration of the perineum. Opioids (fentanyl, pethidine, morphine, buprenorphine) can be added to (or even replace) the local anaesthetic solution in many of these routes of administration (epidural, spinal, caudal). The block can be tailored to the individual's needs and expectations, the stage of labour, the degree of pain and the need for operative delivery. Recent innovations include mobile or ambulatory epidurals, combined spinal–epidural, continuous intrathecal opiates and patient-administered top-ups.

1. Lignocaine (Xylocaine, lidocaine)
    *   Dose: the maximum safe dose of lignocaine is 3 mg/kg (about 200 mg) but this may be raised to 7 mg/kg (450 mg) if the lignocaine is combined with 1/200 000 to 1/400 000 adrenaline. For example, if 2.0% (2.0 g in 100 ml) lignocaine with 1/200 000 adrenaline is used, the maximum safe dose for an adult is 27 ml. Lignocaine is available in concentrations of 0.5, 1 and 2% with or without adrenaline.
    *   Onset of action: 5–15 minutes.
    *   Duration of action: its duration of action is about 45–60 minutes following local infiltration and regional block and up to 90 minutes following epidural block.
    *   Advantage: potent local anaesthetic.
2. Bupivacaine (Marcain)
    *   Dose: the maximum safe dose of bupivacaine is 2–3 mg/ kg (120 mg). It is available in concentrations of 0.25, 0.375 and 0.5% with or without adrenaline and as 0.125% with either 5 µg/ml fentanyl or 2.5 mg/ml pethidine.
    *   Onset of action: 15–30 minutes.
    *   Duration of action: bupivacaine has a prolonged (but variable) duration of action of more than 90 minutes.
3. Ropivacaine
    This agent is very similar to bupivacaine but is less cardio- and neurotoxic than bupivacaine and is reported to have improved sensory–motor split, i.e. it produces less numbness for the same degree of analgesia.

Complications of regional blockade (including spinal subarachnoid and lumbar epidural blockade)

1. Local nerve injury as a result of:
    (a) Adrenaline ischaemia.

(b) Intraneural injection of local anaesthetic.
(c) Direct needle trauma.
2. Toxic reaction: caused by the effects of a high plasma level on the central nervous system (CNS) and cardiovascular system. Characteristics of a mild reaction include pallor, anxiety, nausea and restlessness, which may be difficult to distinguish from simple nervousness. In its more severe forms, CNS stimulation leads to convulsions, followed by drowsiness, unconsciousness, medullary depression, apnoea and vasomotor collapse. Often the first observed indication of any overdosage is a sudden convulsion. Hypotension and cardiac arrest may either be due to direct myocardial depression or to effects on the medullary vasomotor control network. Allergy or sensitivity to local anaesthetics is very rare; reactions are nearly always caused by overdosage.

Prevention of systemic reaction

1. Use of minimum effective concentration and do not exceed the maximum safe dosage. Check the dose and concentration before injecting.
2. Vasoconstrictors (e.g. adrenaline 1/200 000) prolong the action and result in lower plasma levels. Vasoconstrictors may, however, reduce placental blood flow.
3. Avoid intravascular injection by:
    (a) Aspirating the syringe before injecting.
    (b) Using a small, adrenaline-containing test dose.
    (c) Dividing the total bolus into several smaller incremental doses.

Epidural anaesthesia

Epidural blockade is achieved by the introduction of local anaesthetic solution into the epidural space (outside the dura). The epidural (peridural) space is a potential space and lies between the ligamentum flavum and the dura mater. A needle is inserted into this space in the lumbar or sacral (caudal) region. There is diminished or absent perception of pain from the waist down with variable degree of motor paralysis. Uterine contractions continue, but the patient is not aware of them. Attempts have been made to use this form of anaesthesia in surgery and obstetrics since the beginning of this century, but its major development has taken place since 1950.

Indications

1. Maternal distress caused by painful uterine contractions not adequately relieved by simpler forms of analgesia (pethidine, nitrous oxide).
2. Failure of a labour to progress in spite of what appear to be adequate uterine contractions.
3. To provide anaesthesia for a forceps delivery or vacuum (ventouse) extraction.
4. Pregnancy-induced and associated hypertension. Epidural anaesthesia is useful in reducing the amount of sedation required and also is helpful in lowering the blood pressure.
5. Caesarean section. The majority of Caesarean sections are performed under epidural anaesthesia.

Technique

Before an epidural anaesthetic is administered, patients should be preloaded with 1000–1200 ml Hartman's solution to minimize the potential fall in blood pressure that may arise from the vasodilatation produced by the epidural sympathetic blockade.

The patient is positioned in a left lateral position and the trunk is flexed as much as possible to open up the intervertebral spaces. After infiltrating the skin with local anaesthetic, a 16–18G (Tuohy) needle is introduced at right angles to the back in the midline at the L 2–3 or L 3–4 intervertebral spaces. It is advanced through the ligaments until the epidural space is identified by a sudden loss of resistance to injection through the needle. The anaesthetic solution is injected through the Tuohy needle, and an epidural catheter (a fine plastic tube) can be inserted through the needle and left *in situ* for subsequent injections. The needle is withdrawn.

Disadvantages

1. Instrumental delivery rate may be increased.
2. Maternal hypotension.
3. Accidental dural puncture.
4. Epidural haematoma secondary to bloody tap.
5. Post-dural puncture headache.

Contraindications to regional anaesthesia

1. When time does not permit this, i.e. when there is a true emergency (cord prolapse, persistent fetal bradycardia despite cessation of Syntocinon, change of posture and augmentation of inspired oxygen fraction by administration of oxygen by mask).
2. When the patient refuses major regional blockade or it is desirable, for humane reasons, that the patient be rendered unconscious, e.g. delivery of a deformed fetus).
3. Coagulopathy, e.g. thrombocytopenia secondary to pregnancy-induced hypertension, von Willebrand's disease.
4. Local abnormalities of the lumbar area, e.g. herpetic lesions in the lumbar region; extensive previous thoracolumbar laminectomy.
5. Cardiovascular instability, e.g. antepartum haemorrhage causing hypovolaemia; cardiac lesions where decreases in afterload are to be avoided.

Local infiltration of perineum

Advantages

1. Maternal and fetal mortality and morbidity resulting directly from use of this technique is negligible.
2. Simplicity of administration.
3. Uterine contractions are not impaired.
4. No interference with the desire to bear down during labour.
5. Toxic effects are minimal provided safe dosages are not exceeded and the agent is not injected intravascularly.

Disadvantage
Does not help first stage pain.

Technique
The patient is placed in the lithotomy position. The fourchette and the adjoining area are first infiltrated using a 5-cm, 23-gauge needle. The infiltration is then extended in a fan-shaped manner. Alternatively, if analgesia is required simply to perform an episiotomy, only the area to be incised need be

infiltrated – with 0.5% lignocaine without adrenaline, the maximum amount being 40 ml (200 mg).

Pudendal block

The pudendal nerve is formed by branches of the 2nd, 3rd and 4th sacral nerves in the sacral plexus. It lies behind the ischial spine on each side medial to the pudendal artery, where it begins to divide into several branches. As it curves forward to the medial aspect of the ischial tuberosity, it gives off the inferior haemorrhoidal nerves, perineal nerves, the dorsal nerve of the clitoris, and the nerve to the labia majora.

Technique

1. Transperineal
   First, a small skin wheal is raised by injecting local anaesthetic into subcutaneous tissue on each side, midway between the anus and the ischial tuberosity. The index finger of the left hand is inserted into the vagina and the left ischial spine is palpated. A 10-cm, 20-gauge needle is guided to a point just below and beyond the spine. After drawing back (to exclude the possibility of intravascular location), 10 ml of 1% lignocaine are injected to anaesthetize the pudendal nerve. Repeat on the right side. Wait 10 minutes.
2. Transvaginal
   A transvaginal guarded needle is guided to the ischial spine. It is held with the point just posterior and medial to the tip of the spine. The needle is then advanced until it touches the sacrospinous ligament, which is infiltrated with 2 or 3 ml of 1% lignocaine. It is then advanced through the ligament, and about 10 ml of 1% lignocaine are injected. Repeat on the other side. Wait 10 minutes.

Advantages

1. Relatively simple and painless procedure.
2. Anaesthetizes large area of vagina and perineum.

Disadvantages

1. Considerable failure rate; constant practice is necessary.

2. Inadequate for anything except the simplest outlet forceps delivery.

Injectable pharmacological agents

Parenterally injected agents raise the patient's pain threshold (i.e. the level of awareness at which any sensation becomes painful), produce amnesia or sedation or reduce apprehension or anxiety.

Narcotic analgesics

Examples are pethidine (meperidine; Demerol), morphine, papaveretum (Omnopon), fentanyl (Sublimaze), buprenorphine (Temgesic).

All these agents produce good pain relief for a variable period of time usually lasting 1–2 hours but, because of neonatal and maternal side effects they produce cannot be used in full dosage. At these doses, not all patients find narcotics effective and some derive little benefit. Opiates also frequently cause sedation or nausea and, occasionally, an acute confusional state.

Opioids all have the potential for causing respiratory depression in the newborn and, less frequently, in the mother. Narcotic antagonists, e.g. naloxone (Narcan®), can be used to prevent or reverse respiratory depression of the infant. To achieve this they must be given either intravenously to the mother at least 20 minutes before delivery, or to the infant (either via the umbilical vein or intramuscularly). The maximal risk of neonatal depression is 2–4 hours after intramuscular and 1–2 hours after intravenous opiates.

Anxiolytics, sedatives and tranquillizers

Benzodiazepines: e.g. diazepam (Valium), midazolam (Hypnovel).
Because benzodiazepines cause neonatal hypotonia and impaired thermoregulation, these agents, which are good anxiolytics, anticonvulsants and amnestics, are rarely used to reduce anxiety during labour.

Phenothiazines: e.g. promethazine (Phenergan), promazine (Sparine).
These agents can alleviate maternal anxiety and reduce nausea and vomiting but can cause somnolence and disorientation in some mothers. They have no analgesic properties.

Barbiturates: e.g. amylobarbitone (Amytal), thiopentone (Pentothal).
Because of their anti-analgesic properties, they are rarely used as sedatives.

Hypnotic amnestics: e.g. ketamine (Ketalar), hyoscine (scopolamine).
Both agents are potent amnestics but ketamine produces dissociative hallucinations and dysphoria while scopolamine can cause delirium. As a result, both agents are now rarely used to manage uncomplicated labour and delivery.

Inhalational analgesics

The analgesic gas or volatile agent is administered via a mask held by the patient and alleviates the peaks of pain. Inhalation analgesia may be used throughout the first and second stages, especially at the time of delivery. It takes 15–30 seconds for these agents to build up in the brain, so inhalation should be started at the onset of a contraction, rather than when the pain becomes severe. Special filters are placed in the delivery system to prevent the possible transmission of infectious diseases such as hepatitis C or HIV. The filter is replaced and tubing changed and resterilized after use. Popular agents include anaesthetic gases and volatile anaesthetic agents.

Anaesthetic gases

An example is nitrous oxide:

- Delivery: N_2O 'piped' gas is delivered from the Midogas apparatus activated by the patient inhaling from a mouthpiece or closely fitting mask. The patient should be asked to hold the mouthpiece or mask herself, so that if she becomes unconscious it will fall away from her face.
- Action: central nervous system action, producing first

analgesia and later anaesthesia (if a high concentration is inhaled continuously).

- Dose: the Midogas apparatus allows a maximum concentration of 70% nitrous oxide (N_2O) with 30% oxygen (O_2). At this concentration, provided that maternal respiration and circulation are adequate, maternal or fetal hypoxia should not occur. Because onset of effect may not occur for up to 30 seconds, inhalation must start as soon as the onset of a contraction is felt.
- Onset of action: may take up to 30 seconds, especially if concentration less than 70%.
- Duration of action: 60 seconds after cessation of inhalation.
- Advantages: quick action; safe with adequate oxygen; no interference with uterine action; no fetal depression; does not build up in the body – can be used intermittently for several hours; suitable for patients with cardiac or pulmonary pathology.
- Disadvantage: mixture requires adjustment according to individual tolerance; expensive, complicated equipment which must be checked often.

Volatile anaesthetic agents

Examples are isoflurane (Forthane), Methoxyflurane (Penthrane).

These agents are potent anaesthetics with prompt onset of action but they have a pungent odour and must be delivered through sophisticated, accurately calibrated vaporizers.

- Action: used in a vaporizer. Central nervous system effect, producing analgesia. If the concentration is high enough or is inhaled for a prolonged period, anaesthesia may result.
- Advantage: potent analgesic.

'Natural' techniques

One or a combination of regimens are taught during antenatal preparation ('prepared childbirth') and are followed by a large number of women who earnestly desire to have their baby by their own unaided efforts and without the need for drugs. These include:

1. Changing postures in labour, e.g. walking, leaning over a bean bag, rocking, etc.
2. Psychological exercises and conditioned reflexes.
3. Promotion of the belief that childbirth can be a pleasurable experience.
4. Breathing control and mental exercises that focus on the breathing pattern.
5. Hot packs.
6. Soothing music.
7. Warm showers.
8. Massage.
9. A supportive partner who acts as an enthusiastic 'coach'.
10. Exercise to strengthen back and abdominal muscles and relax pelvic joints.

This psychological preparation for labour often results in a valuable reduction in the reaction to pain experienced by a considerable proportion of the women practising them. However, a good 90% will not be able to carry on in labour without assistance and will require some additional pain relief. It is most important that these parturients should not feel frustrated that they have failed.

While painless labour should never be promised to any mother who undertakes to study and practice a method of psychological preparation for labour, pain can be lessened by a confidence approach and a realistic expectation of the birth process. Midwives, obstetricians and medical students should have a general knowledge of the various methods that may be used by these women, and, even if not themselves enthusiasts, should do nothing to destroy the patient's faith in her chosen regimen.

Hypnosis
Hypnosis is a state of altered consciousness in which the profound concentration causes reduced awareness of the pain of labour. Unfortunately, the technique is not successful for all mothers, requires considerable time-consuming antepartum coaching and the results have not been impressive.

Acupuncture
Acupuncture has not achieved widespread use because the pain relief is usually partial. The process whereby subcutaneous

insertion and vibration of needles along 'energy pathways' (meridians) in order to restore energy levels from a particular organ towards normal and the way in which this relieves pain is poorly understood.

Transcutaneous Electrical Nerve Stimulation (TENS)

Electrodes are applied to the skin and deliver a low-voltage current to the skin. While TENS has its supporters, there are many who feel that, for relief of labour pain, it is of limited value with, at best, a 44% patient acceptance and satisfaction rate. The electrodes over the dermatomes of T10–L1 (first-stage stimulation) and over the sacrum (late first and second stage) transmit a 40–150 Hz stimulus of 1–40 mA. TENS seems to be most useful when it is started in early labour and then mostly to relieve pain in the early first stage.

9.5 GENERAL ANAESTHESIA FOR OBSTETRICS

Indications

1. Caesarean section, when a regional technique is contra-indicated.
2. When time does not permit regional anaesthesia, i.e. when there is a true emergency (cord prolapse, persistent fetal bradycardia despite cessation of syntocinon, change of posture and augmentation of inspired oxygen fraction by administration of oxygen by mask).
3. When the patient refuses major regional blockade or it is desirable, for humane reasons, that the patient be rendered unconscious (e.g. delivery of a deformed fetus).
4. Coagulopathy, e.g. thrombocytopenia secondary to preg-nancy-induced hypertension, von Willebrand's disease.
5. Local abnormalities of the lumbar area, e.g. herpetic lesions in the lumbar region; extensive previous thoracolumbar laminectomy.
6. Cardiovascular instability. e.g. antepartum haemorrhage causing hypovolaemia; cardiac lesions where decreases in afterload are to be avoided.
7. Need for full uterine relaxation (e.g. breech extraction; retained placenta; correction of transverse lie by intrauter-ine manipulation) when this cannot be achieved with other pharmacological agents (e.g. glyceryl trinitrate).

Advantages

1. Fast.
2. Reliable and reproducible.

Disadvantages

1. Fetal depression caused by:
   (a) Direct transfer of anaesthetic induction and inhalational agents across the placental barrier.
   (b) A diminution of uteroplacental blood flow secondary to maternal hypoxaemia or hypotension.
2. Risk of intrapulmonary aspiration of gastric contents.
3. All third trimester labour ward patients have a full stomach because raised progesterone levels delay gastric emptying. Also, since the term uterus causes an increase in intra-abdominal pressure, it is best to assume that all labour ward patients are at high risk of 'aspiration'.
4. Little opportunity for immediate maternal and paternal bonding with the baby.
5. Increased haemodynamic sensitivity to intubation in mothers, especially in those with pregnancy-induced hypertension.
6. Increased blood loss which can lead to acute renal failure and (nowadays, rarely) Sheehan's postpartum pituitary necrosis.

Prophylaxis – aspiration of gastric contents

1. No solid foods or hypertonic fluids should be administered during labour.
2. Sodium citrate, 30 ml of a 0.3 M solution should be administered less than 30 min before induction of anaesthesia in order to decrease the acidity (increase pH) of gastric contents rendering them less damaging to the pulmonary alveolar lining.
3. H_2-receptor antagonists (e.g. ranitidine, cimetidine) and metoclopramide should also be administered preoperatively if time permits.
4. A 'rapid sequence induction sequence with cricoid pressure' preceded by preoxygenation should be employed if general anaesthesia is necessary. Cricoid pressure (Sellick's

manoeuvre) should be maintained by an assistant, from the time of induction until an endotracheal tube has been inserted and the cuff inflated. Pressure on the cricoid cartilage will compress the oesophagus and prevent passive regurgitation of gastric contents. This method is only to be used on a paralysed patient.

Management – aspiration of gastric contents
If aspiration does occur, one or both of the following problems may result:

(a) Obstruction of the airway with large particles of food. Treat with suction, posture (head-dependent), O_2 administration under pressure. Bronchoscopy may be needed.
(b) Mendelson's syndrome. After the inhalation of a small volume of highly acid gastric contents, acute inhalation pneumonitis occurs. After a latent period of about 1 hour, cyanosis, tachycardia, dyspnoea and pulmonary oedema supervene.

Aspiration should be treated immediately as follows:

1. Suction of the endotracheal tube and airway. Bronchoscopy (and, possibly, bronchial lavage) may be needed if there are solid food particles in the airway.
2. Continue the general anaesthesia with respiratory support as required using augmented inspired oxygen, intermittent positive pressure ventilation (IPPV) and positive end-expiratory pressure (PEEP).
   (a) Other useful measures may include postoperative ventilation in an Acute Care Centre, continuous airway pressure (CPAP) using a mask, intravenous steroids (i.e. 200 mg of hydrocortisone) and bronchial lavage.

9.6   CARDIAC ARREST

This is failure of the heart to maintain an adequate cerebral circulation in any situation other than that caused by progressive and irreversible disease. The incidence of cardiopulmonary arrest in late pregnancy is estimated at ~1 in 30 000 pregnancies.

Cardiopulmonary resuscitation in pregnancy must be managed differently from that in a non-pregnant woman in a number of ways:

1. Avoidance of aortocaval compression in the supine position assumes considerable importance.
2. Defibrillation paddles are best placed in the anterior–posterior (not apex–sternum) configuration in the left-lateral-tilted term patient with a large gravid uterus with pendulous breasts.
3. Arterial hypoxaemia ensues much more rapidly.
4. Securing the airway can be much more difficult.
5. Pulmonary aspiration of gastric acid is more likely.
6. Pharmacodynamics of drugs is altered in pregnancy.
7. Bretylium becomes a first-line antiarrhythmic when ventricular fibrillation/tachycardia is caused by local anaesthetic overdose.
8. The infant must be delivered expeditiously by Caesarean section if advanced life-support resuscitation is not rapidly successful.

10

The puerperium

Students should understand the normal physiology and psychology as well as the pathological changes that occur in the puerperium so that assistance can be given to the normal mother and baby, as well as recognizing deviations so that appropriate management can be initiated.

10.2 SPECIFIC BEHAVIOURAL OBJECTIVES

1. Define the puerperium and explain the anatomical and physiological changes that occur during normal involution.
2. Identify by history and examination the normal progress of a mother and baby in the puerperium.
3. Discuss the emotional changes and needs in the normal puerperium.
4. Communicate with the mother and baby to provide them with physical and emotional support.
5. Explain the anatomical and physiological changes occurring during lactation.
6. Instruct the mother and assist in the care and feeding of a normal baby in the puerperium.
7. Discuss appropriate advice on sexual relations and family planning for the normal puerperal mother.

10.3 REASONS FOR LEARNING ABOUT THE PUERPERIUM

The puerperium is the time during which the mother's altered anatomy, physiology and biochemistry returns to the normal non-pregnant state. By definition, it commences at the completion of the third stage of labour and is completed 6 weeks later.

There are some variations within each organ system and complications of labour or delivery, exogenous drugs or hormones may alter the normal process.

10.4 NORMAL ANATOMICAL AND PHYSIOLOGICAL CHANGES DURING THE PUERPERIUM

Reproductive tract

Uterine involution

During pregnancy, the uterus increases in size and weight due to the effect of oestrogen, progesterone and chronic stretching on the myometrium by the enlarging fetus. The withdrawal of the sex hormones leads to tissue breakdown (catabolism) due to the increased activity of uterine collagenase and the release of proteolytic enzymes.

There is a migration of macrophages into the endometrium and myometrium. Involution of the uterus occurs as a result of a decrease in the size of myometrial cells and not as a decrease in their number. Following delivery, the uterus weighs about 1 kg and the uterine fundus is at the level of the umbilicus the day after birth. By 10–14 days, the fundus should no longer be palpable abdominally. By 6 weeks, the weight of the uterus has dropped to 50–60 g.

The net result of pregnancy is a slightly enlarged uterus due to the permanent increase in the number of cells, elastin in the myometrium, blood vessels and connective tissue.

Following completion of the third stage, uterine activity continues. For the first 12 hours contractions are well coordinated, strong and regular, but they decrease over succeeding days as involution occurs. Contractions of 150 mmHg or more have been recorded in the early puerperium and are accentuated during breast feeding (afterpains).

Placental site involution

The placenta separates in the decidual layer. Following its delivery, the placental site contracts to 50% of its original area.

This contraction and retraction results in the occlusion of the spiral arterioles (the so-called living ligatures). These processes are more important in the prevention of postpartum haemorrhage than the normal coagulation mechanisms. The placental bed becomes infiltrated by inflammatory cells and the layers superficial to this are shed.

Re-epithelialization occurs from the glands and stroma in the decidua basalis. By 7–10 days, the uterine cavity has been re-epithelialized except for the placental bed which does not completely regenerate until 6 weeks postpartum. The trophoblast and decidua are shed over this time and the uterine discharge is termed lochia. Usually it is blood-tinged (lochia rubra) during the first 2–3 days but then becomes serous and pale (lochia serosa) consisting of some red blood cells, inflammatory cells, decidua plus bacteria and lasts for up to 20 days. After this, the loss becomes thicker, more mucoid and yellowish–white in colour (lochia alba) and may last 4–8 weeks. The lochial discharge usually ceases about the sixth week as healing nears completion.

The lochia provides a good culture medium for bacterial infection but because of the cellular barrier, infection rarely occurs. Persistence of red lochia for more than 10 days or the persistent passage of blood clots may indicate the placental site involution is not occurring properly.

Cervical and vaginal involution

Immediately after delivery, the cervix is patulous and haemorrhagic. It gradually closes down over the first week of the puerperium to a little more than 1–2 cm in dilatation. By the end of the second week the cervical os has closed. Most cervical lacerations will heal spontaneously. The external os is converted into a transverse slit.

The vagina, which as a result of overdistention by the fetus is bruised and swollen, regains its tonicity and rugal patterns and by the end of the third week has almost returned to its antepartum condition. The torn hymenal remnants are termed carunculae myrtiformes.

The perineum, whether torn, incised (episiotomy) or stretched, heals rapidly so that by 5–7 days it is healed.

Pelvic floor muscles

Voluntary muscles of the pelvic floor gradually regain their tone. Tearing or overstretching of these muscles at the time of delivery predisposes to prolapse. This effect is aggravated by interference with neuromuscular function as a result of nerve compression by the presenting part during the latter stages of pregnancy. It may take up to 6 months before the pelvic floor muscles return to their original state and the neurological damage is rarely permanent. Overdistention of abdominal skin may result in persistent striae (striae gravidarum) and divarication of the rectus abdominis muscles.

Urinary tract involution

During a normal delivery, trauma to the bladder base leads to bruising, oedema and some detrusor hyptonia which may lead to difficulty with voiding. Care should therefore be taken to ensure that the bladder does not become overdistended as retention of urine further compounds the loss of tone. These problems may be increased by the use of epidural blockade and forceps delivery. It may be necessary to catheterise the patient to prevent this from occurring. During the first few days, due to a transfer of fluids from cellular to vascular compartments, a marked diuresis occurs. Dilatation of the ureters may remain for up to 3 months after pregnancy.

Cardiovascular changes

1. **Coagulation**
   During pregnancy, concentrations of Factors I, II, VII, VIII, IX and X increase gradually. Following placental separation, consumption of coagulation factors and platelets occur at the placental site with a local intravascular coagulation. There are usually no major systemic changes due to coagulation factors but this predisposes to thrombosis during the puerperium, particularly if the delivery is complicated by trauma, sepsis or immobility.
2. **Blood volume changes**
   (a) Plasma volume. After delivery, the plasma volume decreases by approximately 1000 ml, most of this being

due to blood loss during the third stage. Some patients may show a gradual increase in plasma volume, reaching a maximum of 900–1200 ml above the immediate postpartum values on the third day of the puerperium, suggesting a transfer of extravascular fluid to the intravascular spaces. Plasma volumes have usually returned to the normal non-pregnant state by 6–8 weeks.

(b) Red cell volume. The average red cell loss at delivery is about 14%. The sudden loss of blood leads to reticulocytosis with an increased erythropoietin level for about 1 week. The red cell volume returns to the normal pre-pregnancy level at about 8 weeks.

(c) White cell count. A neutrophil leucocytosis occurs during labour and extends into the puerperium. The white blood cell count may be as high as 25 000/ml with an increased percentage of granulocytes.

3. **Haemodynamic changes**

(a) Cardiac output. Immediately following delivery, cardiac output and stoke volume remain elevated or may even rise for at least 30–60 minutes. (This obviously depends on the duration of the labour and the method of delivery and varies from patient to patient.) These haemodynamic changes have usually returned to normal by approximately 6 weeks postpartum.

(b) Heart rate. The heart rate which normally increases in pregnancy returns to normal by about 6 weeks.

(c) Heart sounds. The physiological changes in heart sounds include increasing intensity of first heart sound with splitting, loud third heart sound, split second heart sound after 30 weeks and systolic flow murmur. These sounds usually disappear early in the puerperium.

(d) Blood pressure. Blood pressure usually returns to normal early in the puerperium.

Hormonal changes

1. Human placental lactogen (HPL) has a half-life of 20 minutes, and reaches undetectable levels during the first postpartum day.

2. Human chorionic gonadotrophin (HCG) has a mean half-life of 9 hours and falls below 100 iu/ml by the seventh day.
3. Oestradiol-17β falls to 10% of the antepartum level within 3 hours, and the lowest levels are reached by the seventh day. Follicular levels are reached by the 21st day in non-lactating women, although it is delayed in lactating women. The onset of breast engorgement at 3–4 days coincides with a significant fall in oestrogens.
4. Progesterone has a very rapid half-life, and is below luteal phase levels by the third day.
5. Prolactin rises throughout pregnancy and reaches levels of 250 ng/ml or more. Postpartum, there is a gradual decline over 2 weeks in non-lactating women. Nipple stimulation causes increased prolactin secretion, although levels are diminished after several months of lactation. Increased levels of prolactin have been associated with the relative refractoriness of the puerperal ovary. This would appear to be an anti-gonadotropic effect of prolactin at the suprasellar or pituitary levels (rather than a direct effect of the ovary), causing a disturbance in a cyclical release of luteinizing hormone (LH).
6. Thyroid-stimulation hormone (TSH) levels are very low in all women during the first 2 weeks postpartum. Levels increase slowly, and reach the follicular phase during the third week. The onset of menstruation varies in lactating and non-lactating women. Usually the first menses follows an anovulatory cycle, and most non-lactating mothers will ovulate by 90 days.

Gastrointestinal tract

The gastrointestinal tract gradually regains its normal absorptive and contractile function. Constipation is common for 3–4 days and the result of dehydration, low oral intake, lack of tone and sometimes reflex inhibition of defaecation as a result of a painful perineum.

Psychological state

About 80% of patients experience some emotional lability (mood swings) in the puerperium, especially in the first week.

Many patients experience depression or melancholia with bouts of crying (postpartum blues). This is regarded as a reaction to the physical and mental stress of childbirth together with the marked physiological changes that occur as a result of tissue breakdown and alteration of the hormonal level. A deep depression is seen in approximately 5% of patients and a frank psychosis in about 0.3%. A preceding history of depression should alert the physician to an increased risk of depression.

10.5 MANAGEMENT OF THE PUERPERIUM

Management in the first 24 hours

Management during the first hour

1. Prevention and control of postpartum haemorrhage. Ten units of Syntocinon are usually given intramuscularly with the delivery of the anterior shoulder of the fetus. As the effects of Syntocinon wear off after a few minutes, ergometrine 0.25–0.5 mg may be given intramuscularly after the delivery of the placenta unless there are maternal complications such as hypertension or cardiac disease.
2. Repair of the perineal trauma that has occurred during the delivery.
3. The parents are both encouraged to handle and touch their baby. This encourages bonding of the new-born infant after which it is carefully examined and the parents are reassured that their baby is structurally normal.
4. The bedding is changed and the mother is given clean, dry clothing and made more comfortable.
5. Provided no complications have occurred, mother may feel like having something to eat or drink and a wash.

Management over the next 23 hours

1. Haemorrhage. Regular observation should be made of the maternal abdomen to ensure that the uterus remains well contracted and that an excess amount of bleeding does not occur.
2. Analgesia. The mother should receive adequate analgesia, particularly if she has had a Caesarean section or has had

an episiotomy or perineal tear. Analgesia may also be required for postpartum contractions (afterpains).

3. Rest. It is essential that the mother has an opportunity to have adequate rest – particularly if she has had a long labour.

4. Urinary tract. Regular observation should be made of the patient's abdomen to ensure that urinary retention does not occur. Should the patient be unable to void then the bladder should be catheterized before overdistention develops.

5. Maternal nutrition. The mother should be given adequate amounts of calories and fluids, particularly if she plans to breast-feed her infant.

6. Breast-feeding. Over the next 24 hours the mother is shown how to put the baby to her breast and encouraged to establish lactation.

Management over the next 6 days

1. Detection and prevention of sepsis.
2. Establishment of breast-feeding.
3. Prevention of deep vein thrombosis.
4. Rest – ensure that the mother gets adequate rest, particularly if the baby is restless at night or she is being plagued by visitors.
5. Psychological support.
6. Physiotherapy – this is necessary if the mother has had an operative delivery.
7. Contraceptive advice – this is usually given before the patient is discharged from hospital.

Conduct of the puerperium

Following their discharge from hospital most patients are encouraged to maintain close contact with nursing staff at their community centre until lactation is successfully established. Rising hospital costs have led to a reduced duration of the traditional lying-in period, but even patients delivered by means of Caesarean section are discharged after approximately 5 days, if there are no complications.

Immediate labour ward management

Patients are kept in the labour ward until their vital signs (pulse and blood pressure) are stable, after which they are transferred from the labour ward provided that there are no abnormalities which require close observation. During this time women should be encouraged to hold and cuddle their newborn infant. Should the mother so desire, she should be helped to suckle the baby for a short period of time. Provided the labour has been uncomplicated, a free choice of fluids is provided. If she has had an epidural anaesthetic, then she is kept in the labour ward until she has voided, at which time her intravenous infusion will probably be removed.

In the postnatal ward

Blood pressure, temperature and pulse are taken 4-hourly for the first 24–48 hours. Thereafter twice-daily observations are sufficient provided all readings are in the normal range. Each day the patient's breasts are checked, and her uterine fundus is palpated to ensure that it is involuting appropriately. Her perineum is checked for evidence of infection and her calves are palpated to ensure that there is no evidence of deep vein thrombosis. The mother's psychological state should be observed, looking for signs of depression and instability.

Prevention of postpartum haemorrhage

Postpartum haemorrhage (PPH) is prevented by the judicious use of oxytocic agents in most pregnancies. Under normal circumstances 10 units of Syntocinon are given intramuscularly with the delivery of the anterior shoulder of the infant. Once the placenta is delivered, unless there are contraindications, she may be given ergometrine 0.25–0.5 mg intramuscularly. Particular attention is paid to ensure that the uterus remains well contracted. Should any bleeding persist, the placenta should be examined for completeness and the fundus may be rubbed up manually to stimulate a contraction. A Syntocinon infusion of 40 units in 1 litre of Hartman's solution may be used to maintain uterine contraction.

Bladder care

Many patients are unable to void postpartum because of bruising to the urethra and the loss of reflex detrusor activity. They may not be able to relax due to perineal or abdominal pain or because of interference of bladder function due to an epidural anaesthetic. If the patient is unable to void, she should be catheterized under aseptic conditions, as overdistention of the bladder must be prevented. If the volume is more than 500 ml, an indwelling catheter should be retained for 24 hours. Most women have a diuresis postpartum and therefore have associated frequency. Frequency may also, however indicate overdistention of the bladder. Should the residual volume be more than 100 ml after the patient has emptied her bladder, then an indwelling catheter should be left *in situ* for a period of 24 hours. If symptoms suggest a urinary tract infection a midstream or catheter specimen of urine should be taken for culture and sensitivity. If the discomfort is due to local trauma, then alkalinizing the urine will usually improve these symptoms.

Psychological state

Soon after the infant is born, a physical examination should be made and the mother reassured that baby has no major structural abnormality. Even though the parents have seen and handled the baby they find this positive observation very reassuring. The sensation of touch, holding and cuddling their baby strengthens maternal ties, as does early suckling of the baby. Observations should be made during this early postpartum period to ensure that there is normal parent-to-infant interaction or bonding. Mothers frequently experience quite marked emotional lability (mood swings) in the first week of the puerperium. Immediate elation of the postpartum period is often followed in a few days by bouts of crying (postpartum blues). This is usually seen as a reaction to the physical and mental stress of labour as well as being related to alterations in hormone levels, together with other marked physiological readjustments that are occurring. These emotional symptoms may be aggravated should the mother be experiencing physical discomfort from operative trauma, breast discomfort or lack of rest. The patient should be encouraged to breast-feed and many new mothers have negative feelings as to whether they will be able to cope with the awesome responsibility of taking care of their newborn child. They often fear that they will be unable to feed their infant appropriately and require a great deal of emotional and physical support from the staff. Postpartum depression is seen in approximately 5% of patients but a frank psychosis develops in less than 0.3%.

Patients who have had a previous history of postpartum mental illness should be referred for psychiatric assessment during the antenatal period as there is a high recurrence rate in the postpartum period.

Analgesia

Patients who have had an operative delivery require adequate analgesia. This may take the form of intramuscular opiates such as Omnopon 10–15 mg or pethidine 75–125 mg intramuscularly, 4–6-hourly. Many women find that twice-daily indomethacin 100 mg administered rectally provides very adequate pain relief. Perineal pain following an episiotomy usually requires either paracetamol or dextro-propoxyphene, compounds which are more potent. A further source of discomfort are afterpains due to uterine contraction, particularly during breast-feeding. These require reassurance and mild analgesics.

Diet

Once the effects of sedation and anaesthesia have worn off, the patients may have a normal diet. Patients are encouraged to increase their fluid intake to overcome the lack of fluid intake and increased fluid losses which occur during labour and the postpartum diuresis.

Perineal care

Patients are encouraged to have perineal showers and sitz baths regularly throughout the day, particularly after defaecation. Episiotomy wounds rarely become infected unless haematoma formation occurs.

Bowels

Patients very rarely experience a desire to defaecate due to the mild ileus and decreased fluid intake that occurs during labour. The postpartum perineal discomfort and fluid shifts also predispose to constipation. Patients may be given oral senna (Senakot) or a rectal suppository on the third or fourth postpartum day.

Rest

Early mobilization after delivery is encouraged, even if the patient has had an operative delivery. This lessens the incidence of venous thrombosis and respiratory complications. Women often have difficulty sleeping as a result of the strangeness of the surroundings, concerns about their home and families or due to physical discomfort from surgical trauma. Appropriate measures should be taken to deal with all of these aspects. A mild hypnotic may be prescribed to ensure that the mother has adequate rest. Rooming-in whereby the infant is in a cot beside the mother's bed for most of the day is encouraged. This has the advantage of improving mother–infant relationships. However, should this proximity exacerbate the lack of sleep, then the infant should be removed to the nursery to ensure the mother gets adequate rest. Some restriction may need to be placed on visitors if they interfere with maternal rest.

Postpartum immunization

1. If the mother's blood group is Rh-negative and she has no antibodies, and the baby is Rh-positive, she should be given 100 µg of anti-D immunoglobulin. Should there be any suspicion of a larger transplacental haemorrhage then the amount of fetal blood in the maternal circulation can be estimated by means of a Kleihauer test and an increased amount of anti-D immunoglobulin can be given.
2. If the mother does not have an appropriate immunity to rubella then vaccination with a live attenuated rubella virus can be undertaken in the puerperium.

Physiotherapy and postnatal exercises

These are usually a continuation of the antenatal exercises designed to improve involution and restore tone to the abdominal and pelvic muscles. Deep breathing and leg exercises help to prevent venous thrombosis and chest complications. These are usually supervised by the physiotherapist and should be carried out on a daily basis.

Puerperal infection

Detection and prevention of postpartum infection

Puerperal pyrexia is defined as a rise of temperature to 38°C on two or more occasions after the first 24 hours of labour. This may be due to a number of different causes so careful physical examination and investigations are required. The most common sites of puerperal infection are:

1. Genital tract infection.
2. Urinary tract infection.
3. Breast infection.
4. Respiratory infection.
5. Thrombophlebitis and venous thrombosis.
6. Other causes of pyrexia.

Due to shorter labours, better labour ward techniques and the availability of potent antibiotics genital tract infections occur in only about 1–3% of patients. The most common pathogens are:

1. Streptococci, both anaerobic and on occasion the β-haemolytic streptococcus.
2. Coliform organisms.
3. Staphylococci.
4. Anaerobic organisms such as bacteroides.
5. Chlamydia.
6. Mycoplasma.
7. Very rarely *Clostridium welchii* can cause serious genital tract infection.

Mode of infection

In most cases infection arises as a result of invasion by normal bacterial flora. If the uterus contains some placental fragments, the growth of these organisms is enhanced. Spread may also occur from the bloodstream or gastrointestinal tract. In the remaining cases the cause may be exogenous – from the attendants or the patient herself.

Clinical features

Infection may be localized in the following sites:

Lower genital tract
Vulva and vagina. The most common site is the episiotomy, which becomes infected usually as the result of haematoma formation. It becomes red and swollen and painful. Treatment usually consists of local cleaning and appropriate antibiotics. Infected wounds usually heal extremely well, but occasionally superficial dyspareunia may result.

Upper genital tract
Endometritis/parametritis/salpingitis. Most patients with puerperal infections have endometritis. This usually occurs at the placental site as this area takes longer to re-epithelialize. The myometrium is also relatively more resistant to bacterial infection. The infection usually occurs between 36 and 72 hours postpartum, and the clinical picture depends on the virulism of the organism. Usually some or all of the following features occur:

- Pyrexia.
- Offensive lochia.
- Malaise.
- Tachycardia.
- Uterine tenderness.

In puerperal infection due to group (A) or β-haemolytic streptococci, the lochia may be scanty and odourless, but rapid lymphatic spread and bacteraemia may occur.

Complications

Delayed complications of puerperal infection are:

1. Pelvic abscess formation.
2. Pelvic thrombophlebitis.
3. Paralytic ileus.
4. Disseminated intravascular coagulation.
5. Septic shock.
6. Subsequent infertility.

Salpingitis, pelvic cellulitis and pelvic peritonitis are seen less frequently now that antibiotics are usually administered much earlier.

Management

This usually consists of obtaining appropriate bacteriological specimens such as endocervical swabs and blood culture for bacterial identification and antibiotic sensitivity. Should chlamydial or myoplasmic infection be suspected, then appropriate swabs should be taken for these. An intravenous infusion may be necessary, both for hydration and administering parenteral antibiotics. Until the organism and its sensitivity are known, a broad-spectrum antibiotic such as amoxicillin, either alone or in combination with metronidazole can be given. If there is excessive uterine bleeding and retained products of conception are suspected, an ultrasound examination can be used to confirm the diagnosis. A digital evacuation of the uterus under general anaesthetic may be required.

10.6 LACTATION

Anatomical structure of the breast (Figs 10.1–10.3)

The mammary glands are specialized skin appendages which have probably developed from sweat glands. Their role is to provide nourishment for the new baby and to transfer antibodies from mother to infant.

Each gland is divided into 15–20 lobes, each of which is further subdivided into a number of lobules. Each of these are made up of masses of milk-secreting units known as alveoli.

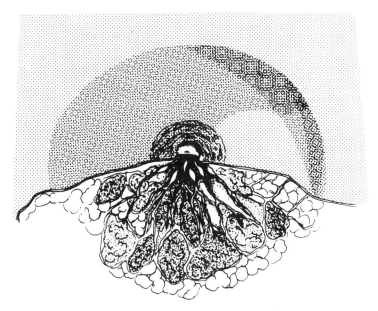

Figure 10.1 Showing a schematic representation of the alveolar system and the collecting ducts draining to the nipple.

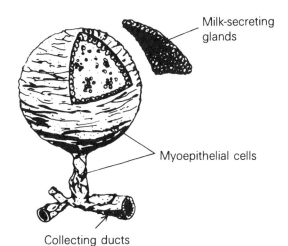

Figure 10.2 Lactating alveolus.

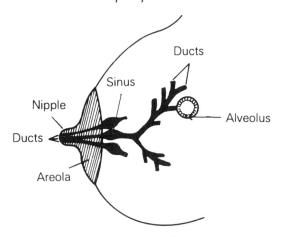

Figure 10.3 The anatomy of the lactating breast.

These cells take up the substance they require to form breast milk from the maternal blood. Intralobular ducts lead from the alveoli and unite to form lactiferous ducts which are the main duct of each lobe. Under the areola, each duct expands to form a lactiferous sinus which opens directly upon the surface of the nipple. The number of these openings varies from 6 to 15. The alveoli and main ducts are surrounded by contractile myoepithelial cells. The remainder of the breast consists of fat and fibrous septa.

Physiology of lactation

Mammary development begins just before the onset of puberty. The duct development is influenced by oestrogen and alveolar cells are under the control of progesterone. During pregnancy, the secretion of oestradiol and progesterone stimulates both duct and alveolar growth. Besides these two hormones, prolactin, growth hormone, insulin, cortisol and an epithelial growth factor as well as human placental lactogen play an important role.

Breast changes in pregnancy

1. Enlargement of both breasts. Each breast may increase by up to 640 g in weight.
2. Increased blood supply. There is an enlargement of the veins over both breasts.

3. Montgomery's glands in the areola became more prominent.
4. The areola becomes more prominent and there is an increase in pigmentation.
5. Colostrum can be expressed. Striae may develop during pregnancy.

Colostrum

The pre-milk (colostrum) is an alkaline, yellowish secretion that may be present in the last few months of pregnancy and for the first 2–3 days after delivery. It has a higher specific gravity, higher protein, vitamin A, sodium and chloride content as well as a lower potassium, carbohydrate and fat content than breast milk. Colostrum contains antibodies which play an important part in the immune mechanism of the newborn.

Milk is a complex fluid; it is a suspension of protein and fat in the solution of lactose and sodium salts. Human milk contains 87% water, the aqueous phase resembling dilute intracellular fluid, although the potassium levels are higher. Milk production is a monocrine process. Milk passes through the apical cell membranes into the acinar lumen (a similar progress to the secretory activity of the pancreas and salivary glands).

Onset of lactation

Many physiological and behavioural processes are involved in lactation. At a local level in the breast it consists of three stages; the production of milk in the alveoli, the flow of milk along the ducts to the nipple and the withdrawal of milk by the baby.

Secretion of milk occurs after delivery (even as prematurely as 16 weeks of gestation) as a result of falling oestradiol, progesterone and human placental lactogen levels as well as the increase in prolactin levels. The milk usually 'comes in' by the third or fourth postpartum day. This may be associated with the breasts becoming full, tense and uncomfortable. Often the baby becomes unsettled for approximately 24 hours when the milk 'comes in' due to the increased volume of milk produced. If suckling is delayed for any reason the onset of lactation may be inhibited. As local nipple stimulation leads to increased pro-

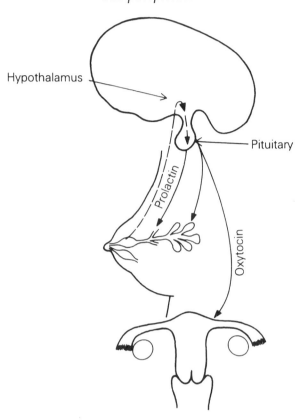

Figure 10.4 The 'let down' reflex.

lactin stimulation, the pain and fullness associated with the coming in of the milk needs to be differentiated from the pain that occurs early in the puerperium due to vascular congestion.

For milk secretion, the breast must elaborate specific milk components (lactose, fat, protein) from the plasma, concentrate and exclude plasma substrates. Regular removal of milk prolongs secretion and some women have nursed for as long as 4 years. Should conception occur, lactation only continues until late in pregnancy.

Nipple stimulation following suckling leads to stimulation of the paraventricular nucleus of the hypothalamus and release of oxytocin from the posterior pituitary gland (Fig. 10.4). This leads to the 'let down' reflex whereby oxytocin stimulates the myoepithelial cells to contract, which in turn assist to express the milk from the alveoli and ducts into the lactiferous sinuses where they are accessible to the infant. Therefore the baby obtains most of the available milk in the first few minutes of suckling.

Oxytocin release also stimulates uterine contractions, encouraging uterine involution and causing 'after-pains'.

Mechanism of sucking (Figs 10.5–10.7)

Sucking produces a negative pressure, which draws the nipple and areola into the mouth of the baby and holds these structures in this position. By compression of the areola, and also the lactiferous sinuses, between the tip of the baby's tongue and the roof of its mouth milk is expressed from the sinuses. At the same time, the let down reflex is initiated and this helps to express the milk from the alveoli and ducts into the lactiferous sinuses.

Pain, fear, discomfort, anxiety, lack of privacy and many other psychological influences may inhibit the milk ejection reflex at the hypothalamic level.

Because of the action of the milk ejection reflex, the baby will obtain most of the available milk in the first 5–7 minutes of sucking. Leaving the baby on the breast for periods longer than 10 minutes results only in the baby swallowing additional air, and may lead to colic.

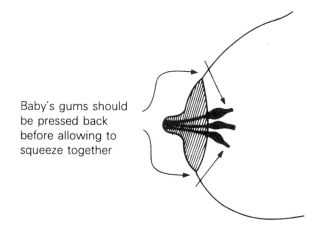

Baby's gums should be pressed back before allowing to squeeze together

Figure 10.5 Demonstrating the technique which allows the baby to express milk from the breast.

The puerperium

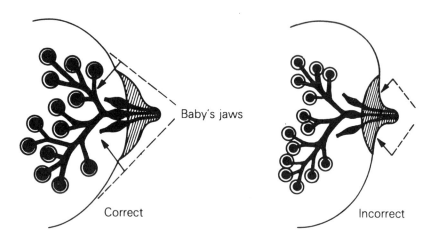

Figure 10.6 The lactating breast, showing the correct and incorrect positions of the baby's jaws.

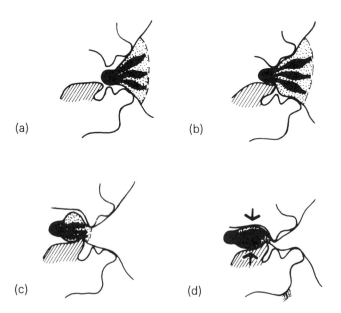

Fig 10.7 Lactation. demonstrating: (a) How the whole nipple is drawn into the mouth; (b) the gums close behind the nipple; (c) to squeeze milk from the sinuses and then; (d) the tongue compresses the nipple to obtain the milk.

With prolonged or excessive sucking, the nipples may crack, and so lead to considerable maternal discomfort.

Antenatal preparation for breast-feeding

During the antenatal period, instruction should be given about breast-feeding to avoid anxiety and fear of failure during the first few days of feeding when the milk production may not be adequate. The advantages and disadvantages of breast-feeding should be discussed with parents, but the ultimate decision should be made by the couple. The advantages of breast-feeding are:

1. Convenience.
2. Economy.
3. Emotionally satisfying to most women and may improve mother–baby relationship.
4. Helps contract the uterus and accelerate involution.
5. Sterile natural food which is easily available.
6. Passive antibody transfer. Protection against infection.
7. Breast food is easily digestible and always at the correct temperature.
8. Errors in formula do not occur.

Disadvantages of breast-feeding are:

1. Disrupts activities.
2. Mastitis may develop.
3. Breast-feeding may not be possible if the infant is pre-term or has difficulty with sucking. However, the mother may express her milk which may be used until the infant is well enough to feed.

There is no convincing evidence that antenatal breast preparation increases the number of mothers who are successfully able to breast-feed. It is doubtful whether the skin of the nipples can be toughened by the application of any particular cream or lotion. Many patients find that exposure of the breast to direct sunlight prenatally and while breast-feeding has a positive beneficial effect on the skin.

Flat or inverted nipples may be gently regularly massaged and with gentle traction the patient may elevate the nipples during the latter part of pregnancy. Some people believe that nipple shields worn under the brassiere for inverted nipples are of value. Patients require a firm, well-fitting and supporting brassiere during pregnancy and lactation to support their enlarged breasts.

There is no evidence that regular manual expression of colostrum during the last few weeks of pregnancy is of any value in the initiation of lactation.

Breast-feeding technique and timing

Breast-feeding usually starts 8–12 hours after delivery, although suckling the baby after delivery may shorten the third stage and give the parents a greater sense of pleasure. The milk usually does not come in until 3–4 days postpartum. The newborn infant should be fed when hungry (demand feeding) if possible. This is not always practical in a busy nursery, therefore rooming-in is encouraged.

Both breasts should be emptied at each feed to avoid engorgement and milk stasis and promote milk production. As soon as the breast is empty feeding should cease so as to avoid nipple problems – 5–10 minutes of sucking on each side is usually sufficient. Before breast-feeding the mother should:

1. Wash her hands with soap and water.
2. Cleanse the nipples with fresh water.
3. Assume a comfortable position for her and her baby.

Demand feeding or 3–4-hourly feeding is the usual aim, but each baby nurses differently so the guidelines need to be varied.

1. Usually 5 minutes at each breast is sufficient, initially increasing by the minute each, not exceeding 10 minutes.
2. Compression of the periareolar area and expression of a small amount of milk, or colostrum into the baby's mouth may provide the stimulation to suck.
3. Place the nipple well back in the baby's mouth, so that it rests against its palate where it can be compressed. The breast should be kept away from the baby's nostrils during feeding.
4. The infant can be removed by gently opening the mouth,

and lifting the outer border of the upper lip to break the suction.

Diet

The maternal diet should be well balanced, with adequate food and fluid intake. There are no special foods that enhance milk production.

Drugs excreted in breast milk

Most drugs are excreted in small amounts in breast milk. Sedatives and analgesics used in normal therapeutic doses in the postpartum period will not affect the infant to any great extent. Antibiotics which are safe during the pregnancy may also be used if the mother is lactating. Alcohol, nicotine and caffeine all cross into breast milk.

Complications of breast-feeding

1. Inadequate lactation. The most common problem encountered is inadequate lactation. Its origins are complex and may be due either to lack of milk production by the breast or the inadequacy of the let down milk reflex in response to suckling. The latter may be psychological, or due to pain or inadequate suckling. If the nipples are painful, manual expression or expression by means of a breast pump may be required until the nipples heal. If the nipples are not painful then more frequent feeding will supply extra stimulation. Oxytocin nasal spray may be used to induce a milk let down reflex. Failure of milk production is very rare and may indicate pituitary failure or systemic disease. Patients should be encouraged to increase their fluid intake. Drugs which increase prolactin secretion such as metoclopramide have been used to try and increase milk production.

2. Engorgement. Tightness and swelling which occur on the second or third day are usually vascular phenomena while their occurrence after that is usually due to milk retention within the breast, as well as lymphatic and venous stasis. This is an extremely painful and uncomfortable condition. The pain and swelling inhibit the let down reflex. Tightness

of the breast flattens the nipples so that the baby is unable to suck, thereby reducing stimulation.

Management consists of emptying the breast either by manual expression or breast pump. It is also useful to use an oxytocin spray or 10 units of Syntocinon intramuscularly, 20 minutes before this. Appropriate analgesia is also necessary.

3.   Mastitis. This is now much less common and affects only 1% of breast-feeding mothers. The usual pathogen is *Staphylococcus aureus*, which gains entry through the nipple fissures or ducts.

The symptoms usually occur between 3 and 14 days after delivery. Signs and symptoms are:
(a)   Unilateral breast tenderness and induration.
(b)   Spiking fever.
(c)   Malaise.
(d)   The affected breast may be inflamed over the area of infection.

Management consists of:
(a)   Culturing the breast milk.
(b)   Antibiotics. Because the infection usually occurs with a hospital staphylococcus (which is usually penicillin-resistant), cloxacillin or methicillin should be the drug of choice. If the infection has been acquired after discharge from hospital, large doses of amoxicillin can be given until the organism's sensitivity becomes available.
(c)   Breast support. Prompt treatment may allow even a fulminating mastitis to resolve without abscess formation. Should an abscess form, it should be drained. The baby may continue to breast-feed if the breasts are not too tender. It is important to empty the breasts and, if necessary, the baby should be fed from the non-infected breast and the milk expressed from the infected one and discarded.

Suppression of lactation

If the mother does not intend to breast-feed or if there has been a stillbirth then lactation can be suppressed. Stimulation of the breast should be avoided and a good supporting brassiere should be worn. Mild analgesic drugs may be necessary should some engorgement occur. This is all that is required in 40% of patients. Should the breasts become uncomfortable then bromocriptine (Parlodel) is the drug of choice. It is given in a dosage of 2.5 mg twice daily for 10 days. Bromocriptine inhibits prolactin synthesis and its release from the anterior lobe of the pituitary gland. Suppression of lactation with bromocriptine leads to an earlier return of fertility; ovulation can occur as early as the 27th day postpartum.

Previously, oestrogens were used to inhibit lactation but because of the increased incidence of thromboembolic disease associated with oestrogen use, they have been abandoned.

10.7 THROMBOSIS AND EMBOLISM

Fatal pulmonary embolism is the major cause of maternal death, other than abortion. Two-thirds of these deaths occur after delivery, and one-third antenatally. Most emboli occur without any clinical evidence of pre-existing venous thrombosis.

Predisposing factors

Infection, venous stasis and altered coagulation predispose to thrombosis during pregnancy and the puerperium.

Infection may be the result of puerperal pelvic infection. If the external iliac vein is invoked, phlegmasia alba dolens (white leg) may occur.

Stasis due to inferior vena caval obstruction is present throughout the pregnancy and may be compounded by enforced rest in bed if there are any obstetrical complications. These factors can be minimized by the use of leg exercises and early mobilization. The increased coagulation has been referred to elsewhere in this chapter. Other factors are:

1. The delivery. Patients delivered operatively (whether by Caesarean section or forceps) have a higher rate of thrombosis.
2. Trauma to leg veins. From pressure by stirrups when the patient is in the lithotomy position.
3. Age. Older patients are more at risk.
4. Anaemia.

Clinical features

Venous thrombosis presents in several ways:

1. Superficial thrombophlebitis. This is probably the most common – and always occurs in varicose veins. It is probably a misnomer, because infection plays only a very small part in its aetiology. It is usually caused by venous stasis. Clinically, a superficial varicose vein is tender and thrombosed, with an area of redness surrounding it.

    Occasionally the long saphenous vein can be involved. Very rarely the superficial thrombosis may spread and be associated with deep venous thrombosis. This must always be investigated.

    Management consists of analgesia and encouragement of physical activity. Careful bandaging (from toe to groin) may give added support.

2. Deep venous thrombosis. This may affect either the vein of the foot or calf initially, but may spread to the thigh involving the iliofemoral vessel. It may also occur in the pelvic vessels. Clinically it may present with some or all of the following:
    (a) Pain in the calf.
    (b) Swelling.
    (c) Pyrexia.
    (d) Painful and swollen, cold white leg. (This is due to secondary arterial spasm.)
    (e) Swollen, warm blue leg. (This is due to unimpeded arterial supply, with occluded venous return.)
    (f) Thrombosis may present with a sudden pulmonary embolism.

Investigation

It is important to examine all puerperal patients for evidence of deep venous thrombosis. However, all signs and symptoms are most imprecise. Almost half of those patients with a positive Homan's sign will not have a deep venous thrombosis – and a similar number will have a false-negative Homan's sign.

To establish a clear diagnosis, special investigations are necessary. The most frequently used are:

(a) Venography. This is the most accurate way of diagnosing venous thrombosis up to and including the common iliac veins. Its accuracy does depend on the experience of the operator.
(b) Ultrasound scanning. This utilizes the Doppler effect to detect blood flow in the vein, and is of greatest benefit above the knee.
(c) Radioactive iodine-labelled fibrinogen (^{125}I). This is taken up by the developing thrombus, and best defines the calf veins. Radioactivity counts from each leg are compared.

Of these tests, the most widely available and useful is venography.

Management
Prophylaxis is important; early mobilization, avoidance of calf pressure, and regular leg exercises should the patient be confined to bed.

In high-risk patients (those that are obese, elderly, have cardiac disease or have had surgical procedures), prophylactic subcutaneous heparin 7500 i.u. twice daily can be given. This does not affect the whole blood clotting time, so does not need to be monitored. Its action is explained by the anti-factor Xa-potentiating effect of heparin. The use of Dextran 70 infusion in surgical patients may also reduce the incidence of deep vein thrombosis, probably by altering the viscosity and platelet function.

Management of the thrombosis is by means of intravenous heparin. This should be given as a continuous infusion, monitored by whole blood clotting times, thrombin times or partial thrombin times. Treatment is usually continued for 10 days. At present, haematologists advise introduction of oral anticoagulants 3–4 days before cessation of heparin. This should be continued for 3 months (for deep vein thrombosis) or 6 months if a pulmonary embolus has occurred. The effects of warfarin are monitored by means of the prothrombin index.

Streptokinase and urokinase have been used in an attempt to dissolve the clot. Oral anticoagulants should be reduced slowly rather than ceased abruptly, because of the risk of rebound thrombosis.

Pulmonary embolism

The immediate effects of pulmonary embolism vary from sub-clinical to cardiac arrest and death and obviously depend on the size of the embolism and the haemodynamic effects. Symptoms are:

1. Dyspnoea.
2. Cough.
3. Pleuritic chest pain.
4. Central chest pain.
5. Haemoptysis.

Signs are:

1. Tachypnoea.
2. Rhonchi.
3. Tachycardia.
4. Pleural rub.
5. Gallop rhythm.
6. Loud pulmonary valve closure.
7. Cyanosis.
8. Elevated venous pressure.
9. Fever.
10. Systolic blood pressure less than 80 mmHg.

Special investigations include:

1. Ventilation – perfusion scan.
2. Electrocardiogram – showing classical S1, Q3, T3 changes, right axis deviation or right bundle-branch block.
3. Chest radiology – showing reduced vascular markings. A normal chest X-ray does not exclude a pulmonary embolus.
4. Blood gases – showing reduced arterial $PO_2 + PCO_2$ with an elevated pH.
5. Pulmonary angiography should be performed before pulmonary embolectomy is considered.

Management of embolism

This depends on the severity and varies from external cardiac massage with oxygen, heparin, vasopressor agents and correction of acidosis with possible pulmonary embolectomy to heparinization alone and subsequent confirmation of the diagnosis. Streptokinase or urokinase may be therapeutic in massive pulmonary embolism. The place of surgery (ligation, plication or thrombectomy) on the venous drainage is uncertain. It is certainly indicated for patients who have recurrent embolism from a proven lower-limb thrombosis.

10.8 SECONDARY POSTPARTUM HAEMORRHAGE

After the first few days, bright bleeding occurring during the puerperium should be regarded as abnormal. Secondary postpartum haemorrhage can occur from 24 hours to 6 weeks after delivery. The amount of bleeding may vary from light to very heavy. The usual causes are:

1. Retention of placental tissue or membranes.
2. Infection of the placental site.
3. In the case of Caesarean section, the dehiscence of the uterine wound.
4. In later cases, choriocarcinoma is a rare condition which should be considered.

Treatment consists of admission to hospital and if the bleeding is only moderate antibiotics can be given in the first instance after an ultrasound examination has excluded retained parts of the placenta and the patient re-assessed after 12–24 hours. If the bleeding continues to be heavy then surgical emptying of the uterus can be undertaken under antibiotic cover after appropriate cervical swabs have been taken. Care must be taken during this procedure, because of the risk of uterine perforation.

10.9 DISCHARGE

Before discharge from hospital, the patient should be thoroughly examined. If involution is occurring normally, the patient can be discharged after advice on normal activities and contraception.

Hygiene should be the same as practised in hospital. On discharge, most women find management of a new infant strenuous and require significant support from their husbands. The usual household activities should be curtailed for the first few weeks until a routine with the infant is established. If possible, the mother should have a few hours sleep during the day. The doctor should be notified immediately of any onset of fever or bright vaginal bleeding.

Intercourse can take place whenever the couple feel so inclined usually after the lochia has subsided and all cuts have healed. Patients are usually advised to return for postnatal check at 6 weeks. At this stage contraception is discussed. The earliest reported time of ovulation as determined by endometrial biopsies is 33 days postpartum in non-lactating and 49 in lactating women. It appears that provided the mother is still doing the early morning feed she will have some protection against ovulation from lactation. If the patient is breast-feeding then the 'mini-pill' (progestogen only) is probably the best form of contraception. It does have the disadvantage that it may be associated with poorer cycle control and a slightly higher pregnancy rate. Oestrogens, however, do suppress lactation and this outweighs the use of a combination oral contraceptive. Mechanical methods (condoms, foams, diaphragms or IUCDs) may be preferred by some nursing mothers.

Some women require permanent contraception. A tubal ligation can be performed easily in the puerperium with minimal disruption to the family, and only minimally increases the length of hospitalization. There is, however, an increased failure rate of sterilization when undertaken following a pregnancy.

10.10 POSTNATAL CARE

Mothers are asked to return at 6 weeks for a postnatal check.

Aims of postnatal visit

- To assess the physical and mental health of the mother and to assist with any problems that have arisen.
- To detect any gynaecological problems that may have arisen from the pregnancy and delivery.
- To assist with any feeding or behavioural problems in the infant.
- To provide contraceptive advice.

Examination of the mother
Routine questions should elicit problems relating to feeding,

sleeping, bowels and bladder function, vaginal discharge or bleeding.

Examination includes weight assessment, blood pressure recording, looking for pallor, examining the breasts and the abdominal muscle tone.

Pelvic examination should be done with special attention paid to the following:

(a) Healing of the perineum.
(b) The presence of prolapse or stress incontinence.
(c) Vaginal discharge or bleeding.
(d) Speculum examination to examine the cervix and take a cervical smear if this was not done at the booking visit.
(e) Uterine size and position.
(f) Adnexal enlargement or tenderness.
(g) Tone of the pelvic floor muscles.

Laboratory test

A Papanicolaou (PAP) smear is taken for cytological examination of the cervix.

Contraceptive advice

This is one of the most important aspects of the postnatal visit (see section 10.9).

11

Abortion, ectopic pregnancy and trophoblastic diseases

11.1 GENERAL INSTRUCTIONAL OBJECTIVE

The students should understand the aetiology, pathology and clinical manifestations of abortion, ectopic pregnancy and trophoblastic diseases so that such conditions can be identified and appropriate management instituted.

11.2 SPECIFIC BEHAVIOURAL OBJECTIVES

1. List the types of abortion and discuss how to differentiate one from the other.
2. List the major causes for early abortion and discuss the possible steps in management.
3. List the possible causes of midtrimester abortion and discuss the management.
4. Examine a pregnant patient who is bleeding during the first trimester and make a diagnosis as to the likely cause of the bleeding.
5. Take a history from a patient who has had previous abortion and discuss the most likely causes for that abortion.
6. Discuss the differentiating symptoms and signs of ectopic pregnancy, acute salpingitis, torsion of ovarian cyst and abortion.
7. Discuss the presenting symptoms and signs of hydatidiform mole.
8. Discuss the complications and management of trophoblastic tumours.
9. List the steps necessary for the emergency management of a woman who presents with vaginal haemorrhage and signs of shock during the first half of pregnancy.

10. Counsel a woman, who has lost an early pregnancy, on the possibility for future normal pregnancies.
11. Discuss the aetiology and pathology of ectopic pregnancy.
12. Differentiate by description of clinical and pathological process how ruptured ectopic pregnancy varies in presentation to unruptured ectopic pregnancy.
13. Discuss the general management of women who have an ectopic pregnancy.

11.3 REASONS FOR LEARNING ABOUT ABORTIONS

Often a woman will present with a history that suggests pregnancy is present but may be in the process of being lost. This may be due to the expulsion of a normally implanted conception from within the uterus (abortion or miscarriage), from an abnormal site (ectopic pregnancy) or because the conception itself is grossly abnormal (hydatidiform mole). The understanding of the pathophysiology, the diagnosis and the management of these problems requires knowledge, skill and personal involvement on the part of the attending physician, otherwise the woman may suffer severe morbidity or even die if the appropriate management is not given at the right time.

Medical practitioners must be able to diagnose and manage women who present with abortion states, ectopic pregnancy or even a rare neoplasia of pregnancy. They will certainly see women presenting for the first time for assistance because of some abnormal pregnancy condition – and it is important to remember that the loss of a pregnancy can have very serious physical and emotional consequences.

Students of obstetrics and gynaecology who are given lectures and tutorials related to abortion, will see women in the outpatient clinics and the wards and will observe and assist in operations on women who are suffering from one or more complications of an early pregnancy. The students thus have the opportunity to observe and note the presenting history and signs, and can then become involved in the practical management of these conditions.

11.4 ABORTION (MISCARRIAGE)

When discussing abortions, nomenclature may give rise to some confusion, because the lay public tend to associate abortion with a criminal procedure, and miscarriage with spontaneous onset of the expulsion of the products of conception. The two terms are in fact synonymous and the definition for both is: 'the expulsion of the products of conception before the 20th week of amenorrhoea'.

Threatened abortion

This is said to occur when a pregnant patient bleeds vaginally. About 75% of women who threaten to abort carry on to a normal delivery.

Inevitable abortion

This occurs when a pregnant patient not only bleeds, but has uterine contractions sufficiently strong and painful enough to dilate the cervix, so that the products of conception will eventually be passed through the cervix.

Incomplete abortion

This occurs when a portion of the products of conception has been expelled through the dilated cervix but some products still remain in the uterus.

Complete abortion

This has occurred when the products of conception have been completely expelled from the uterus.

Missed abortion

This occurs when the fetus dies but the products of conception are retained within the uterus, and either become surrounded with layers of inspissated blood or are gradually absorbed.

A *termination of pregnancy* (commonly incorrectly called an 'abortion') is caused by some interference to the implantation of the trophoblast or the decidua, is usually achieved by applying a negative pressure via a hollow plastic catheter and is more safely done in the first trimester.

A *septic abortion* occurs when organisms invade any retained products of conception. This condition may be life threatening.

1. A threatened abortion typically has the following symptoms and signs: there is amenorrhoea for 5 or more weeks, followed by a vaginal bleed. The bleeding may be slight as a faint brown discharge or as profuse as a heavy red loss

with clotting. Pain is generally not present but there may be a dull ache or discomfort due to congestion of the pelvic organs. Unless the abortion is proceeding, the bleeding subsides and over 75% of cases continue to a normal delivery of a normal infant. The risk of pre-term labour and delivery, however, is three times higher than in women who do not bleed in the first trimester, i.e. 18% versus 6%.

2.   Inevitable abortion. About 25% of women with a threatened abortion proceed to colicky uterine contractions, leading to cervical dilatation. Almost all of these women will lose their pregnancy. The uterine contractions which are normally present from the beginning of any conception become vigorous and painful, the cervix dilates, bleeding continues and the pregnancy separates from its attachment to the decidua.

3.   The next phase in the process is that of incomplete abortion in which the uterine contractions have continued the process of inevitable abortion. The cervix is dilated, there is continuing haemorrhage, uterine contractions persist and on inspection of the material that has been expelled, fetal and placental debris may be recognized. However, some products of conception are still present in the uterus, which is enlarged and soft. During the phase of inevitable and incomplete abortion, the patient may be found to suffer from shock with a low blood pressure and thin, thready pulse. She will be pale, cold and sweating and the degree of shock will be out of proportion to the observed blood loss. One of the rare causes of such a shock-like picture is the vaso-vagal effect of the products of conception passing through the dilating cervix. A vaginal speculum should be passed and, using a sponge-holding forceps, the material should be removed from the endocervical canal. This simple procedure will alleviate the features of shock if dilatation of the cervix is the cause. If despite this manoeuvre the patient remains shocked, then a search for the cause should be made elsewhere, i.e. hypovolaemia or septicaemia.

4.   The final phase in the sequence is that of complete abortion, in which all the products of conception have been expelled. Bleeding slows and ceases, the cervix closes and the uterus becomes smaller and firm.

5. A missed abortion differs from the other stages of abortion
    in that although bleeding and possibly some dull lower
    abdominal pain may be present, the cervix does not dilate.
    Because the trophoblast separates from the decidua, the
    pregnancy dies but remains within the uterus. Layers of
    blood and clot usually form around the dead material to
    produce a hard mass of tissue, which may remain *in utero*
    for weeks, months or even years. When it is expelled,
    heavy bleeding may occur, which may be difficult to
    control.

Epidemiology of abortion

There are a number of facts known about spontaneous abortion
and these are important in the management of this condition.

Recent work indicates that as many as 50% of all conceptions
come to grief. With the advent of radioimmunoassay of the
beta sub-unit of HCG, it has been shown that approximately
30% of fertilized ova failed to survive long enough to cause a
missed menstrual period. Since these very early losses have no
specific clinical implications, it is best to concentrate upon the
estimated 20% of recognized conceptions which terminate as
spontaneous abortions.

The majority of intrauterine deaths occur during the first trimester and are primarily caused by serious genetic abnormalities. Chromosomal abnormalities have been observed in
approximately 60% and 23% of spontaneous abortions occurring during the first 7 and 8–12 weeks of gestation respectively.
The majority of chromosomally abnormal pregnancies lost are
anembryonic (old term – blighted ovum) and are triploid.
Chromosomal abnormalities continue to contribute to fetal mortality during the second and third trimesters but their importance relative to other factors are unavoidable, especially those
which occur early in the pregnancy. However, current data
indicate that the risk of loss is associated with a number of
demographic and behavioural factors, several of which can be
either directly or indirectly influenced by couples contemplating childbearing.

1. **Maternal age.** Many studies have shown that women
    under the age of 20 and over the age of 35 have a dis-

proportionate number of fetal losses (including late fetal and neonatal deaths). Recent studies have shown that if an ultrasound examination is performed at or after 7 weeks of amenorrhoea (when a live fetus of 10 mm should be seen) and a normal continuing pregnancy is found, the risk of subsequent loss is very low, but appears to be related to maternal age. Under the age of 30, the incidence of loss of an ultrasonographically normal pregnancy is under 2% (1.8%) whereas over the age of 35 the incidence is more than doubled at 4.5%. In summary, the general risk of loss of an ultrasonographically normal pregnancy is approximately 3% but maternal age is an independent variable. Paternal age is not believed to play a role.

2. **Parity.** There is evidence that higher order pregnancies are at increased risk of loss and this increased risk is independent of age. This increase in loss rate is applicable throughout the fetal period.

3. **Pregnancy spacing.** Pregnancies preceded by either short or prolonged intervals suffer higher rates of fetal mortality. Current data suggest that the optimal interval appears to be approximately 12–36 months and that the most extreme rate of early loss occurs when the interval from previous loss to next conception is less than 6 months.

4. **Previous fetal loss.** A woman who has had a previous spontaneous abortion is at an elevated risk of aborting her next pregnancy. The most straightforward explanation of this association is that some women are inherently at higher risk of loss, owing either to genetic or physical factors.

Causes of abortion

The simplest method of categorizing the various causes of pregnancy loss is to divide them into maternal, fetal and paternal.

Before doing so it is important to point out the error of a commonly held belief. For the last four decades many studies have been mounted to evaluate the role of various female hormones in cases of spontaneous abortion. To date, no normal pregnancy has ever been shown to have been lost as a result of abnormal hormone production. In addition, no study has been able to demonstrate any beneficial effect of the administration of either oestrogenic or progestational agents. Indeed there is clear evidence of teratogenic effects of such compounds as diethylstilboestrol and the synthetic 19-nor group of steroids. An expert writing in an English textbook in 1972 said, 'The idea of giving progestational agents for recurrent or threatened abortion is as illogical as the giving of hydrochloric acid to correct the achlorhydria of pernicious anaemia'. In 1980, two American authors wrote: 'The use of hormones in pregnancy without substantial evidence of benefit is no longer admissible. The evidence that prenatal exposure to female sex hormones may be teratogenic is strong enough to prohibit the use of such drugs.' Recently, an Australian author wrote: 'No normal clinical pregnancy has ever been shown to have been lost as a result of abnormal hormone production. The giving of powerful female sex steroids to pregnant women has absolutely no scientific foundation, is potentially teratogenic and cannot be condemned too strongly'.

Maternal causes

General

1. Chromosome abnormalities. Balanced translocations may result in gametes with abnormal chromosome complements and therefore chromosomally abnormal conceptuses.
2. Hypertension. Women with chronic untreated hypertension have an increased risk of pregnancy loss when compared with normotensive women. Treatment may result in reduction of this risk.
3. Systemic lupus erythematosus. Women with this condition have an incidence of pregnancy loss as high as 40%. There is no evidence that treatment of the condition will reduce the rate of pregnancy wastage.
4. Thyroid dysfunction. Severe thyroid dysfunction is much more likely to be associated with abnormal ovarian function and resultant infertility. Occasionally spontaneous abortions occur in women with such dysfunction; appropriate treatment reduces the risk of subsequent loss.
5. Infections. Bacterial and viral infections producing systemic effects, specifically a pyrexia, may be associated with the

demise of a fetus in the early part of the first trimester and subsequent abortion. Syphilis has a specific effect upon the pregnancy and in untreated cases results in early loss, then stillbirth and the subsequent birth of an infant with the stigmata of congenital syphilis.

6. Smoking. Although the regular consumption of more than 10 cigarettes daily is more often associated with intrauterine growth retardation, smoking women abort more frequently than non-smokers.

7. Alcohol. Heavy drinking (more than 100 g of alcohol per week) may be associated with the birth of a baby with the fetal alcohol syndrome; there is clear evidence that even moderate consumption of alcohol may be associated with spontaneous abortion. The combined effects of smoking and drinking (social habits often associated with each other) are graphically shown in Fig. 11.1.

Local

1. Cervical. Cervical incompetence is either of a functional or an anatomical nature. In this condition cervical dilatation usually occurs in the second trimester in the absence of

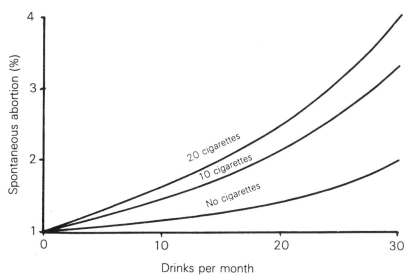

Figure 11.1 The effects of drinking and cigarette smoking on spontaneous abortion.

overt uterine contractions – the so-called silent dilatation. With the support for the membranes at the level of the internal os lost, rupture occurs and is typically followed by a few contractions and expulsion of the fetus.

Cervical incompetence may be congenital (present in 30% of uteri with a congenital fundal abnormality) or acquired. The latter form is usually traumatic as a result of over-vigorous mechanical dilatation, e.g. lateral cervical tears at the time of delivery or dilatation beyond 8–10 mm as is necessary for a second trimester dilatation and evacuation.

2. Uterine. Uterine anomalies are believed to be quite common but most do not result in reproductive difficulties. Nevertheless they are found in some 15% of women who abort more than once and are to blame for both first and second trimester abortions equally. Surgical correction of only some of these congenital abnormalities is possible but should only be attempted by those with expertise in this field since the literature shows that even in expert hands, 30% of such operations are followed by sterility.

Acquired uterine abnormalities such as submucous fibromyomata may also be associated with spontaneous abortion, and the judicious use of myomectomy may effect a cure.

Fetal causes

For practical purposes this is a mixed group of fetal anomalies. Some 60% of spontaneous abortions are chromosomally abnormal. As many as 20% more are structurally abnormal, e.g. anencephaly, etc. The majority of spontaneous abortions are anembryonic (blighted ovum) and in these instances the fate of the fetus remains conjectural.

Paternal causes

Chromosomal translocations in the father may also result in abnormal gametes and therefore abnormal conceptuses, as described for the mother. Approximately one couple in ten with a history of recurrent abortion will have one of its members exhibit a chromosome abnormality.

Over the last decade increasing interest in the immunology

of reproduction has developed. Recent studies have revealed the possibility of an immunological cause for spontaneous abortion. Research has shown that women who recurrently abort, and in whom no other cause can be found, have a significantly different response to their husband's tissue antigens when compared with women who reproduce successfully. The foreign genetic material contributed by the father usually provokes the formation of a series of maternal blocking antibodies. In an apparently paradoxical fashion these antibodies seem essential to the normal continuation of a pregnancy and absence thereof is associated with the loss of an otherwise normal fetus. Studies in progress reveal that this form of rejection may be prevented by the intradermal injection of the husband's lymphocytes. This form of immunotherapy is still best regarded as experimental, although its use is being studied in some centres, because of the inherent potential risks attendant upon such manoeuvres.

Management

The management depends entirely on the stage at which the abortion presents. A woman with a threatened abortion should be reassured that three-quarters of such cases will carry on to deliver a perfectly normal baby, albeit with an increased risk of pre-term delivery. She should have an ultrasound examination performed which will confirm or refute the diagnosis of a continuing pregnancy. In the event that the ultrasound reveals evidence of a continuing pregnancy she should be advised to take it easy for the next few days until the bleeding ceases. The visualization of a fetal heart beat will almost always allay the anxiety associated with vaginal bleeding in early pregnancy. There is seldom an indication for admission to hospital under these circumstances. The ultrasonic evidence of a non-continuing pregnancy indicates the need for admission and evacuation of the uterus. When an inevitable or incomplete abortion is diagnosed, admission to hospital is indicated. Evacuation of the placental and fetal tissues is performed under a general anaesthetic. Blood transfusion may be required if haemorrhage is severe. When the risk of infection is high, antibiotics should be administered to reduce the risk of post-abortal sepsis. If sepsis is already present when the patient is first seen it is wise to treat with broad-spectrum antibiotics both before and after evacuation of the uterus.

Complete abortion needs no active management when diagnosed. However, a missed abortion should be evacuated under general anaesthesia. Care should be exercised when using a curette for a missed abortion, because bleeding may be heavy and transfusion may be required.

Termination of pregnancy

Termination of pregnancy by interference before the 20th week of pregnancy is commonly, though incorrectly referred to as an abortion. The termination of a pregnancy in New South Wales is still illegal, but the ruling given in 1971 by Judge Levine in the *Heatherbrae* case now allows a doctor to perform an abortion if, in his or her opinion, the continuation of the pregnancy is likely to cause harm to the mother or the fetus. Similar legal judgments in the UK and the USA have also liberalized the laws regarding the availability of termination in these countries. The earlier in pregnancy the termination is performed, the safer is the operation. If performed before 12 weeks the risk of major morbidity is only 1% whereas when a termination is performed after 12 weeks the major morbidity rate rises to 4%. The safest time to perform a termination is between 6 and 8 weeks of amenorrhoea; the safest person is a doctor who has an extensive experience in termination procedures; and the safest place is in a large institution such as a teaching hospital which has developed the special skills to handle the abortion procedures and the associated complications.

Complications of abortion (spontaneous or induced)

Haemorrhage

This may be immediate and require blood transfusion, or may occur several days or weeks later due to retained placental tissue. In the latter case, the patient should be re-admitted to hospital, transfused if necessary and then thoroughly curetted to remove any tissue. All such tissue should be examined in a pathology department to confirm that the debris is indeed innocent.

Infection

The most common organisms that may be associated with all types of abortion are the coliform anaerobes: *Escherichia coli*, *Klebsiella* and *Streptococcus faecalis*.

Coliform organisms release endotoxins that cause endotoxic shock. The endotoxin is a lipid released (as a lipopolysaccharide) from the cell wall of a Gram-negative organism, after the death or lysis of that organism. The lipid endotoxin acts as an antigen, in a complex reaction in which complement is utilized, histamine is produced, and lysosomes and kinins are released. This reaction results in increased vascular permeability and capillary dilatation, leading to a peripheral pooling and loss of intravascular fluid, as well as activation of the plasmin enzymes to produce hypofibrinogenaemia. The end result of such a reaction is stagnation and pooling of blood in the periphery, poor return of blood to the heart and eventual cardiac output failure. Shock (and often death) follows.

Because of the cellular reaction to infection, there is also an increase in leucocytosis. This causes cellular phagocytosis and release of lysosomal enzymes, which further increase tissue damage. This combination of hypofibrinogenaemia, capillary damage and phagocytosis leads to haemolysis, shock, cardiac failure, renal failure, bleeding disorders, cellular anoxia, acidosis and death. It is a serious complication and requires urgent and adequate management. The steps in management of endotoxic shock are:

1. Insert an intravenous line and begin transfusion with a volume expander such as blood, dextran or even saline/dextrose.
2. Insert a central venous pressure manometer to ensure that the circulatory blood volume is not increased to the extent where cardiac failure ensues.
3. Improve capillary tone and activity by agents such as cortisone or dexamethasone.
4. Use digitalis/digoxin as indicated.
5. Measure hourly urine output after inserting an indwelling catheter.
6. Take blood, cervical and vaginal, urethral and other appropriate culture material to identify the organism and obtain the antibiotic sensitivity.

7. Only after taking the appropriate swabs for culture should antibiotics be given. It is usual to begin with crystalline penicillin (2 million units every 4–6 hours) and an aminoglycoside such as streptomycin, kanamycin or gentamicin. Care must be taken to ensure that the urine output is adequate when using these drugs.
8. Take blood for analysis of electrolytes and blood gas. Metabolic acidosis produces a very poor prognosis.
9. Remove surgically any focus of dead and infected tissue by D and C or hysterectomy if necessary.
10. Avoid using vasoconstrictors, as these are more likely to do more harm than good to the patient.
11. Check the haemoglobin and bilirubin, and transfuse blood as required.
12. Check the blood urea and creatinine levels. Renal failure may require dialysis.

Trauma

Another major complication of abortion is trauma, and is almost always associated with criminal abortions. The types of trauma may include vaginal lacerations, cervical tears, uterine perforations, avulsion of loops of bowel, and gas or fluid in the abdominal cavity.

In addition to the acute emergency procedures, it is important to remember the likelihood of long-term sequelae that increase morbidity and mortality. For instance, tubal occlusion and cervical incompetence may occur. Cervical incompetence is present when the internal os is forcibly dilated and torn. Future pregnancies may be lost between the 16th and 25th weeks of amenorrhoea.

Recurrent abortion

Formerly a patient was regarded as suffering from recurrent abortions when three or more successive pregnancies had been lost. Once this definition had been satisfied it was suggested that investigations be instituted. Today, however, the expectations of couples intent upon having children is such that this definition should be modified and it is recommended that investigations should begin after two first trimester abortions or one second trimester abortion. A general practitioner may perform some of the more standard tests before referral to a specialist or may choose to effect referral immediately.

The basic investigations are indicated by the causes listed previously and are summarized as follows:

1. Karyotype both parents. $\longrightarrow$
2. Hysterogram. $\longrightarrow$
3. Maternal blood for the presence of the lupus anticoagulant and anticardiolipin antibodies. $\longrightarrow$
4. Serological test for syphilis. $\longrightarrow$

It is wise to remember that many couples who experience spontaneous abortions develop profound emotional problems of which guilt is the most common. They need careful patient handling and counselling, and need to be told that pregnancies are rarely lost because of what they might have done or not done.

11.5 ECTOPIC PREGNANCY

Ectopic pregnancy is the implantation of a pregnancy in a site outside the normal uterodecidual area (Fig. 11.2). It occurs in about 1 in 300 pregnancies. The common site is the tube, but a pregnancy may implant in the ovary, the abdominal cavity or the uterus, and may produce some bizarre symptoms and signs.

Like abortion, an ectopic pregnancy is usually associated with a period of amenorrhoea followed by bleeding and then pain.

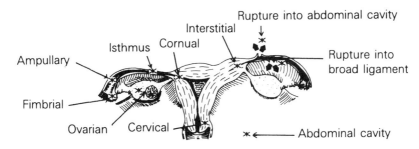

Figure 11.2 Sites of ectopic pregnancy.

The pathophysiological process of tubal ectopic pregnancy is as follows:

1. A normal ovum is fertilized near the site of ovulation and usually passes into the fimbrial end of the tube.
2. The zygote becomes blocked in the tube either by adhesions and agglutination of the endosalpingeal processes, or there is narrowing or spasm of the tube (isthmial implantation), or loss of the cilial processes of the endosalpinx. The zygote then develops into a blastocyst, which implants into the endosalpinx at about the sixth day after ovulation.
3. Following implantation, the trophoblast produces chorionic gonadotrophin. This maintains the corpus luteum.
4. The corpus luteum produces oestrogen and progesterone, which changes the secretory endometrium of the uterus into decidua.
5. The trophoblast produces bleeding and necrosis within the tube at its implantation site, and the ectopic pregnancy begins to degenerate. The levels of chorionic gonadotrophin, oestrogen and progesterone fall, and the corpus luteum regresses.
6. The decreased level of progesterone induces a withdrawal bleed as the decidua breaks up and is shed. This withdrawal bleed from the decidua is the most common presenting symptom in ectopic pregnancy.
7. Occasionally the whole decidua is shed as a cast and the expulsion of this may resemble an incomplete abortion.
8. The trophoblast in the tube usually results in one of three processes occurring:
    (a) The trophoblast may die and be reabsorbed without any further management required.
    (b) It may be disrupted in the same way that an abortion separates from the decidua of the uterus. This leads to bleeding from the fimbrial end of the tube, peritonism and tubal abortion. Like an incomplete abortion, removal, or evacuation, is required. This type of ectopic pregnancy is by far the most common (80% of cases), and it is rarely associated with sudden shock from heavy blood loss.
    (c) The trophoblast may continue to erode into the endosalpinx until it passes right into the muscle surround-

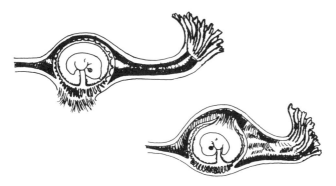

Figure 11.3 Ectopic pregnancy. The trophoblast may invade the wall of the tube or pressure may rupture the tube into the abdominal cavity.

ing the tube. If the pregnancy is still growing and enlarging, then rupture of the tube is likely to occur (Fig. 11.3). This type of case presents with acute pain and shock, requiring urgent operation and transfusion.

Symptoms and signs

An ectopic pregnancy usually presents with vaginal bleeding for several days, accompanied by vague lower abdominal pain. The bleeding is caused by decidua breaking down and the pain is caused by the tube distending and leaking blood (usually through the fimbrial end of the tube) onto the peritoneum. Patients presenting at this stage will be found to have amenorrhoea of up to 6–8 weeks and some symptoms of pregnancy. Examination discloses the cervix to be closed but soft and blood oozing through the os. The uterus may be slightly enlarged and softer. Movement of the cervix or uterus usually elicits an exquisite pain in the pelvis; this is due to the involvement of the serosal surface of the uterus with the peritonism that is associated with the free blood irritating the peritoneum. A small tender mass may be palpated in the tube. Difficulty may be experienced in differentiating these cases from those women who present with a threatened abortion. It may be some days before positive symptoms or signs develop.

If the ectopic pregnancy continues to grow in the tube, it may suddenly rupture. Blood striking the peritoneum then causes severe pain accompanied by shock. Hypovolaemic shock may follow if the intra-abdominal bleeding persists. Although only 15–20% of ectopic pregnancies present in this manner, it is the dramatic picture that most clinicians remember. The woman suddenly collapses with severe abdominal pain and, on recovering from the initial vasovagal shock, develops shoulder-tip pain and eventual hypovolaemic shock. This is a relatively uncommon manifestation of ectopic pregnancy, but one which is easy to diagnose.

Diagnostic procedures

There are several procedures that may assist in diagnosing an ectopic pregnancy:

1. A pregnancy test may be helpful in differentiating between ectopic pregnancy and follicular cysts, but is of no value in differentiating threatened abortion from ectopic pregnancy.
2. A laparoscopy is of immense value before the tube ruptures or bleeds, but is of little help when blood fills the peritoneal cavity.
3. Where free blood is present, an aspiration (using a large-bore needle) through the posterior fornix of the vagina into the pouch of Douglas may be of immense help.
4. Ultrasound, with enhanced resolution, has become an invaluable diagnostic aid.

Management

1. Admit to hospital.
2. Cross-match blood.
3. Transfuse if necessary.
4. Order relevant investigations if indicated.
5. When the diagnosis is confirmed, perform a laparotomy to remove the ectopic pregnancy. This usually involves removal of the tube and may often include an oophorectomy as well.

Sequelae

Following removal of an ectopic pregnancy, there is an increased incidence of infertility and subsequent ectopic pregnancies. Approximately 50% of women who have had an ectopic pregnancy find difficulty in conceiving again, and about 10% of those who do conceive suffer a further ectopic pregnancy in the other tube.

11.6 HYDATIDIFORM MOLE AND CHORIOCARCINOMA

Hydatidiform moles are neoplastic tumours that arise from the placenta. The villi become grossly hydropic and distend to form masses of vesicles resembling bunches of grapes. The trophoblastic tissue is highly active, having invasive properties and high hormonal activity.

The incidence of hydatidiform mole varies geographically. It is 1:600 in Hong Kong and Singapore, 1:1200 in the USA and about 1:800 in Australia. It follows from fertilization of an ovum, so will only be found in reproductive women.

Although hydatidiform mole is considered to be a benign tumour of the placenta, it is pseudo-malignant due to its activity. The mole may invade the uterine myometrium or the parametria or be carried by the blood stream to deposit in a metastatic manner in tissue far removed from the pelvis.

Clinical features

1. The most common presenting symptom is uterine bleeding occurring between the 6th and 12th weeks of amenorrhoea. Other symptoms and signs of pregnancy are also present, so it is often first diagnosed as a threatened abortion.
2. The uterus is enlarged to a size greater than expected in 50% of cases, and may be confused with a multiple pregnancy. However, in 25% of cases the uterus is the size expected, and in the remaining 25% the uterus is smaller.
3. Because of the increased trophoblastic activity, there is an increase in hormonal levels. Nausea and breast changes are thus more marked, the incidence of pre-eclampsia is higher and occurs early in the pregnancy, and uterine contractions are more pronounced.

Diagnosis

This is usually made when a woman presents with amenorrhoea followed by persistent bleeding, usually after the eighth week of amenorrhoea. A search should be made for hydropic villi in the vaginal blood, chorionic gonadotrophin estimations should be ordered (these are usually increased) and an ultrasonic echogram should be performed (this usually gives a typical snow-storm picture pathognomonic of hydatid moles). Radiology and fetal Doppler will give negative results.

Management

Admit to hospital, cross-match blood, and arrange for an evacuation of the uterus under general anaesthesia. A drip containing high doses of Syntocinon must be kept running throughout the procedure, during which sponge forceps, suction curettes and blunt curettes are used to remove all the products of conception.

Following the initial evacuation, beta-chorionic gonadotrophin tests (β-HCG) are performed twice weekly for 4 weeks and then every 2–4 weeks for 12 months. A recurrence of a positive β-HCG during the year is an indication to perform a further curette.

Moles that appear to be invasive or to show metastasis should be treated with a course of methotrexate. A hysterectomy is rarely indicated.

Choriocarcinoma

This is a rare malignant condition derived from trophoblastic tissue. In 50% of cases it follows hydatidiform moles, but only about 2% of moles ever develop in this manner. Choriocarcinoma is an anaplastic, invasive, highly mortal tumour. The use of (methotrexate) and (surgery) has reduced the previously high mortality rate to under 40%.

Any woman who has had a pregnancy that has terminated (whether by abortion, ectopic, hydatidiform mole or a normal pregnancy) and has persistent uterine bleeding should have a curettage and a β-HCG to exclude the possibility of a choriocarcinoma arising in trophoblastic material.

12

Contraception and infertility

12.1 GENERAL INSTRUCTIONAL OBJECTIVE

The students should understand the physiology of conception and the factors that can prevent pregnancy so that they can initiate management of patients with infertility and advise patients about contraception.

12.2 SPECIFIC BEHAVIOURAL OBJECTIVES

1. Describe the structure and function of the human reproductive organs.
2. Describe the physiology of the menstrual cycle.
3. Describe the actions of the female sex hormones.
4. Outline the factors necessary for fertilization and implantation.
5. Outline the factors that may interfere with fertilization and implantation.
6. Discuss variations in the levels of human fertility and the factors that may influence it.
7. Discuss the investigation of an infertile couple.
8. Discuss those factors identifiable by history taking that are relevant to infertility.
9. Discuss the psychological factors and the emotional sequelae of infertility.
10. Outline the management of common causes of infertility.
11. Describe the methods of contraception, their modes of action and their efficiency.
12. Discuss the implications of sterilization and its medicolegal aspects.
13. Discuss the complications of and the contraindications to various methods of fertility control.

14. Discuss counselling of an individual and a couple in the selection of a contraceptive technique.
15. Discuss the problems of counselling a woman with a pregnancy following failure of her method of conception control.

12.3 REASONS FOR LEARNING ABOUT CONTRACEPTION AND INFERTILITY

We live in a global village! By the year 2000 it has been estimated that the world population will increase by 100 million people per year. One million per year will die from AIDS. By the year 2050 it has been estimated that the world population will be 9.2 billion at best and 14.2 billion at worst. The difference in these two figures is the size of the current world population (1995). The good news is that between 1985 and 1990 the fertility rates in developing countries has dropped from 6.1 children per couple to 3.9 (2.1 children per couple equals zero population growth). Today, as you read this chapter, the world population will increase by 250 000.

In contrast to these horrific statistics, approximately one couple in every eight, in Australia, find that they cannot conceive after 2 years of trying. In developing countries, 14% to 32% of couples are unable to get pregnant due to sexually transmitted diseases.

The doctor must have the knowledge and counselling skills to advise patients on contraception and infertility.

12.4 NORMAL MENSTRUATION (Fig. 12.1)

The hormonal control of normal menstruation is fully covered in Chapter 14 but will be summarized here.

The anterior pituitary of a normal young woman will begin to produce follicular-stimulating hormone (FSH) at about the age of 11–12 years. This acts on the maturing ovaries to stimulate the growth of one or more Graafian follicles (Fig. 12.2), which in turn produce oestrogen from granulosa cells and theca interna. The oestrogen has effects on the physical, hormonal and psychological characteristics of maturing women. Breasts, hips, vagina, uterus and supporting pelvic tissue all develop and together give rise to the physical characteristics of

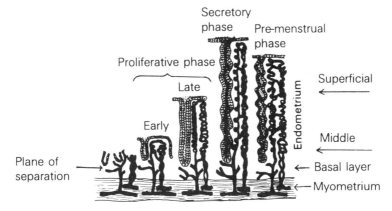

Figure 12.1 The endometrial cycle.

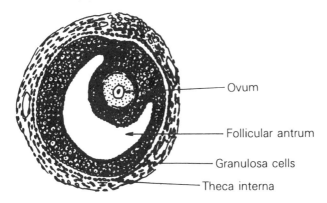

Figure 12.2 Graafian follicle near maturation.

young adult females. Concomitant with this physical develop-ment are psychological changes of femininity and sexuality. Oestrogen also plays an important role in the interaction with other hormone-secreting areas (by feedback on the pituitary and hypothalamus), as well as effecting bone epiphyseal closure and limitation of growth.

The effect of oestrogen on the endometrium and the anterior pituitary is discussed in this chapter.

Briefly, menstruation occurs in the following manner:

1. At the end of a normal menstrual cycle, the plasma level oestradiol reaches its lowest concentration. The plasma pro-gesterone concentration has also fallen to a low level.

2. Under these circumstances the arcuate nucleus in the hypo-thalamus produces pulses of gonadotrophin-releasing hormone (GnRH) every 90 minutes.
3. This releasing hormone activates the basophil cells of the an-terior pituitary to secret FSH and luteinizing hormone (LH).
4. FSH stimulates the growth of follicles in the ovary and increases the protein that binds sex steroids in the ovary.
5. By attachment to cell membrane receptors LH causes the release of adenyl cyclase. This enzyme controls the reaction in which adenosine triphosphate (ATP) forms cyclic adeno-sine monophosphate (cAMP) which stimulates the theca interna cells of the ovary to produce oestradiol. As the folli-cles increase in size, the production of oestradiol increases.
6. These increasing levels of oestradiol act on the pituitary to modulate the level of FSH and LH being produced (nega-tive feedback loop). Eventually, however, the level of oes-tradiol exceeds 40 pmol/l for at least 36 hours. At this level the positive feedback mechanism overrides the negative effect and a surge of gonadotrophin is released from the pituitary.
7. The Graafian follicle responds to this surge of gonado-trophins by full maturation, massive oestradiol secretion, follicular rupture, ovulation, corpus luteum formation and progesterone production. Because progesterone inhibits any new follicular development, a new cycle is not begun (even though gonadotrophins are still being produced in quan-tity) until the corpus luteum undergoes regression. This normally takes 14 days and at this stage a new ovulatory cycle begins again.
8. While this whole system can continue to function in a regular cyclic manner every 28 days, there is no doubt that the midbrain can be profoundly influenced by higher centres as well as by other endocrine systems and hor-mones. These changes are probably initiated by changing the pulsatile release of GnRH by the arcuate nucleus.

Suckling, prolactin section and progesterone production act to inhibit or change the frequency of the pulses of GnRH and so interfere with the production of gonadotrophins by the pituitary. This ultimately interferes with the maturation of folli-cles within the ovary.

12.5 SAFETY OF ORAL CONTRACEPTION

The first oral contraceptive pill was approved in 1959 and it has taken 35 years to establish the safety of the pill. During this time almost three million women worldwide have used combined pills and many large-scale epidemiological studies have demonstrated the safety of their use. The beneficial effects of the pill have far outweighed the relatively few dangers. The well-established protective effects include those against ovarian and endometrial cancer, pelvic inflammatory disease, ectopic pregnancy, bleeding irregularities, benign breast disease, iron-deficiency anaemia and ovarian cysts. There are also possible benefits from reduced chance of thyroid disease, rheumatoid arthritis and uterine fibroids, and an increase in peak bone mass. If the patient has no risk factors for cardiovascular and cerebrovascular disease (smoking, diabetes, hyperlipidaemia and hypertension) then she is safe to take the combined oral contraception until the menopause. Smoking is the main risk factor. At the age of 40 the non-pill using smoker has a mortality rate of 31.3 per 100 000 while the non-smoking pill user has a mortality of 10.7 per 100 000.

12.6 MODE OF ACTION OF ORAL CONTRACEPTIVES

In commercially available preparations, the two oestrogens used are ethinyl oestradiol and its 3-methyl ether, mestranol. On a weight-for-weight basis, ethinyl oestradiol is nearly twice as active as mestranol and has a slightly better therapeutic-to-toxic ratio. In order to produce consistent ovulatory suppression 0.05 mg daily of ethinyl oestradiol has to be given for 7–14 days before ovulation. The effectiveness of suppression of ovulation is highest when tablets are begun on the first day of the cycle (beginning of menstruation). However, oestrogens used alone may produce irregular, prolonged and unpredictable menstrual bleeding patterns. For this reason it is necessary to use a progestogen with the oestrogen.

Synthetic steroids that are capable of producing a secretory change in the endometrium are known as progestogens. A progestogen alone (in a dose equivalent to 0.4 mg of norethisterone) will suppress ovulation if given for a week before the expected date of ovulation. However, it is not commonly used

Table 12.1 Currently available oral contraceptives

Brand name	Oestrogen	Progestogen	Approximate potency*
1. Combined type			
	Ethinyl oestradiol	**Levonorgestrel (d-norgestrel)**	
Nordiol	0.05 mg	0.25 mg	2.5
Microgynon 50:Nordette 50	0.05 mg	0.125 mg	1.25
Microgynon 30:Nordette 30	0.03 mg	0.15 mg	1.5
Biphasil: Sequilar	0.05 mg	0.05 mg (11 days)	0.5
	0.05 mg	0.125 mg (10 days)	1.25
Triquilar	0.03 mg	0.05 mg (6 days)	0.50
Triphasil	0.04 mg	0.075 mg (5 days)	0.75
Logynon	0.03 mg	0.125 mg (10 days)	1.25
		Desorgestrel	
Marvelon	0.035 mg	0.15 mg	1.5
		Norethisterone	
Brevinor	0.035 mg	0.5 mg	0.5
Brevinor 1	0.035 mg	1.0 mg	1.0
	Mestranol		
Norinyl-1	0.05 mg	1.0 mg	1.0
	Ethinyl oestradiol		
Synphasic	0.35 mg	0.5 mg (12 days)	0.5
		1.0 mg (9 days)	1.0
		Ethynodiol diacetate	
Ovulen 0.5/50	0.05 mg	0.5 mg	2.0
Ovulen 1/50	0.05 mg	1.0 mg	4.0
		Cyproterone acetate	
Diane 35	0.035 mg	2 mg	
2. P.O.P. (Progestogen only pills)			
Micronor: Noriday	0.35 mg	Norethisterone	
Microlut: Microval	0.03 mg	Levonorgestrel	

*In terms of norethisterone (1 mg norethisterone = 1.0)

because irregular bleeding, breakthrough bleeding and amenor-rhoea may occur in 25% of patients. When the progestogen is used for more than 7 days, there is an increased frequency of break-through bleeding. To overcome these problems, an oestrogen is combined with the progestogen.

The combined type of oral contraceptive is the most common one on the market (see Table 12.1).

12.7 SIDE EFFECTS OF ORAL CONTRACEPTIVES

Some women who are taking one of the many oral contraceptive preparations suffer from some of the side effects of either the oestrogen or the progestogen component. Table 12.2 summarizes the side effects and the best management of these problems.

The combined oral contraceptive depends on progestogen for suppression of ovulation. The oestrogen is added to prevent breakthrough bleeding and to promote a predictable and satisfactory menstrual flow 2 days after finishing the hormonally active tablets. The numerous commercially available preparations vary in their content of oestrogens and progestogens. Thus a patient who is sensitive either to progestogen or oestrogen may be placed on a preparation containing a lower amount of that particular hormone. However, lowering the dose of either hormone will given slightly reduced reliability.

It is not simply the weight but rather the activity and the amount of the hormone that needs to be taken into account when comparing relative potency of the various brands. Norgestrel derivatives, although low in weight, are 10 times more potent than norethisterone derivatives, while norethisterone is 10 times more potent than medroxyprogesterone (Provera).

The so-called 'tailor-made' contraceptive is reserved for patients who have unacceptable side effects on existing commercial contraception and aims to 'mimic' the natural cycle by using oestrogen alone for the first half of the cycle followed by oestrogen and progesterone in the second half of the cycle. Tailor-made contraception depends on oestrogen for suppression of ovulation and the progesterone provides cycle control.

Other hormonal preparations

Progestogen injections and implants act in the same way as the mini pill, or progesterone-only pill.

Postcoital pills contain high doses of oestrogens and progestogens and are taken within 72 hours of intercourse. This inter-

Table 12.2 Side effects of oral contraceptives

Side effect	Cause	Management
Oestrogen effects		
Fluid retention	Excess oestrogen	Reduce oestrogen
Nausea, vomiting	Excess oestrogen	Reduce oestrogen or increase progestogen
Increased mucous discharge	Excess oestrogen	Reduce oestrogen or increase progestogen
Ectopic columnar epithelium	Excess oestrogen	Reduce oestrogen or increase progestogen
Menorrhagia	Excess oestrogen	Reduce oestrogen or increase progestogen
Skin pigmentation	Oestrogen	Reduce oestrogen
Thrombophlebitis	Oestrogen	Reduce oestrogen or cease the pill
Growth of fibroids	Oestrogen	Reduce oestrogen or cease the pill
Progestogen effects		
Full, bloated feeling	Excess progestogen	Reduce progestogen
Scanty menses	Excess progestogen, deficient oestrogen	Increase oestrogen
Weight gain	Excess progestogen	Reduce progestogen
Loss of libido	Excess progestogen	Increase oestrogen reduce progestogen
Irritability	Excess progestogen	Reduce progestogen
Breakthrough bleeding	Excess progestogen, deficient oestrogen	Increase oestrogen
Depression	Excess progestogen, deficient oestrogen	Increase oestrogen Reduce progestogen
Dry vagina	Deficient oestrogen	Increase oestrogen
Reduced breast size	Decreased oestrogen	Increase oestrogen
Acne	Increased progestogen, deficient oestrogen	Reduce progestogen, increase oestrogen
Hirsuitism	Increased progestogen,	Reduce progestogen, increase oestrogen
Moniliasis	Increased progestogen	Reduce progestogen
Combined effects		
Headaches, migraine	Excess oestrogen or progestogen	Reduce oestrogen and progestogen
Breast engorgement and tenderness	Oestrogen and progestogen	Reduce oestrogen and progestogen or give progestogen alone
Blood pressure increase	Oestrogen or progestogen	Reduce oestrogen and progestogen

rupts implantation of the ovum. Hormonal side effects are very common – 25% of women experience nausea and vomiting.

Prostaglandins in effective doses can be used to produce an early abortion. They are thus abortifacients and not contraceptives. Their side effects of diarrhoea and nausea make them unacceptable generally.

Effect on plasma proteins

The steroid contraceptives act on the liver to alter the metabolism of protein synthesis and thus most plasma proteins are altered. This fact must be taken into consideration when interpreting the results of investigations carried out on women taking the pill. The levels of the plasma proteins altered are:

Albumin	decreased
Ceruloplasmin	increased
Transferrin	increased
Transcortin	increased
Thyroxine	increased

There is also an increased liver production of the substrate angiotensinogen. This results in an alteration in the renin–angiotensin–aldosterone balance, which may lead to hypertension in some women. Fortunately, these hypertensive changes are usually reversed when the pill is ceased. Other adverse effects include an increase in the coagulation proteins, with an associated increased risk of thromboembolism.

Progesterogens such as norethisterone and norgestrerol may increase the production rate of certain lipids, particularly the triglycerides and the lipoproteins. Progestogen steroids appear to be involved in producing an elevation in the blood glucose levels.

All these metabolic changes are significant in relation to the following clinical conditions:

1. Monilial vaginitis is increased.
2. Diabetes may develop or be unmasked.
3. Existing diabetes may become less easy to control.
4. Heart disease and thrombosis appear to be slightly increased in cigarette smokers.

5. Existing liver and gallbladder disease may be aggravated. (When known liver or gallbladder problems exist, the pill should not be prescribed).
6. Blood pressure may be increased and is probably related to the amount of progestogen in the combined pill. Fortunately, only about 3–5% of women develop an increase in blood pressure, and in most cases this is reversible when the pill is ceased.
7. Increase in the incidence of migraine headaches, particularly the premenstrual type. This is probably due to the fall in levels of progestogens before the onset of menstruation, and the resultant increase in aldosterone levels.

Summary

The combined oestrogen/progestogen pills are probably the best and safest to use for the majority of women.

In prescribing any combination of hormones to provide contraception, the risks and complications of the therapy must be balanced against the benefits to be derived. In reaching such a decision, the following factors must be taken into consideration:

1. History of any medical disorders.
2. Prior menstrual history.
3. Feelings and fears expressed by the patient, especially fear that the pill causes breast cancer.
4. Symptoms or signs that develop while on the pill.
5. Development of complications while on the pill.
6. Risk factors due to the pill.
7. Side effects of the pill.

Oral contraceptives, besides providing adequate protection against pregnancy, also have the advantage that they regulate the menstrual cycle, can be used to prevent intermenstrual bleeding of hormonal origin, and can be used to ameliorate dysmenorrhoea due to increased uterine muscle activity. Preparations that contain high levels of oestrogens may also assist in management of acne conditions. Those that contain small quantities of oestrogen and relatively more progestogen may be of great benefit in treating women with endometriosis.

12.8 OTHER FORMS OF CONTRACEPTION

Methods used by both partners

(a) **Continence.** Abstention. Very effective, but not very popular.
(b) **Rhythm method.** This is the avoidance of coitus around the time of ovulation. In a woman with a regular 28-day cycle, ovulation takes place on about the 14th day. Allowing for slight irregularities and sperm survival, intercourse should not take place from day 9 to day 19 of the cycle – or, to be safer still, from day 7 to day 21.
Advantages: acceptable to the Roman Catholic Church. Relatively simple procedure.
Disadvantages: cycles must be regular. Requires an intelligent patient. Requires continence during part of each cycle. High failure rate.
(c) **Billings method**. Ovulation can be anticipated in regularly ovulating women when cervical mucus becomes thinner and more elastic. This is accompanied by a cascade of mucous secretions and indicates ovulation is impending or has just occurred. While it is reasonably reliable when used by intelligent women in conjunction with a temperature chart, it has a high failure rate and is not acceptable for most women.

Methods used by the male

(a) **Condom (sheath, protective, French letter)**
Advantages: Simple to use. Male's responsibility. Mechanical barrier to infection.
Disadvantages: Expensive. Diminished sensation. Lack of spontaneity. Failure rate, most due to faulty technique (defect rate 0.25–0.89). Danger of rupture (1 in 150–300 times).
(b) **Coitus interruptus (withdrawal method)**
This is probably the most common method used.
Advantages: Simple and easy to understand.
Disadvantages: Much self-control needed by both partners. Often unsatisfying. High failure rate.

(c) **Vasectomy**

Surgical removal of a section of the vas deferens, the remaining ends being turned back on themselves. The patient should be warned that sterility is not effective for at least 3 months, in which three seminal analyses, 1 month apart, must show complete absence of sperm.

Advantages: Simple technique that can be done on an 'outpatient' basis under local anaesthesia. Little morbidity. Very effective.

Disadvantages: Surgery is necessary. Male (and female) attitudes towards the procedure often prevent its acceptance. Not totally reversible (only in 30–40% of cases), so reversibility must not be expected. The possible death of a couple's children, or of a couple's possible divorce must be taken into consideration. Long postvasectomy time before 'safe' period is reached. Theoretical possibility of late autoimmune effect to sperm.

Methods used by the female

(a) **The diaphragm**

Once inserted, the diaphragm must be left in place for at least 6 hours after intercourse, but no longer than 16 hours, as the rubber and prolonged retention can cause an unpleasant discharge. The safest technique is to insert the diaphragm nightly. A spermicide should also be used.

Advantages: Relatively simple to use. Woman's responsibility. Inexpensive.

Disadvantages: Doctor is required to instruct the patient how to fit the device (Fig. 12.3). Must be used regularly. Anatomical variations may make fitting impossible. Psychological fear of touching the genitalia and general patient unwillingness may prevent use. Lack of sponteneity unless fitted nightly.

(b) **Cervical cap**

A plastic or metal cap fitting over the cervix and left in place for several days. A spermicide must also be used.

Advantages: May be left in place for days. Cheap and will last. Woman's responsibility.

Disadvantages: Doctor required to instruct patient and to fit the device. Not effective for abnormal cervices. Technique

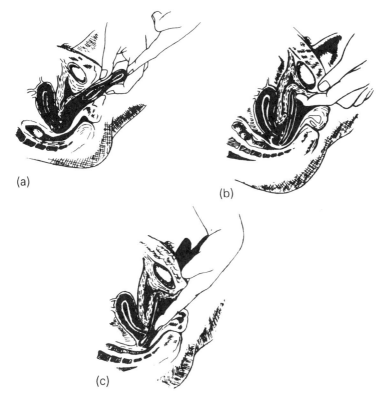

(a)

(b)

(c)

Figure 12.3 Insertion of the diaphragm.

difficult to learn. Psychological fear of touching the genitalia and general patient unwillingness may prevent use.

(c) **Douches (postcoital)**

Water or chemical douching is very unreliable, and often induces pathological infestation of vagina by washing out the normal vaginal flora.

Chemical. The types of preparations are:

- Gels, creams and pressure-pack vaginal foams.
- Vaginal foam tablets.
- Vaginal pessaries.
- Sponge and foam.
- Sponges and tampons with spermicides.

Advantages: Simple to use. Most are inexpensive.

Disadvantages: Often messy. Equipment must be at hand. Some require much preparation. A few are not effective for a time after insertion. High failure rate.

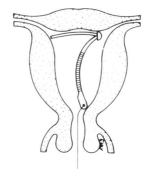

Figure 12.4 Intrauterine contraceptive device 'Copper 7' *in situ*.

(d) **Intrauterine contraceptive devices (IUCDs)** (Fig. 12.4)
This is an age-old technique. For many centuries, the Arabs have placed small intrauterine stones in their camels to prevent pregnancy. Human experience in this century dates back to Grafenberg's first paper in 1928 (a 10-year series); he used rings of silver and gold wire. The IUCDs did not gain popularity until the 1960s, when plastic devices (with flexibility, shape retention, ease of introduction and non-irritability to the uterus) were produced. Nowadays most IUCDs are made of inert plastic and have fine copper wire round the shaft or arms. The copper is thought to enhance the contraceptive effect and reduce the associated bleeding.
Mode of action: The mode of action of the IUCDs is uncertain. They do not cause obstruction to the sperm ascent, hormone imbalance or endometritis. Three theories have been put forward:
- The IUCD accelerates tubal peristalsis, so hindering implantation.
- The encroachment of the IUCD on the endometrium produces a local inflammatory reaction so inhibiting implantation.
- The IUCD may cause a pre-clinical abortion.

The inert plastic IUCDs and even the copper-containing IUCDs do not cause cancer or fetal injury (if accidental pregnancy occurs).
Advantages: Usually easily inserted. Acts immediately after insertion. Complete return to normal after removal. Does not irritate either partner. Very good in those patients with little motivation. Effective contraceptive.

Disadvantages: Must be inserted by a doctor or trained technician. Expulsion may occur (in 10% of cases). Uterine perforation (1 in 2500 cases). Pelvic infection may occur (in 1% of cases). Side effects may be seen (40% of cases), such as:
- Bleeding. Usually after insertion.
- Pain. Abdominal cramps.
- Discharge. Increased normal discharge.

However, 80% of patients will be happy with the amount they bleed each month.

(e) **Surgical sterilization**

Laparoscopic tubal occlusion

The Fallopian tubes are clipped, cauterized or tied in the isthmic region by using a laparoscope.

Advantages: Relatively simple. Little disturbance to the patient, as compared with the formal tubal ligation.

Disadvantages: Requires a general anaesthetic. Peritoneal cavity is entered. Possibility of damage to other organs. Expensive.

Tubal ligation, partial excision or excision

Advantages: Relatively simple. Effective.

Disadvantages: Requires a general or regional anaesthetic. The peritoneal cavity is opened (abdominally or vaginally). There is an associated morbidity and mortality. Expensive.

(f) **Hormonal contraception**

Ovulation may be suppressed either with oestrogens or progestogens. These act at the level of the hypothalamic

Table 12.3 Use and failure rates of methods of contraception

Contraceptive technique	Usage by at-risk population (%)	Failure rate, pregnancies/100 women–years (%)
Combined pill	25	0.5–2.0
IUCD	5	2–3
Condom	20	6–16
Diaphragm and spermicides	10	6–16
Coitus interruptus	20	30
Rhythm	5	30–40
None	15	60–70

centres, suppressing the output of FSH and LH releasing factors.

Usage and failure rates of contraception methods are summarized in Table 12.3.

12.9 INFERTILITY AND SUBFERTILITY

Infertility is the inability to conceive. Subfertility is defined as failure to conceive after 1 year of normal coitus. Of women desiring to become pregnant, 70% do so within 12 months and 85% within 2 years.

About 15% of all married couples will seek advice about fertility. There are only four main questions that need to be answered when investigating fertility:

1. Are there enough sperm? Subfertility in men accounts for at least 30% of infertility problems.
2. Is ovulation occurring? Endocrine factors causing anovulation account for about 15% of infertility problems.
3. Can the egg and sperm meet? Barriers to fertilization account for 40% of infertility.
4. Are there other, more subtle factors, preventing fertility? Unexplained infertility accounts for 15% or more of infertility.

Male infertility

Incidence

About 1 out of 25 men has a problem with the reproductive tract.

Terminology

- Azoospermia – total lack of sperm.
- Oligospermia – decreased number of sperm.
- Aspermia – absence of semen.
- Motility – ability of sperm to move.

Causes of male infertility

1. Testicular atrophy (e.g. mumps orchitis, trauma).
2. Undescended testes.

3. Chromosomal abnormalities (e.g. Klinefelter's syndrome).
4. Epididymal block (e.g. from previous infection or herniorrhaphy).
5. Raised temperature of the testes (e.g. varicocoele).
6. Sperm antibodies.
7. Unexplained or idiopathic is probably the commonest cause for male infertility.

Investigations

Two semen analyses should be performed. The first one (specimen A) is to test the man at his best. The count is done after 4 or 5 days' abstinence from intercourse/ejaculation. The second test (specimen B), to test the man at his worse, is performed within 48 hours of intercourse/ejaculation.

What is a normal count?

Volume: 2–5 ml.
Density: 20–100 million sperms per ml of semen.
Motility: At least 50% should still move after
              4 hours.
Morphology: At least 30% of sperm should appear
              microscopically normal.

Values lower than these do not preclude a normal pregnancy occurring, but if an abnormality is found, then a full urological examination should be performed by an appropriately trained person.

Treatment

Donor insemination (DI)
This is a most successful form of treatment of male subfertility. Fresh DI has a 70% success rate of 12 months, but frozen sperm have a lower pregnancy potential. Sperm donors are usually anonymous to the female recipient, and are screened to ensure that there is no significant family history of genetic disease. Tests are done to exclude venereal disease. Sperm donations are frozen for at least 6 months so that AIDS screening can be performed before the donation is used.

The recipient has her time of ovulation assessed using temperature charts, cervical mucus and daily LH estimations. At her peak ovulatory time a small sample of sperm (usually 0.5 ml) is injected high into the vagina and occasionally through the cervix. The donors are carefully matched to some of the husband's physical characteristics including hair colour, eye colour, body build and race.

Artificial insemination by husband (AIH)
This treatment is less successful, with reported pregnancy rates of about 6–20%. It is used mainly for couples who find donor insemination ethically unacceptable. Highest success rates occur if the infertility is caused by impotence, hypospadias, retrograde ejaculation or cervical mucus hostility. Concentrating the sperm of men with poor counts does not improve pregnancy rates.

IVF
About 20 000–40 000 healthy sperm are used to fertilize ova that have been collected in an IVF procedure. If there are insufficient sperm for this, then intracytoplasmic sperm injection (ICSI) can be used as it requires only a single sperm to achieve fertilization.

Drug treatment
The treatment of male infertility with hormones, anti-oestrogens and zinc has a low success rate unless a hypothalamic–pituitary insufficiency is present and appropriate treatment has been instigated.

Surgery
Varicocoele operations and sperm tube reconstruction have varying published success rates, and probably only improve the success rate in selected individuals.

Antibiotic therapy
If prostatitis or other genitourinary infection is present then antibiotic therapy may improve the potential for fertilization.

Ovulation disorders

Ovulation is the physical rupture of one or more follicles within the ovary, allowing the egg to be released. Problems associated with ovulation account for 15% of infertility.

Provided a woman has a normal uterus, only two things can happen, after ovulation has occurred:

1. Menstruation no later than 16 days after ovulation.
2. Pregnancy.

Causes of anovulation

Physiological causes

(a) Before menarche. The hypothalamus has not yet initiated cyclic hormonal release.
(b) Pregnancy. Amenorrhoea persists due to increasing levels of oestrogen and progesterone.
(c) Lactation. Ovulation is suppressed due to prolactin inhibition of gonadotrophin production.
(d) Postmenopausal. The ovary fails to respond to gonadotrophin.

Local causes

(a) Surgical intervention: oophorectomy.
(b) Chemotherapy.
(c) Hermaphroditism: in this rare condition, both testes and ovaries coexist.
(d) Pseudo-hermaphroditism: female genitalia exist with male gonads.

Genetic causes

Examples are Turner's syndrome, XO genotype, with dwarfism and webbing of the neck.

Endocrine causes

(a) Cerebral. Emotional stress.
(b) Hypothalamic:
   • Postpill amenorrhoea.
   • Anorexia nervosa.
   • Obesity.
   • Marked or relatively rapid weight changes.
(c) Pituitary
   • Hyperprolactinaemia. Excess prolactin is produced during lactation and from certain types of pituitary

tumours. The prolactin depresses the release of the gonadotrophin-releasing hormone.
- Acromegaly.
- Cushing's disease.
- Postpartum ischaemic necrosis of the pituitary due to
  haemorrhage, shock or infection following childbirth and
  sometimes known as Sheehan's syndrome.

(d) Ovary
- Premature menopause. The average age for the menopause is about 52 years. If it occurs when the patient is
  under the age of 35, it is defined as premature. The
  diagnosis is made by high levels of FSH and LH and if
  confirmation is required in doubtful cases, then an
  ovarian biopsy will demonstrate complete absence of
  promordial follicles.
- Polycystic ovary syndrome (Stein–Leventhal syndrome).
  Symptoms may include amenorrhoea or oligomenorrhoea, obesity, hirsutism, infertility and enlarged ovaries.
  (An asymptomatic patient may be found to have polycystic ovaries. This is a normal variation and requires no
  treatment.)
- Arrhenoblastoma of the ovary. This is an androgen-producing tumour which inhibits the hypothalamic centre.
- Granulosa-cell tumour. These tumours produce excess
  oestrogen and, like arrhenoblastoma, are very rare.

(e) Adrenal
- Congenital adrenal hyperplasia. This condition is caused
  by enzyme defects that prevent cortisol synthesis from
  progesterone, so leading to raised ACTH levels. This
  inhibits ovulation.
- Adrenal tumour, producing excess androgens and cate-
  cholamines.

(f) Thyroid
  Both hypo- and hyperthyroidism may lead to abnormal
  feedback responses to the hypothalamus.

Physiology of ovulation

Gonadotrophin-releasing hormone is secreted by the arcuate
nucleus and other areas of the hypothalamus and reach their
target organ, the pituitary, via the pituitary portal venous

system. Follicle-stimulating hormone (FSH) is released and stimulates the development of follicles (which contain the ova). The maturing follicles produce oestrogen, and this has a positive feedback on the pituitary gland. When the follicle reaches a critical diameter, usually about 22 mm, the oestrogen stimulates a luteinizing hormone (LH) surge. This causes rupture of the follicle and so the egg is released. The remnants of the follicle develop into the corpus luteum which produces increasing amounts of progesterone. Progesterone causes the development of a glandular endometrium which becomes ripe to accept the fertilized egg.

Tests of ovulation

1. Menstrual history
   If a woman consistently has regular menstrual cycles of 21–35 days it is almost certain that she ovulates, and that ovulation occurs about 14 days before menstruation.
2. Basal temperature chart
   This is a simple and very useful tool for assessing when ovulation has occurred. Just before ovulation there is a dip in the temperature recording followed by 0.5°C rise in the temperature. This rise is a reflection of progesterone production and indicates ovulation. The best time to have intercourse, if a pregnancy is desired, is just after the dip in temperature (Fig. 12.5).
3. Hormone assays
   (a) Progesterone. If the progesterone level in the blood is greater than 10 nmol/l (3 ng/ml), then ovulation has occurred. For fertile cycles the midluteal level should be above 30 nmol/l (10 ng/ml).
   (b) LH. If tested daily the LH surge may be detected. This can be done by using daily blood samples or by new urinary dip stick methods which are now available to help the timing of ovulation. A blue colour change usually corresponds with the LH surge and indicates that ovulation will follow 24–36 hours later.
4. Endometrial biopsy
   The endometrium demonstrates a secretory pattern if ovulation has occurred. While this is unnecessary for documenting the occurrence of ovulation, a well-timed

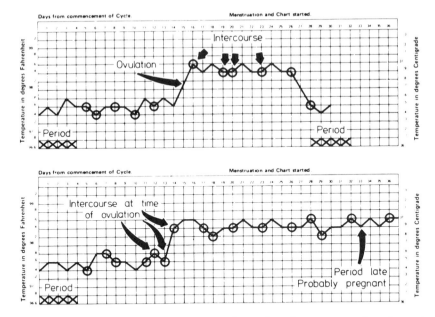

Figure 12.5 Basal body temperature chart showing a normal cycle and the temperature following fertilization.

endometrial biopsy is sometimes done to rule out an inadequate luteal phase, an uncommon cause of infertility.

5. Cervical mucus

This is not a precise way of determining the exact time of ovulation but an increase in mucus production and Spinnbarkeit (stretchiness of the mucus), occurs 2 or 3 days before ovulation. If the cervical mucus is put on a slide and dried, ferning will occur if there is no progesterone present.

Treatment of anovulation

1. Clomiphene

This stimulates ovulation in about 80% of cases but only one-half will conceive. This drug is an anti-oestrogen and acts primarily by blocking the effects of oestrogen on the hypothalamus. Therefore more FSH is produced which stimulates follicle growth. It has the disadvantage of drying up the mucus in some patients because of its anti-oestrogenic effect.

2. Gonadotrophins

   FSH in the form of human menopausal gonadotrophin or human pituitary gonadotrophin can be used to bypass the pituitary gland and directly stimulate the ovaries. The treatment is given by injections, and intensive monitoring with daily blood samples and frequent ultrasound examinations is required. Hyperstimulation of the ovaries can occur which may lead to multiple pregnancies and/or huge cystic ovaries.

3. Gonadotrophin-releasing hormones

   This is successful in patients who have a hypothalamic cause of anovulation and the hormone is delivered via a pulsatile pump. This can be strapped to their belt, with the needle inserted either subcutaneously or intravenously. A bolus of hormone is injected, usually every 90 minutes around the clock. The pump is used until ovulation occurs.

4. Bromocriptine

   This drug achieves an excellent pregnancy rate if anovulation is caused by hyperprolactinaemia. The drug lowers the hormone level, even in cases where there is a micro-adenoma of the pituitary, allowing the return of normal ovulation.

Barriers to fertilization

Tubal disease

Tubal disease accounts for about 35% of infertility problems, despite improvements in prevention and treatment.

Physiology

The Fallopian tubes are amazing organs and have the ability just after ovulation to pick up the ovum and transport it towards the centre of the tube (ampulla). At the same time the sperm swims in the opposite direction towards the egg. Fertilization normally occurs in the ampulla and for about 2 days the fertilized egg stays in the tube where it is supplied with nutrition by the tubal fluid. Then as the progesterone concentration increases, the direction of cilial movements transports the embryo to the uterus for implantation into the uterine lining. For this process to be carried out efficiently the tube must be patent and the cilia intact.

Damage to the fimbrial end of the tube may result in the surface area of the fimbria being greatly reduced, therefore decreasing the chances of picking up the newly released egg. Blockage of the tube will prevent the sperm and the ovum from meeting and this may be caused from within or by adhesions around the outside of the tube.

Causes of tubal disease

1. *Infection*
This is the most common cause of tubal disease. An active tubal infection is called pelvic inflammatory disease (PID). PID is difficult to diagnose and is often confused with many other conditions including appendicitis, endometriosis, ovarian cysts, inflammatory bowel disease, ectopic pregnancy, and even constipation. Therefore it is sometimes necessary to confirm a diagnosis of PID with a laparoscopy. It is a diagnosis that should never be made on history alone.

There are several types of PID, the most damaging of which are gonorrhoea and chlamydia. The latter disease process may be silent and atypical. It can be diagnosed by taking a culture from the cervix or from the tubes themselves if laparoscopy is performed. When diagnosed, treatment should be vigorous and prompt. Even with good care, 10% of women having one episode of gonorrhoea can become infertile. Other infections include chlamydia, mycoplasma, streptococcus and staphylococcus. Tuberculosis these days is rare but devastating, and even if pregnancy does occur, 85% will be ectopic.

2. *Intrauterine contraceptive devices (IUCD)*
Pelvic inflammatory disease is twice as common in women with IUCDs. The risk is greater if she has a history of PID and increases with the number of sexual partners.

3. *Female sterilization*
Between 20 and 30% of women in the reproductive age group use sterilization as a method of contraception. Circumstances change and requests for reversal of sterilization are increasing. Of all the causes of tubal block, reversal of sterilization has the highest pregnancy rate. This depends upon the type of sterilization done initially, but reversal rates as high as 70% are possible with modern methods of sterilization, including clips and rings.

4. *Congenital*
Rare, but occasionally women exposed to diethylstilboestrol
(DES) *in utero* can have non-functioning tubes.

5. *Endometriosis*
Endometriosis of the tube is much less common than endometriosis in other sites, but can cause tubal damage because of the
formation of adhesions around the tube.

6. *Pelvic surgery*
Any pelvic surgery can lead to adhesion formation. Operations
on the ovary should be avoided if at all possible.

Investigations

1.   Laparoscopy and dye insufflation.
2.   Hysteroscopy and endometrial biopsy.
3.   Hysterosalpingogram.

Treatment
Several surgical procedures are performed on the tubes. If the
distal end of the tubes is blocked it may be re-opened by sal-
pingostomy. If the tube is distorted by adhesions, salpingolysis
(freeing of adhesions) may improve tubal function. A midtubal
block may be removed and both ends re-anastomosed. If the
proximal end of the tube is blocked; the tube may be probed
using a hysteroscope and a fine catheter. If this fails then the
block may be removed and the distal end re-implanted into the
uterus.
    Results of surgery may be very poor with a pregnancy rate
of about 10–20%. However, results depend largely on the
extent of disease. Adhesions alone in the presence of otherwise
normal tubes may offer a pregnancy rate of 50–60%. Micro-
surgery, using an operating microscope, improves the accuracy
of the procedure, as does prevention of tissue damage by
gentle handling. An alternative treatment is *in vitro* fertilization,
and this has a pregnancy rate of 15–20% per cycle.

Cervical factor

The cervix is the first major barrier that the sperm must penetrate in order to achieve fertilization. Problems with the cervix
and its mucus account for about 5% of all infertility.

Physiology

Mucus is a normal healthy discharge which is produced by glandular epithelium in the endocervix. The cervix has at least three main functions:

1. Sperm transport.
2. Sperm selection.
3. Sperm storage.

The cervical mucus is a three-dimensional network of linked mucus strands (about 400). Variations in the structure and viscosity of the mucus determine whether the sperm are allowed to penetrate. As the oestradiol secreted from the ovary increases towards the time of ovulation, the water content between the strands of mucus increases, ensuring free movement of the sperm. This allows some to pass through into the uterus and some to be stored in the crypts of the endocervix. The sperm passing through to the uterus take less than 10 minutes to reach the tube while those sperm stored in the crypts have a slower migration towards the tube, thus allowing a constant supply of sperm over the next 24 hours.

It is thought that the cervical mucus also acts as a sieve for abnormal sperm. For every one million sperm deposited in the vagina, only 2000 will be selected to reach the tube.

A knowledge of the normal physiology of cervical mucus production may help the couple decide when the fertile time is near. This is particularly helpful if the female has irregular cycles. If ovulation is delayed the onset of the mucus is usually delayed. If ovulation is going to occur early, the signs of mucus change may begin immediately after the period.

Causes of cervical hostility

1. *Acidity of the cervical mucus*
   The pH of the cervical mucus is important for spermatozoal motility. Motility is inhibited if the pH is below 6.3 or above 8.5. The ideal pH of the mucus occurs 2 or 3 days before ovulation and up until the time of ovulation. After ovulation, under the influence of progesterone, an impenetrable plug is formed in the cervix.
2. *Trauma*
   Trauma from cone biopsy, over-enthusiastic cautery and cervical amputation as part of repair operations can

decrease the amount of fertile mucus and this may decrease the pregnancy rate.

3. *Antisperm antibodies*

   Sperm antibodies are non-sperm specific and form cross-links between the sperm and the glycoproteins of the mucus. This stops forward progression of the sperm. The antibodies can be autoantibodies on the sperm or antibodies within the cervical mucus.

4. *Cervicitis*

   T-mycoplasma and chlamydia are the most common causes of cervicitis, and although these can be easily treated with doxycycline, it is doubtful whether the treatment improves the pregnancy rates.

Investigations

1. *Postcoital test (PCT, Sims–Huhner)*

   The aim of this test is to detect whether motile sperm are present in the mucus. Standardization is difficult but very important because the most common cause of an abnormal test is incorrect timing. An easy way to remember one form of a standard test is 2, 2, 2. The test should be done after 2 days of abstinence from intercourse, within 2 days before ovulation and the mucus should be collected 2 hours after intercourse and examined immediately. A normal postcoital test should disclose at least five motile sperms per high-power field.

   Poor postcoital test. This occurs when no sperm are seen at all in the cervical mucus. Surprisingly this is associated with a 10% pregnancy rate.

   A non-progressive test. This is associated with one or more immotile sperm present in the mucus. This is associated with a 25% pregnancy rate.

   Progressive test. This occurs when one or more motile sperm are seen in the mucus and it is associated with a 40% pregnancy rate.

2. *Hostility test*

   Several tests may be used to detect cervical hostility including the sperm cervical mucus contact test (SCMC) or sperm penetration migration test (Kraemer test). They are all dependent on good timing, good mucus pH, the absence of pus cells and the presence of sperm in the mucus. These tests can detect the presence of antisperm antibodies and demonstrate sperm shaking.

Treatment of cervical hostility

Poor mucus quality can be improved with the use of small doses of oestrogen in the early part of the menstrual cycle, but it is doubtful whether this leads to an improved pregnancy rate. Antisperm antibodies in the cervical mucus may be bypassed with intrauterine artificial insemination of the sperm. More recently treatments using high-dose steroids for a short time have been shown to decrease immunity and improve pregnancy rates, but the side effects of this treatment are unacceptable.

Unexplained infertility

This condition occurs in 10–15% of all infertile patients. It is defined as infertility in a couple who have been trying to become pregnant for at least 2 years, in whom no abnormality has been found with the sperm count, ovulation and tubal assessment including a laparoscopy.

These patients usually see many doctors and the constant refrain from doctors and relatives is 'relax'; 'go and have a holiday' or 'it's all psychological'.

Most patients hate to hear from the doctor that all the tests are normal. They often need to find something wrong, something to explain why they are not pregnant.

Some possible causes of the unexplained infertility

1. *Minimal endometriosis*

   This is a condition in which the tissue lining of the uterus is found in ectopic sites outside the uterus. If severe, it may cause excruciating dysmenorrhoea and dyspareunia. Even in a mild form it can be associated with infertility. How endometriosis causes infertility is unclear. It is very rare for it to cause tubal blockage. The diagnosis of minimal endometriosis is usually made at laparoscopy and treatment is controversial.

   (a) Diathermy of the endometriotic spots is often done at the same time as laparoscopy.

(b) Progestogens used continuously may reduce endometriosis.

(c) Danazol (Danocrine), a synthetic steroid, is the most common drug at present used in the treatment of endometriosis. This is a potent androgen and some patients find the side effects unacceptable.

(d) Gonadotrophin-releasing hormone (GnRH) analogue is given in high doses, suppressing the LH, and therefore stopping ovulation and menstruation. The only recorded side effects of this non-steroid are those of oestrogen deficiency. It can be taken as a nasal spray or as a daily injection.

2. *Deficient luteal progesterone*
   Occasionally in regularly ovulating women, progesterone deficiency can occur and is diagnosed by serial progesterone estimations in the luteal phase, and/or endometrial biopsy. Progestogen supplements have been shown to be of limited value in the treatment of this condition and the use of gonadotrophin has not yet been fully assessed.

3. *Intrauterine adhesions*
   In patients with unexplained infertility and who have questionable findings on hysterosalpingogram, the use of hysteroscopy has demonstrated a higher incidence of intrauterine pathology than in control groups. Pregnancy rates may be improved when these factors have been treated.

4. *Asymptomatic infection*
   Intrauterine T-mycoplasma and chlamydia may cause infertility without obvious macroscopic damage.

5. *Psychological factors*
   Many believe that unexplained infertility is all psychological. This is not true. However, infertility and the investigation and treatment of infertility may itself cause emotional trauma. Many women suffer severely every time a period comes. Most studies, however, cannot find a difference in the basic personalities of infertile and fertile women. Despite this, infertility gives the couple an insoluble problem that strains them physically, emotionally and financially. Suicide is twice as common in childless couples. Despite common belief, adoption does not increase the chance of pregnancy.

Recent advances in the treatment of infertility

1. *In-vitro fertilization (IVF)*

   This refers to the process used to conceive a child outside the body. Ova may be picked up from stimulated ovaries either using a laparoscopic technique or transvaginal ultrasound. The technique was developed by Steptoe and Edwards and the first IVF baby was born in the UK in the late 1970s. By the end of 1994, 40 000 babies have been born by this technique worldwide.

   The technique was developed to overcome infertility in women with damaged tubes, but the indications have broadened to include women with unexplained infertility and men with poor sperm counts.

   The success rate is low (about 15%). The miscarriage rate is high, so the take-home baby rate may be reduced to 10% per cycle.

2. *Gamete Intra-Fallopian Transfer (GIFT)*

   This was developed in 1984 in San Antonio, Texas by Dr Ricardo Asch. This technique involves the placement of gametes (eggs and sperm) separately into the catheter followed by injection directly into the Fallopian tubes during laparoscopy. Fertilization occurs in the Fallopian tube, not outside the body as with IVF.

   GIFT is not suitable for women with damaged tubes, but has higher success rates than IVF in women with other causes of infertility. The main indications for this technique are couples with unexplained infertility or a severe male factor or women with an immunological infertility.

3. *Sperm microinjection*

   This technique is used for men with very low sperm counts.

   - Sub Zonal Injection (SUZI)

     A single sperm is injected into the ovum beneath the zona pellucida. Pregnancy rates are low.
   - Intra Cytoplasmic Sperm Injection (ICSI)

     A single sperm is injected directly through the ovum cell membrane. This is a new technique which holds a great deal of promise and may largely replace donor insemination.

These new techniques have revolutionized the treatment of the infertile couple. Patients can now be treated almost indefinitely. Using donor eggs, patients as old as 65 have become pregnant. We must be careful to allow and encourage adequate counselling and consideration of ethical issues involved with these scientific advances. Patients must be given opportunities to get off the 'merry-go-round' of infertility investigations and treatment.

13

Genital tract infections and discharge

13.1 GENERAL INSTRUCTIONAL OBJECTIVE

The students should understand genital tract infections so that they can diagnose, appreciate the management and initiate the treatment of these conditions.

13.2 SPECIFIC BEHAVIOURAL OBJECTIVES

1. Discuss pathological and physiological vaginal discharge.
2. Discuss the aetiological factors involved in common genital tract infection.
3. Discuss the clinical features of genital tract infections.
4. Examine patient(s) and demonstrate an ability to differentiate between normal vaginal secretion and pathological discharge.
5. Examine patient(s) and demonstrate an ability to elicit and recognize signs of endometritis, salpingitis and pelvic peritonitis.
6. Indicate the appropriate investigations that will aid the diagnosis and management of genital tract infection.
7. Discuss the appropriate therapy of genital tract infections.
8. Explain the public health and the possible social implications of genital tract infection.
9. Discuss the sequelae of genital tract infection.

13.3 REASONS FOR LEARNING ABOUT GENITAL TRACT INFECTION

Vaginal discharge is the single most common presenting complaint of patients attending a general gynaecological clinic. It is frequently associated with other symptoms such as pain, vaginal pruritus and dyspareunia, or presents as a complication of contraception. The discharge may be pathological or be an excessive 'physiological' discharge. The distinction between the various causes of pathological discharge is important so that appropriate therapy may be commenced. Inappropriate therapy will frequently aggravate the presenting problem or produce further iatrogenic problems. Inappropriate treatment of a physiological discharge may create a pathological discharge.

Genital tract infection, if not diagnosed early and treated appropriately, may have extremely disabling long-term effects on both the patient and her partner because of infertility or recurrent acute exacerbation of a chronic infection, which may eventually result in surgical pelvic clearance to relieve her symptoms.

Thus, although vaginal discharge and pelvic infection and common gynaecological problems and the diagnosis and treatment are straightforward, mismanagement can result in aggravation of the patient's symptoms and the initiation of long-term problems.

13.4 ACHIEVEMENT OF SPECIFIC BEHAVIOURS

Students will take part in tutorial discussion groups on the bacteriology, symptoms and signs of pelvic infection as well as methods of confirming the diagnosis and the appropriate treatment for each type of infection. In the clinics and wards, they will be expected to be able to elicit the symptoms and identify the signs of genital tract infection, and to perform appropriate 'office' investigations, take appropriate bacteriological swabs and suggest appropriate therapy.

13.5 VAGINAL DISCHARGE

The vagina of a hormonally active woman is moist, due to secretions from vaginal transudate and cervical mucus, and to a lesser extent from uterine secretion, Fallopian tube secretion and Bartholin's gland secretion.

The volume of this secretion that is accepted as normal by individual women covers a wide range. Excessive normal secretion (called leucorrhoea) is usually associated with staining of

underclothes and vaginal odour due to the heat denaturation of the proteins in the secretions. The secretions are clear to white and range in consistency from the thick mucus before ovulation to a thin watery more profuse secretion (the ovulatory cascade).
  Increased production of secretions is associated with:

1. Increased production of the ovarian steroids (oestrogens in particular), which occurs:
    (a) At the time of ovulation – ovulatory cascade.
    (b) When oestrogenic oral contraceptives are used.
    (c) In pregnancy.
    (d) With cervical ectopic columnar epithelium (also incorrectly called a cervical erosion), hypertrophy of endocervical columnar glands, and their extension from the cervical canal onto the ectocervix (commonly as a result of increased oestrogenic stimulus).
2. Increased vaginal transudate, which is associated with:
    (a) Sexual excitement.
    (b) Vaginal irritation, such as chemical irritation from inappropriate or too frequent douches or vaginal applications or even use of spermicides.
3. Uterine secretion, which occurs:
    (a) Before menstruation. Secretory changes induced in the endocervical and endometrial glands may give a premenstrual increase in vaginal discharge.
    (b) Following menstruation when the last days of menstrual flow may be prolonged.
    (c) Irritation from an intrauterine contraceptive device (IUCD).
4. Pelvic congestion, which may be due to pelvic pathology.
5. Granuloma (arising in the suture line at the vaginal vault following a hysterectomy), which can give rise to a profuse discharge. It is best treated by cautery, either chemically or by diathermy.

Management of leucorrhoea

Adequate history

Make specific enquiries about:

1. Timing of discharge – midcycle or premenstrual exacerbation.

2. Oral contraception – especially oestrogenic type.
3. Use of douches, additions to bath water or deodorizing sprays.
4. Recent medications – especially vaginal applications, spermicides.
5. Recent pregnancy.

Examination

Assess the amount of discharge, whether there is any redness of the vulval, vaginal or perianal skin. Exclude pelvic or vaginal infection (examine a wet preparation of the vaginal discharge and if there is any doubt, take a high vaginal swab and an endocervical swab for culture and sensitivity).

Making a wet preparation
A drop of the discharge is placed on each of two separate glass slides. A drop of normal saline is added to the one and a drop of 10% potassium hydroxide (KOH) is added to the other and mixed with the discharge using a plastic or wooden stick. Each slide is then smelt to see if any odour is released. (In the presence of *Gardnerella vaginalis* an amine is released, giving a characteristic odour positive whiff/sniff test.) A glass cover slip is placed over the discharge and the slide viewed under low magnification using a microscope.

In the saline preparation one notes the presence of epithelial cells, pus cells, bacteria (mainly lactobacilli), motile organisms such as trichomonads or 'clue cells' (see below). KOH results in lysis of much of the cellular debris and results in the epithelial and white blood cells appearing very pale. The 'ghosting' of these cells makes it easier to see fungal elements such as mycelia or spores.

The diagnostic feature of leucorrhoea is that there are no pus cells visible on microscopy in the wet saline preparation.

Treatment

1. Explain the cause – reassurance that it is not due to an infection may be all that is required.
2. Eliminate any aggravating cause (such as high-dose oestrogenic pill or inappropriate vaginal applications).

3. Give general advice regarding hygiene, limiting local heat to the genital area, taking frequent showers during hot weather, avoiding deodorizing sprays, using cotton underclothes that absorb some of the secretions.
4. Ablative therapy (cryocautery, diathermy, laser) to the cervix to reduce the number of endocervical glands. This may be used in a minority of persistent cases. However, if the original precipitating factor is still present (e.g. oral contraception) relief will be short-lived.

Pathological discharges

Presentation (Table 13.1)

These usually present with other symptoms, such as vaginal/vulval pruritus, dyspareunia or pelvic pain. Many of the infective causes of vaginal discharge produce a classical vaginal reaction; however, more frequently, there is a non-specific discharge and a non-specific vaginal reaction. Even experienced gynaecologists can frequently misinterpret the nature of the vaginal discharge. It is important to realize that many women have organisms that can cause a pathological discharge present in their vaginas without having any symptoms at all. In studies of well women attending family planning clinics, 15–30% of women have been found to have monilia or *Gardnerella vaginalis*, 10–15% trichomonas and 10–20% have *Chlamydia trachomatis*.

Monilial vaginitis (thrush)

Cause: This is caused by a yeast-like fungus *Candida albicans*, which appears microscopically (following Gram-staining) or in a wet preparation as long filaments (mycelia) or as spores. It can be found in the vagina of 15–30% of asymptomatic women.

Presentation: The discharge is classically thick white and cheesy, and tends to stick to the walls of the vagina, leaving a reddened area when removed. The vagina may be extremely sore, making examination painful.

Precipitating factors: The organism thrives in the presence of

Table 13.1 Features of vaginal infections

Symptom	Normal	Moniliasis	Gardnerella vaginitis	Trichomoniasis
Discharge	Scant, varies with menstrual cycle	White, often thick. May be absent	Profuse – yellow or green	Profuse, usually yellow or green, often frothy
Itch	Absent	Present, may be the only feature	Present	Present
Odour	Absent	Absent	Fishy, worse after intercourse	Present, fishy odour
Inflammation	Absent	Present	Present	Present, may have urinary symptoms
Tests that can be performed in the surgery				
pH	⩽4.5	⩽4.5	>4.5	>4.5
KOH (10%) Whiff test	Negative	Negative	Positive	May be positive
Wet film or Gram stain of a high vaginal swab				
Polymorphs	Few	Increased	Increased	Few
Specific features	Nil	Mycelia and spores (in KOH prep)	Mobile trichomonads seen in saline prep	'Clue cells'
Lactobacilli	Predominant	Predominant	Reduced	Reduced
Other organisms	Few	Few	Increased	Increased
Further investigations				
Fluorescent microscopy	Absent	Absent	Absent	Positive
Acridine orange culture		Sabouraud's medium	(Rarely indicated)	Feinberg–Whittington medium (rarely indicated)

carbohydrate; thus it is common during pregnancy or the second half of the menstrual cycle, in diabetes and following broad-spectrum antibiotics, which destroy the normal vaginal flora.

Diagnosis: This is made by: (1) examining a wet preparation using either a saline or 10% KOH and seeing the mycelia and spores; and (2) culture using a Sabouraud's medium.

Treatment: This can either be local or oral.

Local therapy

1. Remove any precipitating cause.
2. Imidazole drugs are very effective; for example, clotrimazole, econazole or miconazole in cream or pessaries for 3 to 6 days. The patient should be instructed to place the pessaries or the cream applicator as high as comfortable in the vagina, so that the whole length of the vagina is exposed to the medication. Clotrimazole may be given as a single-dose pessary (500 mg) which is an advantage when patient compliance is a problem. Vaginal applications may be supplemented with local cream for vulvitis.
3. Mycostatin (Nystatin) in the form of pessaries or cream was once widely used. The treatment should be continued for at least 14 days, even if the symptoms have subsided. Because of the long duration of treatment, patient compliance is not as good as for the drugs that can be used for shorter periods of time. Oral Nystatin tablets (usually give as one tablet three times a day) will remove monilia at least temporarily from the gastrointestinal tract, and was thought to lead to a lower recurrence rate by reducing the risk of self-re-infection of the vagina. This has been disputed as 2 weeks of local miconazole cream has been shown to be more effective than a combination of oral and local Nystatin. Oral Nystatin does not treat monilial vaginitis, as it is not absorbed from the bowel.
4. Dihydroxyquinoline (Floraquin) pessaries can be used for both trichomonal and monilial vaginitis. (However, both are not as effective as the more specific therapy of imidazole drugs for monilia or metronidizole (Flagyl) for trichomonas.)

Oral therapy
Many patients prefer to use oral treatment as they are not as messy and this leads to better compliance.

- *Ketoconazole (200 mg)*: this is the only imidazole drug that is significantly absorbed after oral administration and is useful for vaginal candidiasis. It is as effective as local treatments but is more expensive. An 80–90% cure can be achieved with two tablets daily for 5 days, taken with a meal. The drug is excreted onto the skin reaching its maximal level after 2–4 hours. Patients should be advised not to bath or shower for at least 4–6 hours after taking the drug.
- *Fluoconazole (150 mg)*: this is now available as single-dose therapy for monilia. It is as effective as ketaconazole, but is more expensive.

Recurrent monilia
Patients either get recurrent infection as local intravaginal spores germinate or may be re-infected from a sexual partner. Spores are not affected by either local or oral treatment. Re-infection from the patient's own bowel flora is no longer thought to be such an important factor in causing recurrence. Relapse is more likely to occur at the time of the menses probably as a result of changes in the pH in the vagina. Precipitating causes such as antibiotic use, diabetes or even HIV should be sought.

Patients should ideally be given oral ketaconazole for 1 week and then a further 5-day course after another week. This allows any spores present to germinate first. The partner should be treated either with local imidazole cream applied twice daily for 7–10 days or oral ketaconazole.

Monilia in pregnancy
Local treatment with nystatin or chlotrimazole can be used.

Gardnerella vaginitis

Cause: This is caused by a small, non-motile, Gram-variable coccobacillus (*Gardnerella vaginalis*). It can be found in the vagina of 10–30% of asymptomatic women.

Presentation: The typical clinical presentation includes a variable amount of discharge that has a fishy or unpleasant vaginal odour and is often more pronounced after intercourse. The discharge has a homogeneous, thin consistency, which may cause local irritation but not pruritus.

Diagnosis: Vaginal pH > 4.5. When 10% KOH is added to the wet preparation, a fishy amine odour is released (positive whiff/sniff test).

Microscopic examination of a wet preparation mounted on a slide will show large numbers of coccobacilli floating between and attached to vaginal epithelial cells in a stippled manner ('clue cells'). The combination of the typical clinical findings and a positive whiff test is diagnostic of *Gardnerella vaginitis*, even if clue cells are absent.

Treatment: Tinidazole 2 g (four tablets) taken as a single dose with a meal. Alcohol should be avoided as this drug like metronidazole is metabolized in the liver to antabuse and can cause nausea and vomiting. Some 10% of men will be asymptomatic carriers of this bacteria and so should be treated initially or if a recurrence occurs.

Metronidazole (2 g as a single dose or 200 mg three times daily × 7 days) can also be used. This does cause more gastrointestinal problems and leads to poorer compliance. Tetracycline and ampicillin have also been shown to be effective. More recently clindamycin prosphate (Dalacinc) cream has become available and is as effective as the oral treatment.

Treatment in pregnancy: Patients can safely be given amoxicillin 250 mg 8-hourly for 7–10 days during pregnancy or clindamycin phosphate cream locally.

Trichomonal vaginitis

Cause: This is caused by a flagellated unicellular organism with four flagella anteriorly and a terminal membranous stylus similar in size to a neutrophil. It is harboured, usually asymptomatically, in 2–10% of males and can be transmitted as a venereal disease. It can also be found in the vagina of 10–15% of asymptomatic patients, and appears to require more than just its presence in order to become established and to cause symptoms. (Raising the vaginal pH shortly after menstruation may allow the establishment of the infection.)

Presentation: The discharge is classically frothy and yellow–

green in colour, and has a typical fishy odour. The amount of the discharge varies; in acute cases it is usually profuse and commonly associated with pruritus. It is often associated with dysuria. The vaginal walls and cervix may have an inflamed appearance, with punctate 'strawberry' spots. Dysuria is often a feature of this infection due to the involvement of the Skene's tubules in the urethra. The cervix may have a strawberry-like appearance due to punctate inflammatory vessels present on the cervix.

Diagnosis: If these signs are absent, however, the diagnosis can be confirmed by placing a drop of the discharge and diluting it with a drop of saline on a slide, and examining for motile organisms. These are usually easily distinguished from the only other motile 'organisms' commonly found in the vagina – sperm. It can also easily be identified on a PAP smear and on using fluorescence microscopy using acridine orange which stains the DNA of the trichomonads. It can be cultured using the Feinberg–Whittington medium, but this is expensive and less accurate than fluorescent microscopy.

Treatment: Tinidazole (Fasigyn) may be given as a single dose of 2 g (four tablets). Alternatively metronidazole (e.g. Flagyl) 200 mg three times daily for 7 days can be used. Alcohol should be avoided with both these drugs (see above). The male partner should be treated with the same dose, and certainly whenever there is a recurrence. It is advisable to treat an asymptomatic woman in whom trichomonas has been found, before it becomes an established infection.

Treatment in pregnancy: both of the above drugs have been used in late pregnancy without any obvious complications. Their safety has not been established in early pregnancy and so should be avoided. Dihydroxyquinoline (Floraquin) pessaries can be used for trichomonal and monilial vaginitis in early pregnancy.

Chlamydia trachomatis

Cause: Genital tract infection with *Chlamydia trachomatis* (serotypes D–K) is an important and common sexually transmitted disease. It is the most commonly identified cause of urethritis in young men. In women it has been isolated from multiple sites in the genital tract including the cervix (mucopurulent cervicitis), the urethra (frequency/dysuria syndrome), Bartholin-glands (Bartholinitis), the endometrium (endometritis) and the Fallopian tubes (salpingitis). In most western communities chlamydial infection is much more common than gonococcal infection.

Presentation: Infection in women is frequently asymptomatic. Routine screening at family planning and antenatal clinics have shown 10–20% of sexually active women have an unsuspected cervical chlamydial infection. Tubal damage resulting in infertility may result from both acute chlamydial salpingitis or from asymptomatic unrecognized chlamydial infection. Some women may present with a mucopurulent discharge.

In pregnancy, cervical chlamydial infection has been associated with premature delivery, amnionitis and puerperal infection. Chlamydial infection occurs in 60–70% of the neonates born to women with cervical chlamydial infection. Neonatal conjunctivitis occurs in 35–50% of cases and neonatal pneumonia in 10–20% of cases.

Diagnosis: (1) Endocervical swab and using immunofluorescent staining which utilizes monoclonal antibodies detect chlamydial antigens. (2) Cell culture techniques can be used to detect *Chlamydia trachomatis* but are more expensive and not as readily available.

Treatment: Tetracycline and erythromycin are the antibiotic agents most commonly used for treatment of known or suspected chlamydial infection. The current recommendation is doxycycline 200 mg daily for 10 days, abstinence from intercourse during treatment and the concurrent treatment of sexual partners. Erythromycin (500 mg three times daily for 10 days) is an alternative for treatment during pregnancy or lactation.

Atrophic vaginitis

This is associated with the very thin vaginal epithelium of the postmenopausal woman, which is often easily injured or infected. The responsible organisms are usually non-specific (producing a mixed growth on culture) and of low virulence. The discharge is thin, purulent and often blood-stained and the vagina may appear red and have many tiny bleeding points.

Vaginal, vulval and perineal soreness are frequently present and may make an adequate examination of the patient difficult.

Treatment: This consists of oestrogen, locally in the vagina using either tablets (oestradiol 25 µg) or creams (oestriol). Oral oestrogens can be used and if the uterus is still *in situ*, progestogen must be used to reduce the risk of endometrial hyperplasia (see Chapter 15).

Childhood vaginitis

This is uncommon and may be associated with a wide range of organisms, which are usually of low virulence. Whenever a child presents with a vaginal discharge, always suspect a foreign body. However, *Neisseria gonorrhoeae* and *Trichomonas vaginalis* do occur in children and, as in the case of persistent discharges, one should think of possible abuse.

When examining a young child vaginally, a nasal speculum is a good substitute for the speculum, and a paediatric cystoscope is a useful instrument for removing foreign bodies.

Treatment may also include oral antibiotics, according to the sensitivities of the organisms found in a swab from the discharge. In severe cases, 0.2 mg of oestrogen daily, or twice daily, for 7–10 days, may help in improving vaginal resistance to infection.

Chronic cervicitis

This almost never occurs as a single entity. When there is infection in the tissues of the cervix, there is also more widespread infection of the parametrium, endometrium and/or Fallopian tubes. The term 'chronic cervicitis' has been used loosely in many cases to describe ectopic columnar epithelium on the ectocervix. Chronic cervicitis occurs when the stroma of the cervix is involved in a chronic bacterial infection. This may occur when ectopic columnar epithelium becomes infected but more commonly follows a delivery, an abortion or an operation during which the cervix is torn and then becomes infected.

The term 'erosion' is often used to describe any lesion on the cervix that is not normal squamous epithelium. Included under this broad term of erosion may be found such conditions as physiological ectopic columnar epithelium, infected ectopic columnar epithelium, chronic cervicitis, dysplasia of the cervix, neoplasia of the cervix and even true erosions due to loss of epithelium. The term is thus too broad and should not be used when a better description is available.

Ectopic columnar epithelium is a response to oestrogen stimulation, and is thus common during pregnancy and in women using oral contraceptives.

If the discharge is causing distress to the patient, remove the precipitating cause, such as oral contraception, and any factor giving rise to discomfort, such as heat and non-absorbent clothing. Ablative therapy, such as cervical cauterization by diathermy under anaesthesia, or cryocautery without anaesthesia, may be used when the discharge is particularly troublesome. However, if the precipitating cause is not removed, the discharge will return.

Trachelorrhaphy, or cervical amputation, is usually only performed when the cervix has been lacerated or traumatized.

Diathermy and trachelorrhaphy may give rise to primary or secondary haemorrhage, cervical stenosis or cervical incompetence.

When there is a bacterial chronic cervicitis, the bacteria and their antibiotic sensitivities should be determined by a cervical and high vaginal swab, although systemic antibiotics have little effect when used alone, and the main treatment is surgical.

Chemical vaginitis/cervicitis

Repeated inappropriate therapy of a vaginal discharge can precipitate irritation of the vaginal epithelium, causing discomfort, and lead to destruction of the normal flora. Infection should be excluded by means of a wet preparation and a vaginal swab, the inappropriate therapy withdrawn, and the patient reassured. The problem is self-limiting and, if necessary, a bland cream, for example, Aci-jel with an appropriate pH may be administered. Severe chemical vaginitis may result from douches with such substances as undiluted Dettol, PHisohex, lye or Condys crystals. This may be so severe that admission to hospital for pain relief and catheterization may be required.

A foreign body – the most common being a forgotten tampon in the adult patient, or any variety of objects in the infant or child – may produce an offensive discharge. The only treatment required is removal of the foreign body. Any child with a vaginal discharge should be considered as having a foreign body in the vagina, until proved otherwise by an adequate examination which in some cases will require an anaesthetic.

13.6 HERPES GENITALIS

Cause: Acute primary herpes is becoming a more frequent infecting agent of the vulva, vagina, perineum and bladder and up to 10% of the population may be infected. It is usually caused by the type 2 herpes virus but can be associated with type 1 virus as well. Venereal spread of the disease is possible and is predisposed to by a moist environment, such as excessive leucorrhoea, or by any decline in general health.

Presentation: The symptoms are of severe discomfort and pain in the infected area, which may be associated with urinary retention in severe infections. The retention is due to the severe dysuria when urine comes into contact with the infected area, or may be due to infection in the bladder or urethra. The primary and secondary infections have a similar appearance to the vesicles of a cold sore, which is usually caused by the type 1 herpes virus. Recurrent herpes usually occurs at the same site each time and may be preceded by itching and is often associated with times of stress.

Diagnosis: Herpes infection can be confirmed by viral culture and can be suspected from inclusion bodies in the cells taken from a cervical smear (PAP). It can also be rapidly identified using immunofluorescent techniques on swabs taken from the base of the ulcer. Serology can also be used to demonstrate a four-fold rise in antibody titres over a 2–3-week period using paired sera.

Treatment: This is difficult. Acyclovir is active against herpes simplex viruses and can be used for acute and recurrent genital infections. To be effective the drug must be given as early as possible in the acute illness. Prophylactic treatment may be given for recurrent severe disease and reduces both the frequency and severity of attacks.

Severe episodes may require hospitalization, systemic pain relief, catheterization and treatment of secondary infection. Povidone–iodine has been used locally to control secondary infection. Idoxuridine ointment (Stoxil) has been tried in the past and found not to be very effective.

Genital herpes and pregnancy

It is important for medical personnel to be aware that the patient has a history of recurrent herpes. The danger period is during labour after rupture of the membranes. There is a danger that the infant may develop herpes encephalitis. The risk appears to be about 4% with recurrent herpes and 50% with acute primary herpes at the time of delivery. Patients with a history of herpes should be told to come to hospital at the onset of labour. The vulva should be carefully inspected for evidence of infection. If there are any suspicious lesions and the membranes have been ruptured for less than 4 hours then delivery should be by a Caesarean section.

13.7 HUMAN IMMUNODEFICIENCY VIRUS INFECTION

Human immunodeficiency virus (HIV) infection is a newly discovered communicable disease that has become pandemic in less than 5 years. HIV is a blood-borne and sexually transmissible organism and was identified as a retrovirus in 1983.

The routes of infection and infection risk include:

Route	Infection risk
Blood or blood product transfusion	Almost certain
Sharing needles	Very high
Mother to child	50%
Passive (receptive) anal intercourse	Very high
Vaginal intercourse (male to female)	High
Anal intercourse (active partner)	Medium
Vaginal intercourse (female to male)	Medium
Oral sex	Low
Kissing	Hypothetical only

Following infection an acute mononucleosis-like illness may develop within 6 weeks of exposure to HIV. Some people remain symptomless after primary infection although the majority will develop antibodies to HIV within 6 months of exposure. Once a diagnosis of AIDS has been made the patient should be referred to a specialized AIDS unit. These units take a comprehensive approach to the management of the patient with emphasis on medical and neuropsychiatric assessment, patient counselling and education.

Artificial insemination has been shown to transmit HIV when semen is obtained from infected donors. All donors must now sign a declaration regarding risk factors and semen is accepted only if the donor is HIV seronegative. The semen is frozen and stored for 6 months and used only if the donor is found to be seronegative when re-tested after that time.

In pregnancy where the mother is HIV antibody positive the risk of AIDS in the fetus is approximately 30%. The risk of HIV infection in the infant may be higher than 65%, following intrapartum exposure. Careful supervision is required in pregnancy and the infant should be delivered in a unit capable of providing a high level of perinatal support. Currently, Caesarean section is not indicated. Breast-feeding has been associated with postnatal HIV transmission and its presence in cell-free breast milk has been demonstrated.

13.8 PELVIC INFECTIONS

These infections affect the genital organs above the level of the cervix. The infection may extend into the pelvic cavity giving rise to pelvic peritonitis, involve nearby organs or form a pelvic abscess.

Pelvic infections are usually bacterial, the most common bacteria being anaerobic organisms, chlamydia and Gram-negative organisms, especially *Escherichia coli* and *Neisseria gonorrhoeae*. The symptoms vary widely, depending upon the main site of the infection, the extent of the infection and whether it is acute or chronic.

Acute infection

Puerperal and postabortal infections

The placental site and any placental remnants provide good culture media for infection.

Cause: The most common organisms are anaerobic organisms (bacteroides), *Escherichia coli*, *Chlamydia trachomatis*, other Gram-negative bacilli, clostridium and streptococci. Invasion of the tissues is rapid, and general systemic symptoms result from the toxaemia. Bacteraemia may also occur and progress to septicaemia with possible death of the patient from septic shock, unless adequate treatment is commenced promptly.

Pathology: Acute inflammation is found in the endometrium. Acute salpingitis of the interstitium is common, with only minimal involvement of the endosalpinx until late in the disease (unless the gonococcus is involved). A tubo-ovarian abscess may form, and any peritonitis is usually localized to the pouch of Douglas.

Presentation: Clinically, in well-established infection, the patient looks ill, with a marked pyrexia, tachycardia and perhaps rigors. Pelvic pain and tenderness are present after the infection has spread beyond the endometrium. There is usually a brown or blood-stained offensive heavy lochial loss. The uterus may be soft and larger than expected due to delayed involution, and tender as the infection spreads towards the serosal surface of the uterus.

Signs of peritonitis may be present if the infection has involved the pouch of Douglas, although the lower abdominal rebound tenderness and guarding may not be as marked as expected. (Pouch of Douglas infection produces less marked abdominal signs.) Bowel sounds are usually present.

Complications: If septicaemia and endotoxic shock develop, the blood pressure may fall and the pulse becomes weak and difficult to detect. The temperature may become subnormal and the patient's skin is cold and has a cyanosed blotchy appearance. Oliguria or anuria may develop.

The first evidence of pelvic vein thrombophlebitis, induced by the pelvic infection, may be pulmonary embolism. The differential diagnosis must include acute ruptured appendicitis; if there is any doubt, a laparotomy or laparoscopy is indicated.

Treatment: Take steps to identify the infecting organisms by:

1. Taking vaginal and endocervical swabs (for immediate

microscopy of a smear from the swab) and culture for organisms (aerobic and anaerobic).

2. Blood cultures are best taken during the upward spikes of the temperature.
3. Midstream urine specimen for possible urinary tract infection.

Broad-spectrum antibiotic therapy should be started as early as possible, in an adequate dose so as to combat possible Gram-positive or Gram-negative organisms as well as anaerobic organisms. A possible combination is a high-dose penicillin (which may be given intravenously) together with an aminoglycoside, such as gentamicin and metronidazole, for anaerobic cover. These drugs should be continued until the patient has been apyrexial and asymptomatic for 48 hours.

Blood loss is replaced and fluid and electrolyte balance must be carefully controlled. Oliguria or anuria require prompt correction.

If products of conception remain in the uterus, they should be removed carefully after the patient has been resuscitated and an antibiotic cover has been established.

Pelvic inflammatory disease

Acute salpingitis

Presentation: Abdominal pain usually starts after a menstrual period and associated vaginal discharge and fever.

Population at risk:

1. Nuliparous women under the age of 25.
2. Women with multiple sexual partners.
3. Intrauterine contraceptive device (IUCD) users.

Post-surgery:

1. Termination of pregnancy.
2. Insertion of IUCD.
3. Dilatation and curettage.
4. Hysterosalpingogram.
5. Hysteroscopy.

In about 2–4% of cases salpingitis results from spread of infection from surrounding organs and is associated with appendicitis, Chrohn's disease, etc.

Acute salpingitis will develop in 10–20% of women who have cervical gonorrhoea and in 6–10% of women with cervical *Chlamydia trachomatis* infection.

Cause: This varies from country to country:

Chlamydia trachomatis	40–60%
N. *Gonorrhoea*	15–18%
Mycoplasma hominis	10–15%
Anaerobes	3–5%
Unknown	15–20%

Anaerobes and endogenous bacteria are more likely to be found in older females after surgery, associated with IUCDs and re-infections.

Management: Admit to hospital if symptoms severe. If diagnosis unclear – laparoscopy.

Investigations:

1. Cervical swabs for infecting organisms.
2. Blood culture if temperature >38°C.
3. Full blood count and erythrocyte sedimentation rate (ESR).

Treatment:

1. Antipyretics – paracetamol.
2. Analgesics.
3. Nurse in modified Fowler's position (semi-upright) to reduce the risk of subphrenic abscess.
4. Drug treatment. Commence intravenous broad-spectrum antibiotics. Combination of amoxicillin, tetracycline or aminoglycoside and metronidazole. Must give adequate doses. Continue for 48 hours after temperature and clinical signs have settled before starting on oral treatment which should be for at least 2 weeks. If symptoms do not improve after 24 hours the diagnosis must be reviewed as patient may require laparoscopy.

Progress of the disease can be followed by twice-weekly white blood cell (WBC) and ESR measurements. Failure to improve suggests unresolved disease.

Long-term sequelae:

1. Chronic abdominal pain from adhesions or hydrosalpinx.
2. Subsequent tubal ectopic pregnancy rate increases seven-fold.
3. Risk of re-infection.
4. Infertility depends on the severity and numbers of attacks 15% after first attack, 30% after the second attack and >60% after three attacks.
5. Curtis–Fitzhugh syndrome (peri-hepatitis) with resulting adhesions round the liver usually associated with *Chlamydia trachomatis*.

Gonococcal infection

This is one of the most common venereal diseases, after chlamydia infection. It frequently is not detected in the female by either the patient or doctor, as it is commonly asymptomatic unless it produces an acute pelvic infection. The organism is fragile and will not be detected by normal bacterial swabs or cultures.

Pathogenesis: Gonorrhoea commonly spreads from the cervix via the endometrium to the endosalpinx, with possible exudation into the pelvic cavity with involvement of the ovary and peritoneum.

As the endosalpinx is the first affected part of the tube, adhesive occlusion of the tube (particularly at the fimbriated end) is common, forming a pyosalpinx.

Presentation: Clinically, the patient may present with symptoms of urethritis or salpingitis, cervicitis being asymptomatic apart from some discharge. If pelvic infection develops, the vaginal discharge precedes the elevation of the temperature and abdominal pain. There is bilateral adnexal tenderness and severe excitation pain on moving the cervix. Swelling or thickening of the adnexa may be present but examination usually provokes so much pain that these are difficult to detect. The systemic upset is not marked, despite the pyrexia.

Diagnosis: A differential diagnosis must consider ectopic pregnancy, a complicated ovarian cyst, appendicitis and peritonitis. The bilateral nature of the lesion and the history is likely to indicate the diagnosis. If there is doubt, a laparoscopy should be performed. If the diagnosis of salpingitis is confirmed, the opportunity should be taken to obtain a swab of the pus.

Before treatment, bacteriological swabs should be taken to confirm the diagnosis. The sites to be swabbed should include endocervix, urethra and, depending on history of sexual contact, the pharynx and anus.

An endocervical swab for culture taken with an ordinary cotton-wool swab-stick will probably not produce any growth, for the gonococcal organisms are destroyed quickly if they are allowed to dry. The best method of collecting a specimen for identification of organisms is to use a charcoal-impregnated swab-stick or a calcium alginate (Calgi) swab-stick. These allow the discharge to be absorbed into the swab, keeping them moist at the correct pH. By plating the swabs immediately or transporting them in Stuart's transport media, a high recovery rate for culture is obtained. On Gram staining the Gram-negative intracellular diplococci can be seen. The organisms are grown on a chocolate-agar medium in a carbon dioxide-enriched atmosphere.

Treatment: Antibiotics in large doses are indicated and penicillin is the antibiotic of choice. This treatment should be continued for 10 days or until the patient has been afebrile and asymptomatic for at least 38 hours. If the patient is allergic to penicillin, spectinomycin (Trobocin), erythromycin (EES) or tetracycline may be used.

Secondary infection by other organisms is not uncommon. When this occurs, a regime similar to that for post-abortal pelvic infection is commenced.

Peritonitis should be treated with the patient in a sitting position; with attention to fluids, electrolytes and urinary output. Tubo-ovarian abscess may develop with severe infection and is managed by surgical drainage, usually at laparoscopy.

Chronic pelvic infection

Chronic pelvic infection is an important cause of dysmenorrhoea, dyspareunia, menstrual disturbances and infertility. It usually arises because of inadequate, inappropriate, delayed or too short a course of treatment. The uterus is not usually involved, except in the rare event of pelvic tuberculosis.

Chronic salpingitis and oophoritis

The main changes are associated with occlusion of the Fallopian tubes and (with the gonococcus) destruction of the endosalpinx. Distortion of the tubes with peritubal adhesions is also common. If both the fimbral and isthmic ends of the tubes are blocked, a pyosalpinx may form. Extension of the infection from the tube to the ovary results in chronic inflammatory changes or abscess formation (usually as a tubo-ovarian abscess).

Clinically the patient may complain of dysmenorrhoea, which is characteristically a prolonged pelvic ache. Backache is also common.

Menstrual irregularity, with frequent periods and menorrhagia, is probably related to ovarian involvement in the inflammatory process, and consequent hormonal dysfunction.

A surprising number of patients with chronic inflammatory changes have no symptoms but present with infertility.

Signs

It is sometimes possible to detect a mass or bilateral swellings in the pelvis. The uterus is often enlarged and fixed in retroversion, and attempts to antevert it are unsuccessful.

Management

The treatment depends on age, parity, desire for further pregnancies, the nature of the lesions and their extent and response to treatment.

In general, the management is conservative by medical therapy – although surgical treatment is indicated if there is no improvement.

Medical treatment includes correction of anaemia, analgesics, heat and antibiotic therapy. Antibiotics are not as effective in chronic disease as in the acute condition, and there is also the difficulty of obtaining organisms for culture and sensitivity.

Surgery is indicated if:

1. There is no response to intensive therapy and the general health of the patient continues to deteriorate.
2. There are acute exacerbations of chronic inflammatory disease.
3. Local tenderness persists without improvement.
4. Masses in the adnexa or pouch of Douglas increase in size or show no diminution.
5. Menstrual disorders continue and cause incapacity.

Laparotomy should be undertaken during antibiotic therapy and, where possible, material for culture should be obtained at operation. The operation may vary from a simple sal-pingostomy or salpingectomy to a salpingo-oophorectomy. Rarely a complete pelvic clearance may be required.

Pelvic tuberculosis

This is usually secondary to pulmonary tuberculosis. The Fallo-pian tubes are commonly affected. Many patients are asympto-matic, the diagnosis only being found when specially looked for during investigation of infertility, oligomenorrhoea, vaginal discharge, anaemia, high temperatures or weight loss.

Endometrium obtained at curettage (which must be done premenstrually) should be examined histologically and sent for culture.

Intensive and prolonged anti-tuberculosis therapy is required. The prospects of a successful pregnancy, even after successful treatment, are not great and the risk of an ectopic pregnancy is high.

Venereal disease

See trichomonas, gonorrhoea, chlamydia and herpes as descri-bed earlier in this chapter. Syphilis should be suspected in any patient in whom gonorrhoea has been diagnosed. Like gonor-rhoea, it is commonly asymptomatic in the female, the primary chancre not being observed in the vagina or inner aspects of the vulva.

Treponema pallidum is a slowly multiplying spirochaete, which requires moisture and tissue for survival, and is transmitted by blood or exudate, entering via lacerations or abrasions in the vagina. The incubation period averages 3 weeks. The primary or chancre stage lasts 1–5 weeks. The typical chancre is a single ulcer (commonly with a rolled edge and a chamois leather-like base), often accompanied by a non-suppurative lymphadeno-pathy. It is usually painless, except when secondary infection occurs in a vulval chancre. The secondary syphilis stage may last 2–6 weeks and is the most contagious stage. The eruption may take many forms and mimic many types of rashes. The areas commonly affected are the oral cavity ('snail-track' ulcers), palms, soles and genital area. Condylomata lata may develop, and these are accompanied by generalized adenopathy.

There may be a prolonged latent phase following the second-ary stage before the tertiary stage develops. The tertiary stage may affect any part of the body, producing neurosyphilis (including general paralysis of the insane), cardiovascular changes and gumma.

Congenital syphilis may only be acquired by the fetus after the 16th week of gestation. If the infection occurs early in the pregnancy, the fetus will usually die *in utero*; if later in preg-nancy, the fetus will be born with the stigmata of congenital syphilis; if the infection is acquired late in pregnancy, the stig-mata may occur after birth. Congenital syphilis can be pre-vented by adequate treatment of the mother.

Diagnosis: This is by adequate investigation of those at risk or at special risk, such as the pregnant patient. There are two basic types of test:

1. Sensitive screening tests, such as the Reiter protein comple-ment fixation (RPCF) test; the Wassermann reaction (WR); the venereal disease research laboratory (VDRL) test; *Trepo-nema pallidum* haemagglutination assay (TPHA). All these tests give false-positive results. They may take 9–90 days to become positive.
2. In order to confirm the diagnosis, more specific tests such as the fluorescent treponema antibody test (FTA) or the *Treponema pallidum* immobilization test (TPI) should be per-formed.
3. The diagnosis can also be confirmed by dark-ground exam-ination of exudate from the chancre to detect the spir-ochaetes.

Treatment: Procaine penicillin (1.2 million units daily for 10 days). Long-acting penicillin in adequate doses (e.g. Bicillin 2–4 million units intramuscularly on two occasions, several days apart) can be used for primary disease if the patient is unreliable.

Serological tests should be repeated at least 3-monthly for 2 years to confirm the cure. If there is any doubt about the cure, the cerebrospinal fluid should also be examined.

Social implications of pelvic infections

Venereal diseases (both chlamydia and gonorrhoea) are increasing in frequency in our community. Social groups that form the largest untreated pool of carriers are prostitutes and male homosexuals. The asymptomatic female carrier may only be found by tracing male contacts. Failure of notification of one diagnosed patient may allow a wide spread of the infection. The natural reticence to notify partners must be overcome for public health measures to be effective. Appropriate swabs should be taken of any undiagnosed vaginal discharge of any genital tract infection.

14

Gynaecological endocrinology

The students should appreciate variations from the normal function of the female reproductive system so they can identify patients who have symptoms of gynaecological disorders, usually without corresponding abnormal physical signs and the initiate management.

14.2 SPECIFIC BEHAVIOURAL OBJECTIVES

1. Discuss the symptoms and signs of normal menstruation.
2. Discuss the investigation of a patient with abnormal uterine bleeding.
3. Discuss the hazards of giving hormonal therapy for abnormal vaginal bleeding.
4. Discuss those factors that may cause abnormal uterine bleeding without demonstrable physical causes.
5. Indicate factors that may cause amenorrhoea without demonstrable physical causes.
6. Discuss the aetiology, clinical features and management of dysmenorrhoea.
7. Discuss the causes and management of pelvic pain without demonstrable physical cause.
8. Discuss the management of a patient with hyperprolactinaemia.

14.3 REASONS FOR LEARNING ABOUT GYNAECOLOGICAL ENDOCRINOLOGY

Endocrine problems of the female genital tract are extremely common. Often a woman will present to her doctor complaining of symptoms such as pain, irregular bleeding, dyspareunia, vaginal discharge, hot flushes, loss of libido, or depression, which may appear to have no obvious pathological basis. These symptoms may be due to problems such as oestrogen deficiency, premenstrual tension or primary spasmodic dysmenorrhoea. Before accurate diagnosis and therapy can be offered, it is essential to understand the basic mechanisms that produce these symptoms. An accurate history is essential to sort out gynaecological endocrine problems. Many of these problems will only be recognized by the pattern of symptoms. The logical starting place for most menstrual orders is menarche and a careful menstrual history should be sought from this time. Often the pattern of symptoms will indicate the likely cause of the problem so that only a few specific investigations need to be performed.

14.4 THE HORMONAL CONTROL OF THE NORMAL MENSTRUAL CYCLE

The oocyte

Unlike males, who constantly produce sperms after puberty, women are given their life-time compliment of eggs in fetal life. From a high of around 7 million eggs at 20 weeks gestation oocytes are then continually lost. By birth the number declines to around 2 million and after 400 to 500 ovulations over her life-time by the time of the menopause, none are left. The production of sex steroids is linked to the cyclical release of an oocyte each 28 days or so. Ovulation occurs about 13 times a year and once released, the egg lives for about a day. Before the oocyte can be fertilized to form an embryo, sperms have to reach the cervix, penetrate the cervical mucus and travel up the uterine cavity to meet the egg in the Fallopian tube where fertilization occurs. The control of ovulation is an extremely complex process which is influenced by many factors. However, most of the control is mediated at three levels – the hypothalamus, the pituitary and the ovary.

The hypothalamus

The main central control for menstrual cyclicity resides in the arcuate nucleus which is located in the medial basal hypothalamus. Multiple neuronal connections around the area of the arcuate nucleus are responsible for the tonic control of pulsatile release of gonadotrophin-releasing hormone (GnRH). GnRH is a decapeptide released into the pituitary portal circulation in pulses. Mini-pulses occur frequently and appear to prime the pituitary gonadotrope to produce luteinizing hormone (LH) and follicle-stimulating hormone (FSH). During the follicular phase major pulses occur every 90 minutes and these act on the pituitary to release stored LH and FSH. Before ovulation, GnRH pulses increase in frequency and amplitude whereas in the luteal phase GnRH pulses occur around every 3 hours. The effect of GnRH on the pituitary is influenced by GnRH priming as well as the pituitary content of LH and FSH. These changes in GnRH pulsatility do not appear to be responsible for 'fine tuning' of the menstrual cycle. Women with Kallman's syndrome are GnRH-deficient and usually present with primary amenorrhoea. Treating such patients with a GnRH pump, set to deliver pulses every 90 minutes will produce a menstrual cycle indistinguishable from normal. In other words, the pulse rate does not need to be increased to induce ovulation or slowed in the second half of the cycle to produce a normal luteal phase. This experiment of nature teaches us that to produce a normal 28-day menstrual cycle requires a pulse generator delivering GnRH pulses every 90 minutes and an intact pituitary ovarian axis. One of the ways the oral contraceptive pill (OCP) works is by inhibiting the arcuate nucleus. The pituitary hormone prolactin (PRL) also inhibits the arcuate nucleus and as such hyperprolactinaemia is usually associated with amenorrhoea.

Pituitary ovarian dialogue

As previously stated, the anterior pituitary produces and releases LH and FSH in response to GnRH pulses. LH and FSH, like thyroid-stimulating hormone (TSH) are sialoglycoproteins. They contain an alpha and beta subunit, and in all three hormones the alpha subunit is very similar and it is the beta subunit that delivers hormone specificity. Human chorionic gonadotropin (HCG) is produced by the trophoblast and is in essence an LH analogue. Both LH and FSH have two prime ovarian functions – the production of sex steroids and the control of ovulation. Within the ovary, the basic unit of steroid production is the follicle. Each follicle contains an oocyte which is surrounded by granulosa cells and on the outside of the follicle, the theca cells. Under the influence of LH, the theca cell produces androgen, principally androstenedione (AD) and testosterone (T) which are then converted by the granulosa cell into oestrogens, principally oestradiol (E2) under the action of FSH. FSH also stimulates follicles to grow (hence its name).

Each month or so, about 20 or 30 follicles become sensitive to FSH, but only one is destined to ovulate. The complex relationship between the gonadotropins, LH and FSH, and the ovarian follicle is best understood by examining a normal menstrual cycle. By convention, day 1 of the menstrual cycle is taken to be the first day of menstrual bleeding. By the end of the first week a number of small follicles (up to 6–7 mm in diameter) can be seen with ultrasound. Once one of these follicles has achieved a follicular diameter of about 10 mm, it will double in size in five days. In the early follicular phase these follicles, principally the dominant follicle, produce E2 and, as serum E2 levels rise, a classic negative feedback loop is established. The granulosa cells also make a protein called 'inhibin' which selectively inhibits pituitary FSH release. By the late follicular phase, serum FSH levels are about half that of earlier in the cycle. The dominant follicle continues to grow, despite falling serum levels of FSH whereas its cohort or surrounding follicles will regress. Once the dominant follicle has achieved a size of around 18–20 mm in diameter it signals the pituitary that it is ready to ovulate. Two factors appear to be necessary to induce ovulation – 36 hours of rapidly rising serum levels of E2 as well as 12 hours of rapidly rising levels of LH. Both these events are required to induce a positive feedback loop which results in the LH–FSH surge. The high levels of LH activate the oocyte making it fertilizable and, secondly, induce ovulation. Ovulation is a low pressure event and involves enzymatic digestion of the follicular wall as well as prostaglandins. Immediately after ovulation serum E2 levels fall. The collapsed follicle is transformed into the corpus luteum which produces large amounts of E2 and progesterone. Serum progesterone levels peak about 7 days after ovulation. The corpus luteum appears to have a genetically predetermined life of around 14 days and, if it is not rescued by pregnancy-secreted HCG, it degenerates. Serum E2 and progesterone levels fall and menstruation ensues.

If pregnancy ensues, then trophoblastic HCG stimulates a corpus luteum to produce E2 and progesterone until the placenta is able to take over this function at around 8 weeks' gestation.

Prolactin, the thyroid and the adrenal axis

Prolactin is released from the anterior pituitary and is primarily under tonic inhibitory control. The main inhibitory factor for prolactin is probably dopamine, but it is likely that there are other inhibitory control mechanisms. Thyrotropin-releasing hormone (TRH) is at least one other factor which is known to directly stimulate prolactin release. The main function of TRH is to stimulate the pituitary to release TSH to regulate thyroid gland function. Corticotrophin-releasing factor (CRF) releases pituitary ACTH as well as other peptides from the anterior pituitary. ACTH regulates adrenal cortex function. Stressful stimuli are well known to impact on the menstrual cycle and with stress, CRF increases. This in turn not only stimulates ACTH and cortisol but also elicits the release of opioid peptides which can directly inhibit GnRH secretion.

Sex steroid–endometrium interaction

In general, the effect of oestrogen on the genital tract is to stimulate proliferation and mitotic activity. Thus, in the follicular phase, the unopposed oestrogen effect is to induce proliferation of the endometrium. Oestrogen also stimulates the endocervix to produce clear, watery mucus which is essential for aiding sperm transport into the genital tract.

Oestrogen is also a vasodilator and as serum oestrogen levels rise, uterine blood flow increases. Progesterone's effect on the endometrium is largely that of an anti-oestrogen. It stops proliferation and reduces mitotic activity and transforms the endometrium into a secretory tissue. High levels of oestrogen and progesterone are required to produce decidua which is hypersecretory endometrium, characteristic of the late luteal phase and pregnancy. When levels of oestrogen and progesterone fall in the late luteal phase the upper layers of the endometrium are disrupted and menstrual flow ensues. The first defence against heavy menstrual loss are platelets, so platelet disorders are a potent cause of menorrhagia. Progesterone also alters the cervical mucus, making it thick and impenetrable to sperms. Progesterone is also thermogenic and responsible for a half-degree Celsius rise in basal body temperature, during the luteal phase of the menstrual cycle.

General body aspects of steroid requirements

The sex steroids have important extragenital effects. Bone mass rises through the first 20 years of life and if a young woman becomes sex steroid-deficient (e.g. anexoria) she may fail to achieve her peak bone mass; this has important implications for the development of osteoporosis. Both oestrogen and progesterone are also required for normal breast development. Oestrogen is largely responsible for duct development, whereas progesterone induces alveolar development. Complete breast development is only seen after the first pregnancy.

Tests of the hypothalamic pituitary axis and oestrogen state

The investigation of menstrual cycle abnormalities is usually straightforward and does not require complicated tests. This will be discussed in detail in the following paragraphs. Much information will be gained in many clinical situations by measuring LH, FSH, prolactin (and possibly thyroid function), performing a high-quality ultrasound scan and giving a patient a progesterone challenge. The ovary is a dynamic structure and will change its shape and appearance according to the endocrine milieu. Ultrasound also allows measurement of the uterine size and endometrial thickness, which are useful measures of biological oestrogen activity. To obtain the best quality pictures it may be necessary to perform trans-vaginal scanning. A 5-day course of a progestogen such as medroxyprogesterone acetate (MPA) 10 mg daily will give clinically useful information about the oestrogen state of a patient. Any bleeding, including brown discharge that occurs in the week following, indicates that some biologically active oestrogen is present. A negative progestogen challenge test indicates an oestrogen-deficient state.

When drawing blood to measure in particular, prolactin, it is important that the blood sample is collected before 10.00 a.m.

and in a rested state, as prolactin is a stress hormone. An elevated result should always be repeated. A significantly elevated prolactin usually necessitates imaging of the pituitary gland via computed tomography (CT) scanning or magnetic resonance imaging (MRI). Pituitary function tests are rarely indicated, although a Synacthen test may be required to distinguish polycystic ovary syndrome from late onset congenital adrenal hyperplasia, as described later.

A well-performed basal body temperature chart is an important and simple first-line test of ovulation. The chart should be commenced on day 1 of the menstrual cycle and the patient should record her oral temperature first thing in the morning before rising from bed. Her basal body temperature should rise around half-a-degree Celsius after ovulation and this temperature rise should be maintained until just before menstruation. If pregnancy occurs then the temperature rise is maintained.

14.5 ABNORMAL UTERINE BLEEDING

As discussed previously, the key concepts in understanding the physiology of endometrial growth and shedding are:

1. Oestrogen causes growth and proliferation of the endometrium.
2. Progesterone transforms the proliferative endometrium into secretory endometrium.
3. Platelet plug formation is the first line of defence for cessation of shedding.
4. Prostaglandin interaction is important for uterine haemostasis.
5. The normal cycle length is 21 to 35 days with one to seven days of bleeding. Menstrual fluid also contains its own thrombolytic system so that normally menstrual blood does not clot. If menstrual bleeding is heavy, then this system is overridden and clots may form.

Definitions of abnormal bleeding

1. Menorrhagia   Excessive bleeding at regular intervals (generally >80 ml per month).

2. Hypermenorrhoea   Prolonged bleeding at regular
                     intervals (1 and 2 are sometimes
                     used interchangeably).
3. Metrorrhagia   Variable amounts of bleeding at
                     abnormal and frequent intervals.
4. Metromenorrhagia Excessive bleeding, often prolonged,
                     at abnormal and frequent intervals.
5. Polymenorrhoea   Bleeding at regular intervals less
                     than 21 days.
6. Oligomenorrhoea   Bleeding at irregular intervals of
                     greater than 35 days.
7. Hypomenorrhoea   Decrease in amount and duration of
                     menses.

In clinical practice, menorrhagia may be difficult to prove. Measurement of menstrual blood loss is not a practical clinical test. However, the following may be considered reasonable signs of menorrhagia:

1. Iron deficiency (not due to another cause).
2. If the patient passes clots when she menstruates.
3. If the patient soaks sanitary pads and tampons several times a day.

Abnormal uterine bleeding may be conveniently divided into three sub groups – pregnancy states, pelvic pathology and dysfunctional uterine bleeding (DUB). DUB (Table 14.1) is an imprecise term which may be conveniently defined as 'abnormal uterine bleeding in the absence of pelvic pathology'.

Systemic disease is an important cause of DUB. Thyroid over or under-activity may interfere with the menstrual cycle. Women on anticoagulants usually have normal menstrual loss but those with even minor degrees of platelet dysfunction will often suffer very heavy periods. Liver disease may influence the cycle because of a failure to conjugate endogenous oestrogen and rarely due to coagulopathy.

Ovulatory DUB
This is commonly associated with oligomenorrhoea and the most common cause of this is polycystic ovary syndrome, which will be discussed later. Polymenorrhoea is common at puberty and around the time of the menopause. Typically

Table 14.1 A summary of one approach to subdividing DUB

Systemic causes	Ovulatory DUB	Anovulatory DUB
	Abnormal follicular phase	Metropathica haemorrhagica
Thyroid disease	Too short: Oligomenorrhoea	Polycystic ovary syndrome
Polycystic ovary syndrome	(usually polycystic ovary syndrome)	Follicular cyst
Prolactin excess (and other	Too long: Polymenorrhoea	
causes of oligoamenorrhoea		
Perimenopause	*Abnormal luteal phase*	
	Too short: Irregular ripening	
Platelet disease	Corpus luteal insufficiency	Threshold bleeding
Liver disease	Too long: Irregular shedding	
	Corpus luteal prolonged activity (rare)	

about 5 years before the last period most women notice a shortening in their menstrual cycle. About 1 to 3 years before the last period they may then notice that their periods are 'skipping a month or more'. The perimenopause is a time when low oestrogen months may be associated with menopausal symptoms such as hot flushes and then followed by a light period, only to be followed by a high oestrogen month when menopausal symptoms disappear but breast pain and menorrhagia are common. Low-dose HRT is not potent enough to inhibit ovulation and so often results in break-through bleeding. If not contraindicated, a contraceptive pill is one simple short-term therapy that will control menopausal symptoms as well as irregular cycles. Once the woman is postmenopausal, then HRT is appropriate. Corpus luteal insufficiency is an ill-defined condition and many infertility experts still dispute whether or not this entity really exists as a persistent abnormality. Corpus luteal prolonged activity is extremely rare and is characterized by persistent progesterone secretion by the corpus luteum.

Anovulatory DUB

This is common and is particularly associated with obese women with polycystic ovary syndrome (PCO, described later). These women typically have one or two periods a year and have a significant risk of endometrial hyperplasia which left untreated may progress to carcinoma. A follicular cyst should be considered in a patient who has previously had regular cycles but then misses a month. The patient may think that she is pregnant. She may have some dull pelvic pain at this stage. An ultrasound scan typically shows a 4–6 cm follicular cyst. Severe pain may ensue when the cyst ruptures and then typically a day or two later an unopposed oestrogen withdrawal bleed occurs which can be very heavy. Prolonged unopposed oestrogen action may result in metropathia haemorrhagica, or so called 'Swiss cheese endometrium', a hyperplastic endometrium which is commonly associated with very heavy bleeding.

Clinical management

This is best considered according to the age of the patient.

The young perimenarchal women

The first few periods a woman has are associated with low levels of unopposed oestrogen and therefore should be light and painless. A teenager with heavy bleeding should be referred for haematological assessment and a platelet disorder sought. Juvenile hypothyroidism should also be considered. In this age group dilatation and currettage (D & C) or hysteroscopy are rarely indicated.

Reproductive age women (late teens to 40)

Unless the patient has been virtually amenorrhoeic for much of her reproductive life, then endometrial hyperplasia and carcinoma are uncommon. Hysteroscopy may be indicated to exclude endometrial pathology such as polyps or a submucus fibroid. Transvaginal ultrasound is a useful investigation to exclude pelvic pathology. Few of the women require D & C under an anaesthetic.

The women over 40

For the woman over 40, endometrial pathology and in particular hyperplasia or carcinoma become increasingly common and therefore the physician should be considering hysteroscopy and endometrial biopsy more often. As the woman becomes older, pelvic pathology is also increasingly common and so again transvaginal ultrasound in conjunction with hysteroscopy are useful investigations.

Treatment

The treatment of DUB may be divided into acute and long-term phases.

Acute phase

Moderate doses of progestogens such as norethisterone (NE) 5 mg three or four times a day typically takes 2 to 4 days to start to work, but are worth trying. A 50 mcg contraceptive pill taken twice daily for 3 or 4 days and then once a day for the rest of the packet is also a useful and simple regimen. If a progestogen is used then the dosage should be continued for at least 2 to 3 weeks. High-dose intravenous oestrogens (e.g. Premarin IV, 25 mg) are rarely used in Australia. If heavy bleeding continues in spite of hormone treatment or when associated with anaemia then a hysteroscopy and D & C is useful to exclude intrauterine pathology and to stop the bleeding.

Long-term management

If there are no contraindications, then a monophasic contraceptive pill taken 12 weeks on, 1 week off, is often a simple and reliable therapy for controlling irregular and heavy periods. The Family Planning Association (FPA) of Australia has found that up to 75% of women taking a contraceptive pill will miss tablets. Missing one or two tablets on a 3-week on, 1-week off, regimen is far more likely to result in pregnancy than tablets missed on a 12-week on, 1-week off, regimen. Breakthrough bleeding is common for the first few months but then usually settles down. Another alternative is to use progestogens. It has been commonplace to use luteal phase cycles of progesterone such as NE 5 mg three times a day. Recent clinical trials have shown that these do not significantly reduce measured menstrual blood loss. However, NE 5 mg or MPA 10 mg taken daily without a break, inhibits ovulation and usually result in amenorrhoea by 2 to 3 months. About 10% of women will develop 'premenstrual stress' (PMS)-type side effects on these regimens. Low-dose Danazol (200 mg/day) is another alternative with few side effects.

When medical therapies have failed then a surgical option may be sought. Endometrial ablation using diathermy or laser is becoming increasingly popular. This may result either in amenorrhoea or reduced bleeding. If significant prolapse is present, then a vaginal hysterectomy may be a very suitable alternative for some patients. Abdominal hysterectomy has been the usual surgical option.

14.6 DYSMENORRHOEA

Pain just before and during menstruation is a common cause of time off school or work for many women. The magnitude of the problem has been greatly reduced over the last few years by the widespread availability of non-steroidal anti-inflammatory drugs (NSAIDs). These are very effective therapies for dysmenorrhoea and so the General Practitioner today is likely to be presented with a woman whose pain has not settled with mefanamic acid (Ponstan) or naproxen sodium (Naprogesic).

Dysmenorrhoea may be secondary to pelvic pathology such as fibroids or endometriosis, which will be considered elsewhere. Primary dysmenorrhoea is caused by uterine contractions resulting from the production of prostaglandins by the endometrium. Proliferative endometrium does not produce much prostaglandin, unlike secretory endometrium on the other hand, which produces large amounts of prostaglandin. Prostaglandins, if they enter the circulation, may produce systemic effects such as nausea and diarrhoea.

Clinical features of primary dysmenorrhoea

Age
When menstruation first commences, bleeding is usually painless because the cycles are anovulatory and there is no secretory endometrium producing prostaglandins. Most women *are* having painful periods, however, within 2 years of their first period.

Parity
After the first confinement, dysmenorrhoea is often less severe, possibly because of softening and dilatation of the cervix and its response to uterine contractions.

Pain
The pain typically starts some hours before the onset of menstruation. The distribution of pain is suprapubic, often extending into both iliac fossae, and may extend down the inner thighs and round to the back.

Secondary dysmenorrhoea

If the dysmenorrhoea appears for the first time later in life, it is considered 'secondary' and usually has an organic aetiology. Careful history and examination are necessary to rule out pathological conditions. These need to be supplemented by ultrasound studies and/or direct visualization at laparoscopy. Pelvic infection, adhesions, ovarian masses or tubal pathology, fibromyomata, endometriosis and adenomyosis are some of the more common causes of secondary dysmenorrhoea. If any of these conditions are present treatment is directed specifically at the disorder.

Treatment

The NSAIDs are primary therapy for dysmenorrhoea. They are most effective when taken in full dosage before the onset of menstruation. Contraceptive pills are also effective by producing endometrial atrophy and thus reducing the production of prostaglandins. Continuous moderate dosage of progestogen, sufficient to produce amenorrhoea, are also useful therapies, particularly for young women who have important life events like examinations to sit. If the dysmenorrhoea does not settle with NSAIDs and contraceptive pills then consideration should be given to performing a laparoscopy to exclude endometriosis. Dilatation of the cervix or pre-sacral neurectomy are rarely indicated for dysmenorrhoea.

Pelvic congestion syndrome

This is an ill-defined condition characterized by chronic pelvic pain not associated with menstruation often described as bloating or a 'congested' pelvic sensation, associated with a normal laparoscopy. Some authors have claimed that pelvic varicosities are the cause of the pain although this remains controversial. Two important conditions to consider in the differential diagnosis are a psychosexual problem (and so a referral to a clinical psychologist may be of benefit) and irritable colon. This latter condition is particularly common in young women and considerable benefit may be obtained by appropriate dietary manipulation and the use of antispasmodics.

14.7 PREMENSTRUAL SYNDROME (PMS)

All regularly ovulating women notice some adverse symptoms which relate to their menstrual cycle but in about 5% of women these symptoms are severe and interfere with their lifestyle. Physical symptoms include breast tenderness and swelling, abdominal bloatedness, oedema, weight gain, headache, altered bowel habit and reduced coordination. Psychological symptoms include altered sleep, appetite, libido, irritability, anxiety, depression and tiredness. The non-controversial facts about PMS are summarized below:

1. Most healthy women report some adverse symptoms before menstruation.
2. The syndrome is associated with cyclical ovarian activity and does not occur before puberty, during pregnancy or after the menopause. It does not occur in women who are not ovulating.
3. Menstruation itself is incidental and cyclic symptoms continue after hysterectomy if the ovaries are preserved.
4. Extensive metabolic and psychological studies have failed to find a specific abnormality in PMS. Women who suffer from severe PMS typically find their problem becomes worse in their late 30s and entering their 40s. Some women date their problem to an episode of postnatal depression and then find that their mood swings become particularly harsh as they enter the perimenopause.

Treatment

Vitamin B_6 and oil of primrose have not been shown in clinical trials to work any better than a placebo. High-dose progesterone suppositories have been advocated by many, but it is difficult to show any response better than placebo. Natural progesterone also has a marked sedative effect. Fluid retention symptoms may be alleviated by a mild diuretic and severe breast pain may be effectively treated with continuous progestogen, bromocriptine or Danazol. Many women will obtain great relief of their symptoms by using non-drug therapies such as increasing their exercise, relaxation therapies, yoga or meditation. Cycle suppression with oestrogen implants or high-dose patches ($100/200 \mu g$ twice weekly) have been advocated by some European authors but are generally not practical solutions. If a patient develops menorrhagia with an oestrogen implant it is usually not possible to remove it. Another alternative is to suppress the ovarian cycle with a contraceptive pill, although many women who suffer from severe PMS seem to develop worsening of their symptoms with androgenic progestogens such as levonorgestrel. Some women may find benefit by using some of the newer contraceptive pills containing different progestogens. One important and practical point to consider is that if a woman has decided to have an abdominal hysterectomy for a gynaecological problem such as fibroids, and she suffers from severe PMS, then consideration should be given to removing the ovaries. As previously stated if the ovaries are left behind the severe PMS symptoms will continue.

14.8 AMENORRHOEA AND ANOVULATION

Primary amenorrhoea may be diagnosed if menstruation has not occurred by the age of 16. Oligomenorrhoea has been previously defined as a cycle length of more than 35 days and secondary amenorrhoea is generally defined as the absence of menstruation for 6 months. In general, the problem of amenorrhoea may be largely considered according to three concepts:

1. Is the patient completely sex-steroid deficient or does she have an unopposed oestrogen condition?
2. Does she have a high FSH or a low–normal FSH condition?
3. Does she have an outflow obstruction?

Primary amenorrhoea

In general, the division between primary and secondary amenorrhoea is largely arbitrary. All the conditions that can cause secondary amenorrhoea can also cause the primary condition. There are, however, some special problems associated with the young woman who has not yet menstruated by the age of 16. The first question a clinician should ask is whether or not the patient is sexually infantile or not.

If the patient is sexually infantile then her height should be sought. In general, a sexually infantile teenager should be tall because of a lack of fusion of her long bone epiphyses. If she is short, (under five foot) then this implies that some other condition has intervened to produce short stature. Conditions that produce short stature and sexual infantilism include genetic problems (classically Turner's syndrome), concomitant growth hormone deficiency and thyroid hormone deficiency.

If the sexually infantile patient is tall, then she is likely to be gonadotropin-deficient on the basis of hypothalamic or pituitary problems. Premature menopause remains a possibility. Useful tests to distinguish among these conditions include a serum FSH, thyroid function, karyotype, pelvic ultrasound and pituitary CT or MRI scanning.

If puberty is proceeding and breast tissue is present than consideration should be given to either an endocrine disorder or an outflow obstruction. Pelvic ultrasound is extremely valuable at determining whether or not the uterus is present. If the uterus is absent, then the differential diagnosis is between testicular feminization and congenital absence of the uterus. Testicular feminization is associated with a normal male level of testosterone and by finding a male karyotype, 46 XY. Congenital absence of the uterus is more common and is confirmed by a female-range level of testosterone, normal female karyotype 46 XX and usually a temperature chart confirms ovulation. The young woman with primary amenorrhoea but some breast development and her uterus intact should also be investigated for all the causes of secondary amenorrhoea, including prolactin excess.

These patients need specialist investigation and may have a relatively straightforward problem such as polycystic ovary syndrome, but can also rarely have congenital adrenal hyperplasia or a variant of masculinizing intersex.

Treatment

Gonadal dysgenesis is treated with oestrogen replacement. If Y chromosomal material exists in the karyotype then the streak gonads need to be removed to prevent the development of a neoplasm. CNS lesions in patients with hypogonadotrophic hypogonadism are treated as required by the neurosurgeon.

Testicular feminization is treated with oestrogen replacement, and removal of the gonads is required by the time of maturity to avoid a neoplasm. This is usually carried out by the age of 18. Congenital absence of the uterus requires an explanation and screening for associated skeletal and renal abnormalities. A vaginoplasty may be required or dilation therapy for patients with testicular feminization or congenital absence of the uterus (and vagina). Women who are sexually infantile require sex steroid replacement. It is prudent to start with extremely low doses of oestrogen and increase the dosage only slowly to allow normal breast development. This should be undertaken by an appropriate specialist.

Secondary amenorrhoea

Outflow obstructions of the uterus should be considered here as well. If there is a history of prior instrumentation of the uterus of any kind then a hysterosalpingogram or hysteroscopy should be performed. The minimum investigation of a patient with secondary amenorrhoea should include measurement of her serum LH, FSH and prolactin and a progesterone challenge test. Five days of MPA 10 mg will produce a withdrawal bleed in women with some biologically active oestrogen present. If LH and FSH are low or normal and the progesterone challenge test is negative, then the patient has hypothalamic amenorrhoea. If FSH is high then the diagnosis is premature ovarian failure (if the patient is under 40). Karyotypic abnormalities are common in women under 25 and so women in this age group should have their karyotype carried out. There is no role for ovarian biopsy as it does not change the treatment of these patients. It is important to rule out polyglandular auto-immunity in this group. Thus, autoantibodies such as anti-microsomal, antinuclear antibodies, antiparietal cell antibodies and ovarian antibodies should be sought.

The patient with normal FSH and normal or slightly elevated LH who bleeds after a progesterone challenge usually has poly-cystic ovary syndrome (this will be discussed later). Hyperprolactinaemia should be confirmed by repeating the prolactin estimation and ensuring that the sample was collected before 10.00 a.m. and in a rested state. It will be discussed shortly as a separate condition.

Treatment

If patients respond to progesterone challenge, then anovulation is either treated with intermittent progestogen withdrawal (or a contraceptive pill) or induction of ovulation using clomiphene (if the patient wishes to conceive).

Hypo-oestrogenism in patients with secondary amenorrhoea is treated with oestrogen replacement or with a contraceptive pill. If a patient with hypothalamic failure wishes to conceive then she can either be treated with FSH therapy or pulsatile GnRH.

14.9 HYPERPROLACTINAEMIA

Galactorrhoea is an inconsistent feature of hyperprolactinaemia. Only around 50% of patients with pathological hyperprolactinaemia will have it and most women with galactorrhoea have a normal prolactin. Drug ingestion (e.g. tranquillizers and anti-nauseants) is a common cause of galactorrhoea and a careful drug history is required. Hypothyroidism is an important and treatable cause of prolactin excess and thyroid function (TSH) testing is mandatory. If the prolactin level is greater than 60 ng/ml then a CT scan of the pituitary should be ordered to exclude an adenoma. Most abnormalities of the pituitary are a prolactin-secreting microadenoma (<1 cm) although occasionally macroadenomas will be detected. With larger tumours, visual field evaluation and a more complete endocrine and neurological assessment are necessary. A microadenoma may not require treatment unless oestrogen deficiency exists or a pregnancy is desired. Autopsy studies have suggested that from 5 to 25% of the population have a small asymptomatic microadenoma of the pituitary. Amenorrhoea and oestrogen deficiency in hyperprolactinaemia is associated with significant osteoporosis.

Treatment

After ruling out drug exposure and hypothyroidism, indications for treatment of hyperprolactinaemia are:

1. Macroadenomas.
2. Oestrogen deficiency.
3. Fertility.

Other patients may be followed clinically and with prolactin (PRL) assays at 6-month intervals. In most patients, bromocriptine is used to suppress PRL. A starting dose of 2.5 mg daily is increased up to 10 mg or more in order to suppress PRL levels to normal or until symptoms and signs disappear. Side effects of dizziness, nausea, hypotension and nasal congestion may be significant and bromocriptine should be administered with caution in small incremental doses. Normal oestrogen status and ovulatory function are important end-points of therapy.

In patients with macroadenomas, depending on the response to bromocriptine, neurosurgery may be advocated as an additional measure. Once bromocriptine is stopped, rapid re-growth can occur. In patients with microadenomas, repeat pituitary scans are only requested every 2–3 years, or after a pregnancy has occurred. Although there is no consensus, we do not advocate the use of bromocriptine in pregnancy for microadenomas unless symptoms occur. For patients with macroadenomas, the maintenance dose of bromocriptine during pregnancy may be prudent, because of the danger of pressure damage to the optic nerves from the enlarging gland and possible resulting blindness.

14.10 ANDROGEN EXCESS – POLYCYSTIC OVARY SYNDROME (PCO)

Excessive androgen secretion in women may lead to anovulation as well as acne and hirsutism. Androgen may be secreted in excess by the ovaries, adrenals or peripheral tissues, including fat and skin. The best blood markers of androgen excess are:

1. Testosterone. This is the main serum androgen. About 25% is made directly by the ovary, 25% by the adrenals and 50% by peripheral conversion of precursors.
2. Dehydroepiandrosterone sulphate (DHEA-S), which is principally an adrenal gland product.
3. 17-hydroxyprogesterone, which is a marker for 21-hydroxylase deficiency. This is the most common manifestation of late-onset congenital adrenal hyperplasia.

When a patient presents with clinical signs of androgen excess the following differential diagnosis should be considered:

1. Iatrogenic or drug-related hirsutism.
2. Abnormal gonadal or sexual development.
3. Idiopathic (familiar hirsutism).
4. Polycystic ovary syndrome.
5. Stromal hyperthecosis.
6. Androgen-producing ovarian tumours.
7. Cushing's syndrome.

8. Adult manifestation of congenital adrenal hyperplasia.
9. Androgen-producing adrenal tumours.

Some 8% of Australian women complain of excess body hair during their reproductive years. Between 90 and 95% of women with hirsutism have polycystic ovary syndrome (PCO) and the other causes are all rare. Tumours of the ovary and adrenal gland are excessively rare and their diagnosis is straightforward. Their history is one of a rapidly progressing virilizing disorder associated with a total testosterone level more than twice the upper limit of normal, or a DHEA-S level more than double the upper limit of normal.

Late-onset congenital adrenal hyperplasia (CAH) is suspected when basal levels of 17-hydroxyprogesterone are elevated and is confirmed by performing a Synacthen test. It is treated with low-dose dexamethasone. Cushing's syndrome is rare but an important diagnosis not to miss. A simple screening test is to measure 24-hour urinary free cortisol. This can be elevated in cases of simple obesity and if elevated should be followed up by a short dexamethasone suppression test.

PCO is a heterogeneous group of disorders which is characterized by a late menarche, cycle irregularity which commonly dates from puberty, and skin manifestations of androgen excess such as hirsutism and/or acne. The term PCO refers to the morphological appearance of the ovaries. The polycystic ovary is on average, twice the size of a normal ovary and characterized by a peripheral ring of small 2–6-mm follicles (more than 10). Often the ovarian capsule is thick and the ovarian stroma increased. It is still unknown why the polycystic ovary has this appearance, but using high-resolution ultrasound at least one in five women have this ovarian appearance and only half of them have symptoms. Women with PCO usually find that their periods become more irregular as they put on weight. Women with normal ovarian function on the other hand behave in the opposite manner, that is, their periods tend to become irregular as they lose weight. There is some evidence to suggest that the woman with PCO simply represents a variation of normal, perhaps even a survival mechanism, and it has been postulated that these women may have biological advantages when thin, even pathologically thin. The cardinal biochemical features of the PCO syndrome are high serum LH, normal FSH level and often one or more of the following are also abnormal – testosterone, DHEA-S and sex hormone-binding globulin (SHBG). Obese women with PCO should be encouraged to lose weight.

Management

Treatment should be directed at the symptom most bothering the patient. If cycle control/irregularity is the problem, then they are best managed by a low-dose contraceptive pill. Obese subjects should be encouraged to lose weight. Patients should be reassured that they will rarely, if ever, require surgical intervention for ovarian cysts. Should they want to conceive, they may require ovulation induction with either clomiphene citrate or gonadotrophins.

Treatment

Hirsutism is best managed with either spironolactone 100–200 mg combined with a contraceptive pill. The oestrogen in the contraceptive pill increases the levels of SHBG, and this results in a reduced amount of circulating unbound androgens. Aldactone is generally safe and hyperkalaemia is rarely encountered with these dosages used with healthy individuals. Used alone, spironolactone can aggravate menstrual irregularities in about one-quarter of patients and may have adverse fetal effects and so is best used with a contraceptive pill. Cyproterone acetate combined with ethinyl oestradiol is also an extremely effective combination for excess body hair. Both these therapies generally need to be used for suppressing moderate elevations in adrenal androgens without major effects on cortisol secretion.

15

The menopause

15.1 GENERAL INSTRUCTIONAL OBJECTIVE

Students should understand the changes that occur at the time of menopause so that they can identify its onset and counsel women about the best way of dealing with the results of the hormonal changes they are having and offer the appropriate management.

15.2 SPECIFIC BEHAVIOURAL OBJECTIVES

1. Discuss causes and management of postmenopausal problems.
2. Be familiar with the advantages and disadvantages of hormone replacement therapy.
3. Counsel women with postmenopausal problems.

15.3 REASONS FOR LEARNING ABOUT THE MENOPAUSE

Approximately 12% (1:8) of any Western community is composed of postmenopausal women. They live longer than men and in the process consume a disproportionate amount of the health care budget of most developed countries. Because older women are utilizing so much of the available medical sources, it is imperative that any action, which improves the long-term health of women, should be instituted. In this regard, oestrogen deficiency is one of the most significant contributing factors to rising costs among older women.

The menopause occurs when women run out of viable ova or have their ovaries removed or damaged at surgery. In either case, the production of oestrogen, progesterone and androgens from the ovary is reduced below the level necessary to maintain good cellular responses. In those women who pass the menopause and enter a sex hormone-deficient state, the ensuing problems can be numerous and include both short- and long-term cellular malfunction. Long-term dysfunction ultimately leads to profound and irreversible damage to the total organism.

In Australia, there are about 2 300 000 women who are post-menopausal, with about 80 000 new cases occurring every year. It is by far the most common hormone deficient condition in the world and is the one which until now has been treated least effectively by the medical profession or else, ignored as being a 'natural event'.

The problems associated with oestrogen deficiency can be divided into short-term symptoms and long-term effects:

Short-term symptoms: These occur at or about the time that oestrogen levels begin to fall and include vaso-vagal symptoms such as hot flushes, sweats and formication. There may be bewildering mood changes, loss of self esteem, loss of energy, drive and libido as well as increasing headaches and confusion.

Long-term effects: These include an increase in osteoporosis, atherosclerosis, myocardial infarcts, cardiovascular abnormalities and non-genital cancer.

15.4 PHYSIOLOGICAL ACTIVITY OF SEX STEROIDS

The ovary is responsible for producing a number of sex steroids, including oestradiol, progesterone and testosterone. Oestradiol, like all hormones, will only act on a cell if that cell contains a receptor for the hormone. Oestrogen receptors are found in the vagina, cervix, uterus, tubes, ovaries, bladder, breast, skin, arteries (endothelium as well as muscle), heart, liver, bone, gut and brain. Progesterone receptors have been found in the uterus, ovary, breast, gut and brain while testosterone receptors have been found in the vulva, clitoris, endometrium, ovary, breast and brain.

Oestrogen: This appears to be responsible for growth and maintenance of cells which contain a receptor. It maintains normal cellular activity of osteoclasts in bone. In the arteries (particularly of the coronary vessels) oestrogen appears to prevent oxidation of low density lipoprotein–cholesterol (LDL–C) thus reducing the risk of plaque formation, as well as increasing the production of prostacyclin and nitric oxide, thus inducing vasodilatation. Oestradiol is also responsible for increasing growth of duct cells in the breast and is thought to play a part in reducing degradation of neurotransmitters in the brain.

Progesterone: This is an anti-oestrogen. Within the endometrium, it is responsible for increasing the production of enzymes (oestradiol dehydrogenase, oestrone sulphotransferase) which degrade oestradiol. It also induces secretory activity, inhibits mitosis and reduces the production of a number of growth factors. Within breast cells, it has several actions including suppression of cell mitosis. It is initially stimulatory to alveolar cells but prolonged exposure to progestogens results in suppression of mitosis. Progestogens can induce depression, mood changes, and will inhibit smooth muscle activity (constipation and bloating) and may increase the appetite.

Testosterone: This increases osteoblastic activity, stimulates the dermal papillae of hair follicles, increases labial sensitivity and has a stimulatory effect on certain cells in the brain, particularly in the limbic system.

When the ovary runs out of viable ova, the ability to produce the three major sex hormones is markedly reduced. Initially, anovulation occurs with failure to produce progesterone leading to an irregular bleeding pattern (dysfunctional uterine bleeding). Eventually, even follicular development ceases and this results in low levels of oestrogen. Some 3–5 years later the production of ovarian androgens also decreases.

Clinical features and diagnostic considerations

1. As well as vaso-vagal symptoms such as hot flushes (80% of patients), sweats (70%), generalized skin itching (formication) (17%) and palpitations (30%), at least 60% of women also suffer from vaginal atrophy and bladder problems such as frequency and urgency.
2. Accentuation of psychiatric or neurotic problems is often experienced but a larger number also suffer from fatigue,

tiredness, loss of purpose, feelings of despair, or of being unwanted and unloved.
3. Vaginal discomfort is often accompanied by a loss of libido and disruption of interpersonal relations.

Other changes

1. Apart from the above immediate changes, an increased incidence of myocardial infarction, stroke, osteoporotic fractures and cancer is also seen in later years. However, women who take oestrogen following the menopause have been found to have an incidence of osteoporotic fractures which is less than half that found among women not on hormones. The incidence of myocardial infarction is only about 40%, that of stroke is halved, and that cancer of the uterus, ie. both endometrical and cervical as well as ovarian cancer are all significantly reduced in women on hormone replacement. There is a possible slight rise in breast cancer.
2. Recent evidence has also shown that women taking hormones from the time of the menopause will live 4 years longer than women who have never received hormonal replacement therapy.

Initial assessment

History
It is important to obtain a good history. As women approach the menopause, there may be irregular menses due to anovulation and fluctuating levels of oestrogen. Not only will the menstrual cycle be irregular but symptoms such as irritability, anger, depression, emotional outbursts and mood changes are also common. Some women have intermittent bouts of flushes, sweats and insomnia.

Information on family history of osteoporosis, cancer and cardiovascular disease should be sought.

Physical examination
This should include blood pressure measurement, breast palpation, and examination of the abdomen and pelvis. The vaginal epithelium should be noted for moisture, acidity and epithelial texture. Uterine and adnexal features must also be noted.

Investigations

1. A Papanicolaou (PAP) smear, full blood count, and a mammogram should be performed on every woman who attends for a menopausal evaluation.
2. FSH levels will be high, oestrogen may be low, and progesterone is often non-recordable, indicating anovulation.
3. A dual beam bone mineral analysis is appropriate to determine the calcium status of bone. Evidence of low bone density may help a woman decide on taking hormone replacement therapy.

Management principles

1. Recognize impending hormonal dysfunction early in women presenting for menopausal evaluation.
2. Take a careful history and conduct a thorough physical examination (see above).
3. Provide appropriate advice and education, and institute hormonal replacement therapy. (N.B. No other form of therapy but hormones will stimulate cells to reactivate or function again.)
4. Monitor patients regularly to assess the efficacy of treatment and detect any complications. Adjust treatment accordingly.

15.5 PHARMACOLOGICAL AGENTS AVAILABLE FOR TREATMENT

Oestrogens

Hormonal therapy regimens in the menopause are generally based on use of 'natural oestrogens' (i.e. those that are metabolized in humans in manner similar to that of endogenous oestrogen).

1. Oral 'natural' oestrogens (and their minimal dosages to inhibit osteoporosis) include conjugated equine oestrogens (0.625 mg daily), oestradiol valerate (2 mg daily), and piperazine oestrone sulphate (1.25 mg daily).
2. Transdermal oestrogen patches are also available and deliver oestradiol across the skin (25, 50 100 mg daily).

3. Implants provide oestradiol for up to 6 months from insertion.

The benefits of oestrogens administered from the time of the menopause include:

- Prevention of vaso-vagal symptoms, psychological changes and genital tract changes.
- A reduction in the risk of atherosclerosis and myocardial infarction by 60–70%.
- A reduction in the risk of osteoporosis by 60%.
- A reduced risk of non-genital cancer.
- An increase in life expectancy by 4 years.
- An improvement in the quality of life.
- A fall in blood pressure (via a vasodilating effect).

However, long-term unopposed oestrogen therapy increases the risk of endometrial cancer by 5 to 10 times; thus when the uterus is intact, it is advisable to administer a progestogen to prevent adverse changes to the endometrium. Other adverse effects of oestrogens include gastrointestinal disturbances, fluid retention and sore breasts.

Progestogens

These agents are given in conjunction with oestrogens for a minimum of 12 to 14 days each cycle but a significant number of women are now being given progestogens in a continuous combined regimen with improved results and less side effects. The major beneficial effect is inhibition of mitotic activity in the endometrium, thereby reducing the risk of endometrial cancer. Adverse effects of progestogens include weight gain, constipation, a bloated sensation, break-through bleeding, headaches and depression. In a small percentage of women, progestogens have been shown to be responsible for hypertension and adverse lipid changes, especially when given in a high dosage.

15.6 OPTIMUM TREATMENT

There are many suitable treatment regimens and the choice is influenced by the patient and her response to the regimen being administered.

Always give sufficient oestrogen to control symptoms and prevent osteoporosis. The oestrogen is generally given continually. The longer the progestogen is given in each cycle, the lower the dosage of progestogen required to inhibit mitotic activity in the endometrium. It is normal to advise medroxyprogesterone acetate 5–10 mg daily or norethisterone 0.35–2.5 mg daily for 12 to 14 days per cycle. Many women taking progesterone for 12 days each month will have a withdrawal bleed when they cease the progesterone.

An alternative regimen is to administer the oestrogen and progestogen concurrently without any 'break'. Women taking hormones like this usually do not menstruate but may have some break-through bleeding initially when they start treatment.

Another regimen which has received support is the use of continual oestrogen for 3 to 4 months followed by 12 to 14 days of progestogen to induce a secretory change.

In different women, any of the above regimens may be the preferred option. Cyclical oestrogen therapy followed by 12 to 14 days of progestogen usually induces a withdrawal bleed. Continuous oestrogen and progestogen therapy will usually inhibit endometrial growth, but 'break-through' bleeding may be a nuisance in the first 3 months of therapy.

To obtain the optimum benefit and avoid the risk of cardiovascular or osteoporotic changes, hormone replacement therapy should be continued for at least 15 years. However, in advising women on the length of time to take therapy, they may be assured that they can continue while they are physically, mentally or sexually active. However, as with the administration of all therapy regimens, they must have regular monitoring.

Principal contraindications

Because 'natural' oestrogens are metabolized in an identical manner to endogenous oestrogens, the need to cease administering hormones to postmenopausal women is slight. If there is an oestrogen-dependent tumour which has evidence of metastases or secondary spread, then oestrogen therapy should be ceased. When there is hepatic damage or oral oestrogens have induced an abnormal hepatic response such an increased clotting factor or elevation of sex hormone-binding globulin

(SHBG), then an alternate route of administration such as the skin or vagina should be sought. Conditions such as hypertension, gallbladder disease or thrombosis are not now considered to be a reason for ceasing oestrogen therapy.

Overcoming problems in treatment

If oral oestrogen therapy is contraindicated or is poorly tolerated (e.g. because of gastrointestinal disturbances), intravaginal or transdermal administration may be tried. Piperazine oestrone sulphate, 1 oral tablet of 2.5 mg inserted into the vagina each night, is absorbed readily and blood levels adequate for inhibition of hot flushes and other menopausal symptoms are achieved.

Transdermal oestradiol patches (Estraderm) or impregnated plaster strips are available. Good absorption is obtained and over 75% of women find this form of oestrogen is very satisfactory.

If there is a reluctance to use the vaginal route, oestradiol implants may be inserted under the skin to provide an adequate level of oestrogen.

When an oestrogen-dependent tumour is present some relief of symptoms and reduced risk of osteoporosis may be achieved by using a progestogen such as norethisterone 10 mg daily or medroxyprogesterone acetate 30 to 100 mg daly. However care must be taken that these high doses of progestogens do not induce hypertension or have an adverse effect on the blood lipid status.

In patients experiencing problems with progestogens, use of continuous low-dose regimens such as levonorgestrel 0.30 mg, norethisterone 0.35 mg or medroxyprogesterone acetate 2.5 mg per day will inhibit mitotic activity in the endometrium.

The benefits of hormonal replacement therapy so outweigh any minor discomforts or problems that it is imperative that clinicians devote time, patience and educational activity to allay the fears and myths which have surrounded this hormonal deficiency for so long.

16

Prolapse and urinary incontinence

16.1 GENERAL INSTRUCTIONAL OBJECTIVE

The students should understand the nature and significance of utero-vaginal prolapse and urinary incontinence so that they can diagnose these conditions and appreciate the management of such patients.

16.2 SPECIFIC BEHAVIOURAL OBJECTIVES

1. Discuss the applied anatomy of the uterus, vagina and supporting structures.
2. Discuss the aetiological factors of utero-vaginal prolapse.
3. Explain the meaning of urethrocoele, cystocoele, enterocoele, rectocoele and the degree of uterine prolapse.
4. Demonstrate an ability to examine a woman with utero-vaginal prolapse and relate the history to the physical findings.
5. List the types of management of utero-vaginal prolapse.
6. Discuss urinary continence in the female.
7. List and define the types of urinary incontinence.
8. Discuss the aetiological factors of each type of urinary incontinence.
9. Demonstrate an ability to diagnose the type of urinary incontinence by taking a history and performing an adequate physical examination.
10. Have some knowledge of the available treatments for incontinence.

16.3 REASONS FOR LEARNING ABOUT PROLAPSE AND URINARY INCONTINENCE

Women who have had children, or who have passed through the climacteric, may often present to their doctor with complaints that suggest the bladder, uterus or rectum is involved in a prolapse. It is important to be able to take a history, examine and correctly diagnose these conditions, to then initiate management, or to refer to an appropriate person who can manage the problem.

16.4 INTRODUCTION

Prolapse is one of the most common gynaecological complaints. The diagnosis and management of this condition should be understood by all medical graduates.

Urinary incontinence was long regarded as a shameful condition that many women were too embarrassed to discuss and that many doctors regarded as untreatable. However, with recent advances in the diagnosis and treatment of this condition, no woman should be left to suffer the misery of urinary leakage in silence.

Prolapse often coexists with incontinence but each may occur independently as well.

16.5 UTERO-VAGINAL PROLAPSE

The prevalence of utero-vaginal prolapse is not accurately known but approximately 20% of all patients having gynaecological surgery are undergoing some form of prolapse repair.

Anatomical classification

Vaginal prolapse is defined as descent of the urethra (urethrocoele), the bladder (cystocoele Fig. 16.1), the small bowel (enterocoele Fig. 16.2)) or the rectum (rectocoele Fig. 16.3) into the vagina or even beyond the vaginal introitus. After hysterectomy, the vaginal vault may also prolapse and usually contains small bowel, but the term vault prolapse is generally applied here.

Vaginal prolapse conditions are usually graded as slight,

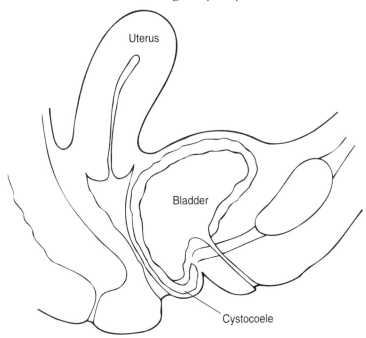

Figure 16.1 Cystocoele.

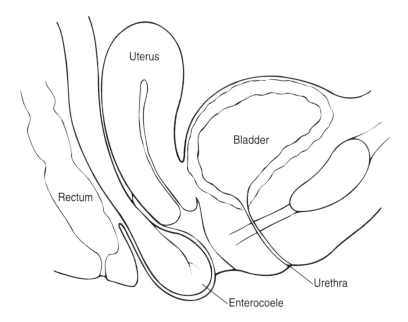

Figure 16.2 Enterocoele.

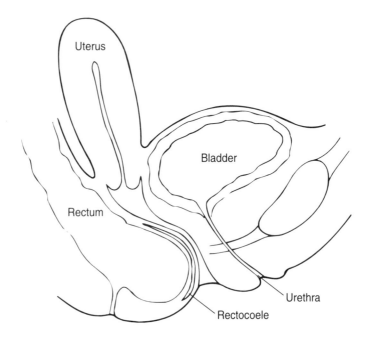

Figure 16.3 Rectocoele.

where there is some descent with cough; moderate, where the prolapse balloons out to the introitus; or severe, where the prolapse protrudes well beyond the introitus.

Uterine prolapse is graded differently. A first-degree uterine prolapse refers to descent within the vagina. When the cervix protrudes through the introitus, this is a second-degree prolapse and when the entire uterus has also come outside the vagina, this is a third-degree prolapse, also called procidentia (Fig. 16.4).

16.6 ANATOMICAL CONSIDERATIONS

The uterus, bladder and rectum are supported by the pelvic floor, which includes the levator ani, the coccygeal, internal obturator and piriform muscles, along with the two transverse perineal muscles.

Students should refer to previous anatomy texts, but essentially the levator ani consists of the pubo-coccygeus and the

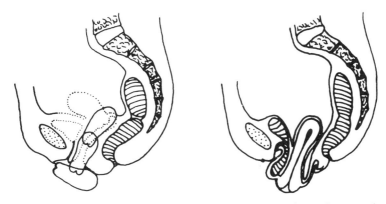

Figure 16.4 Illustrating the stages in descent and prolapse of the uterus. Shows how as the uterus prolapses, the bladder is dragged out as well to produce a cystocoele.

ilio-coccygeus muscles. The pubo-coccygeus comes from the inner aspect of the pubis, decussates around the vagina and passes to the perineal body. The ileo-coccygeus comes from the coccyx and runs down to the median raphe that encircles the anus posteriorly.

Anteriorly the superficial and deep transverse perineal muscles arise from the undersurface of the pubis and encircle the urethra and vagina to insert onto the perineal body.

Within the pelvis, the uterus is mainly supported by the transverse cervical ligaments (also called the cardinal ligaments or Mackenrodt's ligaments) which run laterally from the cervix to the pelvic side walls. Secondary support is provided by the uterosacral ligaments, running from the back of the uterus to the sacrum. Some support is also given by the pubocervical and pubourethral ligaments (from the back of the pubis to the cervix and to the front of the urethra) (Fig. 16.5). These two ligaments are also important in maintaining continence.

The round ligament (actually a muscle) runs from the cornu of the uterus, through the inguinal canal to the labium majus. It does not support the uterus but helps to keep it anteverted. The broad ligaments are a thin filmy collection of fascia above the transverse cervical ligaments, and enclosed by peritoneum anteriorly and posteriorly. Like the round ligaments, they give no support to the uterus (Fig. 16.6).

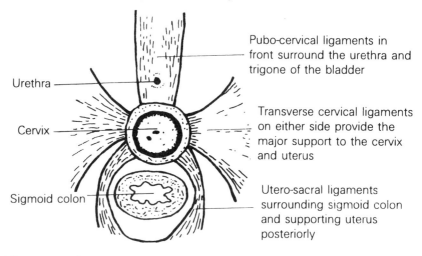

Urethra

Cervix

Sigmoid colon

Pubo-cervical ligaments in front surround the urethra and trigone of the bladder

Transverse cervical ligaments on either side provide the major support to the cervix and uterus

Utero-sacral ligaments surrounding sigmoid colon and supporting uterus posteriorly

Figure 16.5 Ligamentous supports of the cervix and uterus.

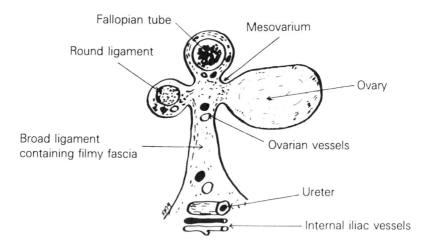

Fallopian tube

Mesovarium

Round ligament

Ovary

Broad ligament containing filmy fascia

Ovarian vessels

Ureter

Internal iliac vessels

Figure 16.6 Anatomy of broad ligaments.

16.7 CAUSES OF UTERO-VAGINAL PROLAPSE

Obstetrical factors

In the labour ward you will observe the tremendous bearing down efforts which may be involved in childbirth, and the resultant strain on the above ligaments is a major aetiological factor in prolapse. Prolonged labour, bearing down before full dilatation, difficult forceps, obstetric lacerations, delivery of the placenta by fundal pressure, and inadequate repair of the perineal body/transverse perineal muscles are all implicated in the genesis of prolapse.

In addition there is some evidence that the pressure of the fetal head can damage the pelvic floor directly or secondarily as a result of nerve compression, leading to a neurapraxia. This in term will impair the function of the pelvic floor muscles.

Following delivery, the elastic tissue returns to normal, but if the tissue is weakened by atrophy (oestrogen lack or by

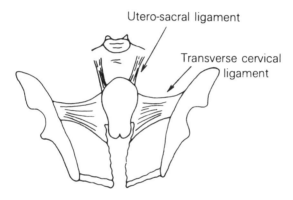

Figure 16.7 Diagram to illustrate the ligamentous supports of the uterus.

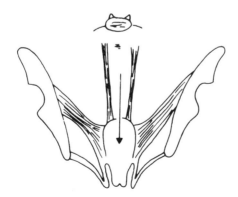

Figure 16.8 Diagram to illustrate how the utero-sacral ligaments and the transverse cervical ligaments become stretched during prolapse of the uterus. Not only does this cause a dragging pain, but the uterus begins to descend through the vagina.

increased intra-abdominal pressure (fat, coughing, ascites, etc.) the fascial supports give way and allow the bladder, uterus or rectum to prolapse (Figs 16.7, 16.8).

Hormone deficiency

Oestrogen deficiency after the menopause is associated with atrophy and weakening of the supportive ligaments, hence prolapse most commonly presents in the 50–70 year age group.

Raised intra-abdominal pressure

Any long-standing cause of raised intra-abdominal pressure such as heavy lifting, obesity, chronic cough or chronic straining to defaecate, increases the risk of prolapse (and should be dealt with preoperatively, else the prolapse may recur).

Post-surgery

Prolapse of the vaginal vault may occur post-hysterectomy if insufficient attention has been paid to attaching it to the supporting ligament.

16.8 SYMPTOMS AND SIGNS OF PROLAPSE

The presenting symptoms vary according to the structure that is prolapsing. The most common symptom is a feeling of 'something coming down' in the vagina, e.g. a lump or bulge. This lump may be the cervix/uterus, the bladder or the rectum.

Low backache or dragging pain is a common non-specific symptom, usually worse at the end of the day.

Cystocoele and/or urethrocoele may cause urgency and frequency of micturition. Stress incontinence may be a major symptom. If the bladder neck region is prolapsing down but the urethra is not kinked then incontinence may result. If the urethra is kinked by the prolapse, then initial hesitancy, poor stream and residual urine (with risk of cystitis) occur but stress incontinence will be absent.

A rectocoele may cause difficulty in defaecation and on direct (tactful) questioning, patients may admit to pushing the lump back digitally in order to empty their bowels.

Any prolapse may cause dyspareunia (or apareunia).

In procidentia, the lump is felt hanging down between the legs and will usually rub on the underwear, causing a decubitus ulcer and haemoserous discharge. This may present as post-menopausal bleeding.

Examination

Many multiparous women have some evidence of prolapse which causes no symptoms and requires no treatment.

The labia are parted and the patient asked to cough (when a severe prolapse is present, it will project well beyond the intro-itus). Visualization is best obtained using a Sims' speculum with the patient lying in left lateral position and the right leg held partly upwards by the assistant. If neither the Sim's speculum nor the assistant is available, withdraw a duckbill speculum slowly and observe both vaginal walls during cough. Observe the presence or absence of the vaginal rugal pattern and if postmenopausal the degree of oestrogenization of the vagina. The presence of an enterocoele should be sought.

The degree of prolapse can be observed by partially withdrawing the Sims' speculum and getting the patient to strain down.

The size and position and mobility of the uterus should be noted. The adnexa are palpated to exclude ovarian pathology.

A rectal examination (PR) is done in all cases to check for the presence of a rectocoele. Occasionally a rectovaginal examination may be needed to exclude the presence of an enterocoele.

Investigations

All women should have a PAP smear taken if one has not recently been performed.

A midstream urine should be cultured to exclude cystitis in cases of cysto/urethrocoele. Other gynaecological tests will not usually affect management (unless incontinence exists, see section 16.9). However, the patient's general status may indicate need for chest X-ray, ECG, etc., before suitability for surgery can be ascertained.

16.9 MANAGEMENT OF PROLAPSE

Conservative treatment

The first step is to correct any cause of raised intra-abdominal pressure. Too often, obese patients with prolapse undergo surgery, only to find that the condition recurs. Chronic cough may require referral to a respiratory physician and preoperative chest physiotherapy, else the cough may worsen after general anaesthesia and endanger the integrity of the sutures. Such patients benefit from spinal anaesthesia for this reason. Patients who strain to defaecate because of constipation should be advised to take unprocessed bran (three tablespoons daily) or Metamucil.

In patients with a mild cystocoele or rectocoele, pelvic floor exercises conducted by a physiotherapist may lessen the prolapse and certainly prevent it worsening.

Women who are postmenopausal will benefit from the administration of topical or systemic oestrogens.

If there is any uncertainty about the diagnosis, a ring pessary may be used as a therapeutic trial to see if it relieves the patient's symptoms. If the symptoms resolve, then one can be certain that these will be cured by surgery.

Patients who are unfit for surgery, or who do not want surgery, may be treated by insertion of a polyethylene ring pessary. However, this must be removed, the vagina inspected for ulceration, and replaced every 4–6 months for the duration of the patient's life. Ulceration may be prevented by the use of topical oestrogens. If the perineum is severely deficient, a ring pessary (which normally sits behind the symphysis pubis and rests on the perineum posteriorly) may not remain *in situ*.

Surgical treatments

1. Anterior colporrhaphy (repair) is used to treat cysto-ure-throcoele. The vagina is incised in the midline, the bladder dissected off the vaginal skin, then the pubocervical ligaments and pubo-coccygeus muscles are brought together in the midline, to provide new support for the bladder. Redundant vaginal skin is excised and the vagina closed.

Because peri-urethral oedema often causes urinary retention, a suprapubic catheter (SPC) is inserted. The patient begins voiding per urethra on the third day; the SPC is removed once two consecutive residual volumes are less than 100 ml.

2. Posterior colporrhaphy is used to treat rectocoele and/or enterocoele. The same principles apply as in 1), except the ischeo-coccygeus and transverse perineal muscles are brought together to provide new support for the rectum. Suprapubic catheterization is not mandatory but patients may not void because of perineal pain, so many surgeons use a SPC here too.

3. The Manchester repair comprises an anterior repair and a posterior repair (with repair of enterocoele if present), with amputation of the cervix and suturing of the cardinal ligaments to the cervical stump. The stump is recovered with vaginal skin, keeping the uterine os patent.

   The Manchester repair is faster than a vaginal hysterectomy. Thus it is often reserved for frail elderly women with only a first- or second-degree uterine descent (in whom cystocoele or rectocoele is the main reason for surgery). It is also used for treating prolapse in younger women who wish to have further children. Subsequent deliveries may need to be by Caesarean section.

4. Vaginal hysterectomy is used for all third-degree uterine prolapse and most second-degree prolapse. Appropriate anterior or posterior repair is undertaken as required.

Postoperative complications include:

1. Prolonged inability to void may require the patient to be sent home with a suprapubic catheter *in situ*.

2. Bruising of the perineum with pain and constipation are quite common after posterior repair.

3. After a Manchester repair it may be impossible to visualize or take PAP smears from the cervical stump.

4. Bleeding from the vaginal vault after vaginal hysterectomy may lead to vault haematoma with abscess formation. Prophylactic antibiotics are usually given to prevent this.

16.10 URINARY INCONTINENCE

The definition of urinary incontinence recommended by the International Continence Society is 'the involuntary loss of urine which is objectively demonstrable and a social or hygienic problem'. A postal study of 22 000 people showed that it affects 8.5% of women aged 15–64 and 11.6% of women aged 65 or more.

Anatomical and physiological considerations

The bladder is a dome-shaped bag of muscle (the detrusor): at the base lies the trigone, which is bounded by the ureteric orifices and the internal urethral orifice. The bladder is supplied by parasympathetic nerves that stimulate detrusor contractions, and to a lesser extent by sympathetic nerves that inhibit detrusor contractility. Unlike any other autonomic viscera, the bladder is also under voluntary control from the cerebral cortex.

The human bladder, by virtue of its viscoelastic properties, normally distends to a volume of 500 ml without any rise in intravesical pressure; that is, the detrusor muscle accommodates this increased volume without any contractile activity. Only when the subject decides (by cortical activity) that micturition is socially convenient, does the command come down the spinal cord telling the parasympathetic nerves to initiate a detrusor contraction (and the urethra to reflexly relax) and thus the patient voids.

The female urethra is short (4 cm length) and directly contiguous with the anterior vaginal wall. The main factor that keeps the urethra closed during bladder filling is the skeletal muscle surrounding it, called the rhabdomyosphincter (in older texts, the external urinary sphincter). This is a rather special muscle, in that it has a postural component (like the erector spinae of the back muscles) which exert a resting tone. In addition, this muscle has a voluntary component, so that patients can learn to contract it at will.

Furthermore the junction between the bladder and the proximal urethra (called the bladder neck, or the zone of continence, and in older textbooks it was incorrectly called the internal urethral sphincter) is normally positioned above and supported by the pelvic floor muscles. When a subject coughs, the pressure of the cough is normally transmitted equally to the bladder and to the bladder neck, so that the bladder neck does not fall open.

The arrangement of the anatomy of the bladder and urethra and their fascial supports results in pressures being generated in both the bladder and urethra. Continence is maintained as the intraurethral pressure is higher than the intravesical pressure.

In patients with a weak pelvic floor, coughing or straining causes the full bladder to press down upon the pelvic floor and the bladder neck descends through what is essentially an intermittent 'hernia' through the levator ani muscles. Once the bladder neck is pushed out through the pelvic floor then the compressive forces of this muscular support are lost and the urethra falls laxly open during cough, allowing urine to escape.

Types of incontinence

Stress incontinence
This is incontinence arising from a weakness of the pelvic floor muscles and the rhabdomyosphincter.

Urgency incontinence
This is incontinence arising from over-activity of the detrusor muscle ('detrusor instability').

Overflow incontinence
This may be associated with neurological disorders leading to sensory abnormalities and overfilling of the bladder. On occasion, the female bladder becomes 'acontractile', usually in association with an over-distension insult, and the patient cannot void at all.

Continuous incontinence
Here the patient is incontinent all the time. This type is usually associated with fistula formation from either surgery or malignancy.

Unfortunately, these problems may occur in combination with one another, hence the need for accurate diagnostic tests.

16.11 SYMPTOMS AND SIGNS OF URINARY INCONTINENCE

Only since the advent of urodynamic testing has it been rea-
lized that symptoms and signs are not always a true indicator
of the underlying diagnosis.

Nevertheless, in the general practice environment, there are
certain constellations of symptoms that may guide one towards
a rational provisional diagnosis and allow initial conservative
treatment. This is worthwhile because urodynamic testing is
not entirely pleasant or non-invasive.

1. If a patient complains only of leakage when she coughs or
    runs, and has no 'urge' symptoms, then it is likely she will
    have genuine stress incontinence.
2. If a patient complains only of frequency (more than eight
    voids per day), nocturia (more than one void per night),
    urgency (rushing to the toilet whenever the desire to void
    is felt) or urge incontinence (leakage when the toilet cannot
    be reached quickly) then she is likely to have detrusor
    instability. However, if she has both leakage with cough
    and any 'frequency/urgency' symptoms then the diagnosis
    is uncertain.
3. If there is initial hesitancy, a poor stream, a feeling of the
    need to return to the toilet shortly after voiding, or a
    history of recurrent proven bacterial cystitis, then she may
    have an acontractile bladder with persistent residual urine
    ($>100\,\text{ml}$).
4. If the patient has symptoms of cystocoele, then either the
    bladder neck may be included in the prolapse, which may
    be associated with stress incontinence, or the urethra may
    be kinked, which may be associated with voiding difficulty.

Examination

Physical examination gives some clue to the diagnosis. If the
bladder is full and the patient coughs, an immediate short
spurt of urine is typical of stress incontinence and a delayed,
prolonged stream of urine is typical of detrusor instability. If
the bladder can be percussed above the umbilicus, an atonic
bladder is likely. Anatomical details of any cysto-urethrocoele
should be determined at this examination.

16.12 UROGYNAECOLOGICAL ASSESSMENT

In the general practice setting, much information can be derived from the frequency–volume chart (FVC). The patient records the times when she voids ('frequency'), and must take a measuring jug to the bathroom so as to measure the amount passed ('volume'). Episodes of leakage are marked with an asterisk. Approximately 72 hours of a FVC are needed for reliable information.

Those who void at half-hour–2-hourly intervals with small (<150 ml) amounts, more than eight times daily, are likely to have detrusor instability. Such patients bladders seldom hold more than 300 ml.

Those who void at 3–4-hourly intervals, four to six times daily, with volumes of >300 ml, are more likely to have stress incontinence.

In addition, urine should be sent for bacteriological culture by the general practitioner. This is because bacterial cystitis cannot be predicted reliably by dipstick testing, and cystitis is associated with frequency and urgency that may cloud the diagnostic picture. Furthermore, it is most unwise to diagnose cystitis on the basis of dipstick proteinuria. On one hand, renal disease may be missed. On the other hand, patients who are incorrectly diagnosed by this qualitative method are often told to drink plentiful fluids and void frequently. Nothing could be more unhelpful to the patient with detrusor instability (as will be seen in section 16.13).

Urodynamic tests

Before urodynamic testing, the urine should be sterile.

1. The pad test quantifies the amount of urine leakage. Patients commence with a comfortably full bladder, then drink 500 ml of water and wear a pre-weighed pad for 1 hour. Provocative manoeuvres such as climbing stairs and the sound of running water are undertaken, then the pad is weighed and urine loss determined. Unfortunately the pad test is costly in terms of nursing staff time and many units cannot afford it.

   The pad test is helpful because patients differ in their

appreciation of incontinence. Slight dampness may be totally unacceptable to some whereas others will be using three to four soaked pads each day before they seek help.

2. Urine flow rate is measured. The bladder should be comfortably full because volumes less than 200 ml make the flow rate difficult to interpret. The patient sits on a commode over the flowmeter, which must be located in private. As a rule of thumb, an average flow rate of more than 15 ml/sec is normal. Abnormal patterns such as an atonic detrusor or abdominal straining can be seen on inspecting the flow tracing (Fig. 16.9).

3. Residual urine volume is measured, either by catheter or by ultrasound. Residual urine >100 ml is abnormal.

4. Twin-channel cystometry is performed by placing a pressure-monitoring line in the bladder (either fluid filled, as in a CVP line, or by microtransducers mounted on the catheter, which is very expensive equipment), and a second line in the rectum, covered with a small rubber balloon which is filled with 10 ml of fluid. As long as the procedure is explained to the patient, most experience minor discomfort but no pain. The risk of introducing urinary infection is estimated at 0.5–2%.

    The two channels are needed because intravesical pressure is composed of the intrinsic detrusor pressure and the

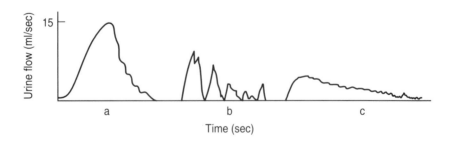

Figure 16.9 Urinary flow rate measurements. (a) normal flow pattern; (b) abdominal straining; (c) atonic detrusor.

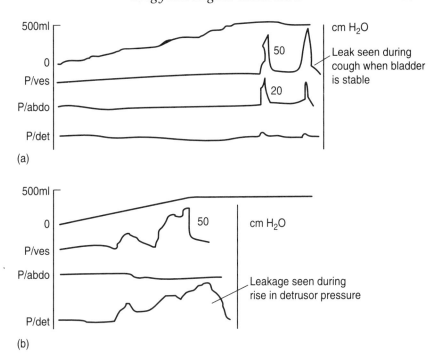

Figure 16.10 Twin-channel cystometry. (a) Stable bladder, stress leak seen; (b) Unstable bladder. P/ves, intravesical pressure; P/abdo, intra-abdominal pressure; P/det, detrusor pressure (=P/ves – P/abdo).

extrinsic (or transmitted) abdominal pressure: both must be measured. When a patient coughs, the rise in her intra-abdominal pressure will be transmitted to the bladder. But this is quite different to the rise in bladder pressure that occurs when the detrusor muscle contracts (Fig. 16.10).

During cystometry, the bladder is filled with warm saline, usually to a maximum of 500 ml. The patient is asked to indicate her first desire to void (normally about 250 ml). She is then asked to inhibit micturition until she cannot tolerate any more fluid – the maximum cystometric capacity (normally about 500 ml). Various provocative man-oeuvres such as standing up, coughing and heel bouncing are then performed.

The following additional tests are performed to a varying extent in different urodynamic units:

5. Voiding cystometry: the patient voids with the pressure transducer lines *in situ*. This is useful in suspected voiding difficulty/atonic bladder, since the pressure generated by the detrusor during voiding is measured.
6. Urethral pressure profile: initial cystometry is performed using a double-lumen catheter; one lumen is at the tip, the other about 6 cm distal so that it lies in the urethra. The catheter is withdrawn from the bladder and the pressure in the bladder and urethra are compared during cough. In continent women, the urethral pressure exceeds the bladder pressure.
7. Video-cysto-urethrography (VCU): cystometry is done in the X-ray department and the bladder is filled with radio-opaque dye. The bladder neck is screened during cough via an image intensifier. The position of the bladder neck is seen in relation to the symphysis pubis.
8. Transvaginal ultrasound of the bladder neck at the end of filling also gives good anatomical information and is becoming more popular as access to an X-ray suite is not needed.

Urodynamic diagnoses

Genuine stress incontinence (GSI)
Leakage of fluid is observed during cystometry when the bladder is stable (not contracting).

Detrusor instability (DI)
Detrusor contractions are seen during filling or provocation that the patient is unable to suppress.

Sensory urgency
Early first desire to void (<150 ml) and small capacity (<400 ml) but the bladder is stable. The patient should go on to have a normal cystoscopy.

Voiding difficulty
Low flow rate with a pattern of abdominal straining, usually accompanied by residual urine >100 ml. This may occur after surgery for stress incontinence.

Atonic bladder
Late first desire (>400 ml) and large capacity (>500 ml) with prolonged voiding phase.

16.13 MANAGEMENT OF URINARY INCONTINENCE

Treatment of genuine stress incontinence

Conservative management

1. Causes of raised intra-abdominal are attended to (as for prolapse).
2. Trial of conservative treatment is usually worthwhile:
   (a) Pelvic floor exercises, making sure by digital examination that the patient knows which muscle to contract and have a target number of contractions to do each day.
   (b) Physiotherapy, i.e. electrical stimulation of the pelvic floor muscles by faradism or interferential treatment.
   (c) Vaginal cone weights to increase postural tone of the pelvic floor muscles.
   (d) Oestregens (toporal and/or systemic) in post-menopausal women.

A specially trained Nurse Continence Advisor or a physiotherapist provide valuable assistance in these treatments.

Surgical management

Surgery is undertaken for severe incontinence or those who have failed to respond to conservative treatment.
Surgical options are as follows:

1. Vaginal procedures
   Anterior repair (as described in section 16.9) with the addition of sub-urethral Kelly buttress sutures. Because the cure rate is only 65–75%, this operation is no longer regarded as the best choice unless prolapse is the major complaint and stress incontinence is minor.
2. Abdominal procedures
   Colposuspension: The anterior cul de sac is dissected through a transverse suprapubic incision and sutures are placed in the para-urethral vaginal fascia, and tied to the ileo-pectineal ligament. The cure rate is 88–92%.
3. Combination procedures (slings)
   These use a combination of an abdominal and vaginal approach using either fascia, synthetic, material or sutures

to elevate the bladder neck. For details of needle suspension procedures (Stamey, Peyrera and Gitties) and sling operations, refer to lecture or postgraduate texts. Variable cure rates are 70–85%.

Postoperative complications

1. Voiding difficulty occurs in approximately 0.5–10%, with a risk of prolonged need for suprapubic catheterization. About 1% risk of temporary or permanent intermittent self-catheterization.
2. Postoperative detrusor instability may arise if a relative outflow obstruction has been created. The detrusor 'over-works' to compensate for the obstruction and becomes unstable. The risk is not fully known (18% in one series of 100 colposuspensions).
3. Long-term failure of the operation.

Treatment of detrusor instability

1. The mainstay of treatment is bladder training. The patient is taught to defer micturition by concentrating on inhibiting the desire to void. The voiding intervals are gradually prolonged and progress is gauged by successive frequency–volume charts.
2. Pelvic floor exercises may also be helpful here since ability to shut the bladder neck will prevent drops of urine escaping into the urethra (that trigger severe urgency).
3. Anticholinergic drugs inhibit the effect of parasympathetic nerves upon detrusor contractors. Most commonly used are:
   - Propantheline (Probanthine) 15 mg t.d.s.
   - Imipramine (Tofranil) 25 mg mane and 50 mg nocte.
   - Penthienate bromide (Monodral) 5 mg b.d.
   - Oxybutynin (Diptropan) 5 mg t.d.s.

Bladder neck surgery is **not** indicated for detrusor instability. Patients with combined GSI and DI should have conservative treatment for their GSI until the DI is treated.

Cystodistension, whereby the bladder is distended to maximum capacity under general anaesthetic and left full for

3–5 minutes can improve bladder capacity in approximately 65–75% of cases.

Sensory urgency can usually be managed by bladder training without recourse to anticholinergic drugs. Cystoscopy can be accompanied by cystodistension.

Treatment of voiding difficulty

First the patient is trained in the technique of 'double empty-ing', e.g. once voiding is finished, she stands up and moves about so that the afferent nerves appreciate the residual urine, then sits down, relaxes the pelvic floor and leans forward, to expel all urine. If recurrent cystitis exists, prophylactic anti-biotics (e.g. Macrodantin 100 mg nocte for 3 months) are given since bladder function may be impaired in the presence of infection.

If these techniques fail, and residual urine is persistently >100 ml and either causing symptoms or is associated with recurrent infections despite prophylactic antibiotics, then the patient is trained to perform intermittent self-catheterization.

17

Benign and malignant tumours of the female genital tract

The students should understand the nature of benign and malignant lesions of the female reproductive system and the significance of pre-malignant conditions of that area so that they can identify those patients requiring further investigation and can appreciate their management.

17.2 SPECIFIC BEHAVIOURAL OBJECTIVES

1. Indicate possible aetiological factors involved in malignancy of the reproductive systems.
2. Describe the macroscopic features of benign and malignant neoplasms of the female reproductive system.
3. Describe the common pre-malignant lesions of the reproductive system and discuss their significance.
4. Discuss the clinical features and complications of the common benign lesions of the female reproductive system, such as endometriosis, adenomyosis, fibromyoma, ovarian tumours, uterine polyps, Bartholin's cysts and cervical lesions.
5. Discuss the clinical features and complications of common malignant lesions of the female reproductive system, such as ovarian carcinoma, adenocarcinoma of corpus, squamous cell carcinoma of cervix, squamous cell carcinoma of vulva.
6. Discuss the clinical differences between benign and malignant lesions of the female reproductive system.

7. Identify by history and examination a patient with a malignant or pre-malignant lesion and record the findings.
8. Take a cervical smear and indicate a knowledge of other techniques available to make a diagnosis of malignant and pre-malignant lesions of the female reproductive system.
9. Describe the symptoms and signs that would arouse suspicion of the presence of a malignant neoplasm of the female reproductive system.
10. Outline the possible management of benign, malignant and pre-malignant lesions of the female reproductive system.
11. Discuss counselling of a patient with a benign, malignant or pre-malignant lesion of the reproductive system.
12. Discuss the clinical behaviour and prognosis of common malignant neoplasms of the female reproductive system.
13. Discuss the clinical behaviour of common benign neoplasms.

17.3 REASONS FOR LEARNING ABOUT BENIGN AND MALIGNANT TUMOURS OF THE FEMALE GENITAL TRACT

Women attending a doctor or a clinic may present with symptoms or signs that may be due to a benign or malignant lesion. It is important that doctors should not only understand the basic disease process, but they should also be aware of how it may present, what steps should be taken to diagnose the problem and how it may be managed. Failure to diagnose and initiate management may lead to a delay that will increase morbidity or mortality. Doctors should also be able to differentiate most benign from most malignant diseases and when the latter is suspected, they should be able to direct the patient to the most appropriate institution for early treatment.

The details of management are not necessary, but a broad concept of what is involved is essential so that counselling and post-treatment advice can be properly directed. The symptoms or signs may lead to an early and accurate diagnosis of the underlying disease; and failure to detect such a disease may lead to an erroneous management plan.

Patients attending the gynaecological clinic and those admitted for surgery will often be found to have some form of genital tract tumour. Most of these patients will have benign tumours, such as ovarian cysts, fibromyomata, adenomyosis,

Handwritten margin notes:
Simple cyst
physiological cyst — follicular / CL
Endometrioma
Epith. cyst
Granulosa/stromal tumours
fibroma
Cystic teratoma

endometriosis, polyps or Bartholin's cysts. Benign lesions of the cervix, such as ectopic columnar epithelium and polyps, must be differentiated from cancer of the cervix. Abnormal uterine bleeding due to fibromyomata, polyps or dysfunctional uterine haemorrhage will often mimic carcinoma of the endometrium, and tumours in the pelvis due to benign follicular cysts or endometriosis may be confused with malignant ovaries.

17.4 TYPES OF TUMOURS OF THE GENITAL TRACT

The common benign tumours of the genital tract are:

1. Physiological ovarian cysts, such as the follicular and luteal cysts.
2. Dermoid cysts.
3. Mucinous and serous cystadenomas of the ovary.
4. Fibromyomas of the uterus and ovaries.
5. Adenomyosis of the uterus.
6. Endometriosis.
7. Endometrial and endocervical mucous polyps.
8. Bartholin's cysts and abscesses.

The common malignant tumours are:

1. Mucinous and serious cystadenocarcinomas of the ovary.
2. Carcinoma of the endometrium.
3. Carcinoma of the cervix.
4. Sarcoma of the uterus.

17.5 PHYSIOLOGICAL OVARIAN CYSTS

The ovary is composed of stroma in which rest the primordial germ cells, both of which are derived from the common mesenchymal cells of the primitive gonad. As development occurs, the stromal or mesenchymal cells that surround each primordial germ cell differentiate into granulosa cells and theca cells.

Under the influence of follicle-stimulating hormone from the anterior pituitary, one (or more) germ cell and the surrounding granulosa cells begin to grow and form a follicular cyst. The granulosa cells normally produce oestradiol, which reaches a peak of production about the 12th to 14th day and stimulates the production of releasing factor from the hypothalamus. This in turn causes the pituitary to release luteinizing hormone in large quantities and thus precipitates the rupture of a follicle. The resultant ovulation leaves a corpus luteum which continues to produce oestrogen and progesterone for a further 5–8 days, followed by a gradual decrease in levels (leading to menstruation) unless pregnancy eventuates.

If the delicate balance of hormonal levels is disturbed in any way a number of dysfunctional actions may occur. If the developing Graafian follicle produces low levels of oestrogens, then the induction of a surge of luteinizing hormone fails to occur and ovulation may not eventuate. In this case follicle-stimulating hormone continues to be produced (as well as low levels of luteinizing hormone) and the follicle continues to grow. Normally a follicle reaches about 2 cm in size before ovulation, but it may grow to the size of a golf ball (4 cm) or occasionally even larger under the continued influence of follicle-stimulating hormone. The patient will present with a history of amenorrhoea (due to sustained levels of oestrogen), followed by irregular bleeds for some weeks afterwards. Because of the prolonged influence of oestrogen, the endometrium is hypertrophied, may become cystic or even polypoidal, and will eventually produce heavy blood loss (metropathia haemorrhagica). On examination, the uterus is usually not enlarged, the cervix is closed and a round mobile mass can be palpated in the region of the ovary. It is sometimes difficult to differentiate such cases from an ectopic pregnancy or even a normal early pregnancy, so when doubt exists, order a pregnancy test. Most cases of dysfunctional uterine haemorrhage due to anovulation occur in women aged over 35, or in girls who have not yet established their cycle. In all these cases there is no need to operate on the ovarian cyst as it will usually spontaneously regress.

Physiological ovarian cysts of follicular origin are so common that they probably account for 80–90% of all identified tumours of the ovary; they are typically less than 5 cm in diameter, and most follicular cysts disappear spontaneously within 60 days without treatment. The size and growth of the cyst can be monitored by means of an ultrasound scan over a 2 months period, and only if it is more than 5 cm in diameter or remains unchanged, particularly if a normal menstrual period intervenes, should a surgical approach be made. An oophorectomy is not required, the cyst can be simply punctured or shelled out of the ovary. The follicular cyst is usually easily identified, as it is 1–5 cm in diameter, thin-walled and filled with clear fluid. The only symptom directly referable to the cyst is haemorrhage or torsion of the cyst, which gives an ache or pain referred to the iliac fossa, or medial side of the thigh.

Other physiological cysts are corpus luteum cysts, which produce progesterone, and the polycystic ovaries associated with the increased production of luteinizing hormone.

17.6 BENIGN OVARIAN TUMOURS

Mucinous ovarian tumours

Benign mucinous cystadenomas account for 10% of non-physiological ovarian tumours. They are usually a semi-solid mass present in one region. Occasionally these cysts are bilateral. They may grow to a huge size, filling the whole abdomen and producing marked pressure effects. The cyst is lined by a tall columnar epithelium, which produces a glycoprotein secretion resembling mucin. If the cyst is accidentally ruptured at removal or ruptures spontaneously, the epithelial cells of the cyst may seed onto the peritoneum and produce a pseudomyxoma peritonei. This leads to the abdominal cavity becoming filled with mucin – eventually leading to repeated bowel obstruction and gradual deterioration and death from malabsorption.

Approximately 5–10% of mucinous cystadenomas are found to be malignant at removal.

Serous cystadenomas of the ovary

These cysts account for 35–40% of ovarian tumours. They are usually thin-walled, unilocular cysts with many intracystic papillae. About 30% are found to be bilateral. They usually are not very large – only 5–10 cm in diameter. The secretions that fill the thin-walled cyst are generally clear or straw-coloured. The lining epithelium is columnar and is said to resemble the epithelium of the endosalpinx. About 30% of these cysts are thought to undergo malignant change.

Other benign ovarian tumours

Fibromas and luteomas of the ovary are rare solid tumours. They are derived from ovarian stroma and depending on the amount of active tissue within each type of tumour, may secrete excessively large or very small amounts of oestrogen. Some 20% of fibromas are associated with the presence of ascites or hydrothorax – a condition known as Meig's syndrome. A pseudo-Meig's syndrome with similar presentation is sometimes seen in malignant as well as benign ovarian tumours other than a fibroma.

Dermoid cysts make up about 10–15% of all ovarian tumours and are often found to be the cause of cystic enlargement of an ovary. The benign teratomas contain skin, hair, sebaceous glands, teeth and bone. Because of the sebaceous glands, they contain thick, greasy, yellow secretions, which have a very distinct appearance and are highly irritant to the peritoneum.

17.7 OVARIAN MALIGNANCY

Any tumour may present as a malignancy and it is often difficult to determine whether the lesion is a primary malignancy or whether there is a change from a benign epithelial stage. However, it is generally conceded that both events may occur.

The common malignant ovarian tumours are ovarian epithelial carcinomas, namely serous cystadenocarcinomas, mucinous cystadenocarcinomas, and occasionally secondary ovarian carcinoma (from bowel, lung or breast – Krukenberg tumours) and sarcoma. Ovarian tumours arise from the sex cord stroma and are classically hormone-producing tumours like granulosa cell tumours, Sertoli–Leydig cell tumours and other allied stromal tumours. About 25% of granulosa cell tumours behave as malignant tumours. They also produce oestrogen and therefore may be associated with endometrial hyperplasia, atypical hyperplasia or even an increased incidence of carcinoma of the endometrium.

Germ cell tumours contain germ cells as the predominant elements which are either embryonic or extraembryonic or a combination of these components. Dysgerminomas, embryonal carcinomas, immature teratomas and endodermal sinus cell tumours constitute the majority of germ cell tumours which occurs principally in young females. These tumours are very aggressive and their recurrence rate after removal of the primary growth is high. The presence of available tumour markers in these lesions and their good response to chemotherapy justify a conservative treatment in young girls, preserving their menstrual and reproductive functions.

Malignant epithelial tumours of the ovary usually have a poor prognosis because they are not detected until late in the course of the disease.

Clinical features of ovarian tumours

Ovarian tumours are notoriously difficult to diagnose early in their course, and they are usually detected when a patient presents for a routine check-up. However, they do have some symptoms and signs that are important indications of a potential tumour.

Symptoms and signs (Table 17.1)

1. **Vaginal bleeding**: Postmenopausal women often have an episode of bleeding when an ovarian tumour is present. This bleeding occurs from the endometrium, which may

Table 17.1 Differentiation between malignant and benign ovarian tumours

	Benign	Malignant
Consistency	Usually smooth walled and cystic	Solid, nodular or part solid/part cystic, with irregular papillae
Fixation	Usually freely mobile	May be fixed, with extension or adhesions
Number of tumours	Only 15% are bilateral	75% are bilateral
Ascites	Usually not a significant amount	Often very copious, with blood staining
Presence of vessels on tumour	No significant increase	Large dilated vessels coursing over the surface, leads to frequent haemorrhage and blood-stained ascites

become proliferative under the influence of oestrogen. The oestrogen is derived from ovarian stromal cells (surrounding any tumour of the ovary) that differentiate to produce theca-like cells, which have the potential to produce oestrogen. Pre-menopausal women may present with irregular vaginal bleeding from the same source.

2. **Pain**: If a cyst undergoes torsion or a vessel bleeds into the cyst, then moderate to severe pain may be experienced. Generally the pain from an ovarian tumour is referred to the iliac fossa and the inner aspect of the thigh.

3. **Abdominal swelling, nausea, vomiting and cachexia**: These are found when the tumour produces metastases to the bowel, the diaphragm or the omentum.

4. **Urinary frequency**: This is a common symptom when the tumour is large enough to encroach on the capacity of the bladder.

5. **Ascites**: A number of tumours of the ovary produce an increase in irritation of the peritoneum (fibromas, carcinomas), and thus produce an increase in ascitic fluid.

6. **An ovarian mass**: This is always dull to percussion in the middle and resonant in the flanks. This sign helps to differentiate an ovarian cyst containing fluid, from ascites in the abdomen.

7. **A palpable mass**: This is within the pelvis or arising from the pelvis into the abdominal cavity.

8. **An ovarian tumour**: This is within the pelvis and will generally not move when the cervix is moved up and down. This sign helps to differentiate fibromyomas of the uterus (which are attached to the uterus) from solid ovarian tumours.

9. **Irregular nodularity**: In the pouch of Douglas, this suggests the presence of malignant deposits.

Staging of carcinoma of the ovary

FIGO (International Federation of Gynecology and Obstetrics) staging of carcinoma of the ovary

Stage I – growth limited to one or both ovaries.
Stage II – growth involving one or both ovaries and pelvic extensia.

Stage III   – growth involving one or both ovaries with
              peritoneal implants outside the pelvis
              and/or positive retroperitoneal or inguinal
              nodes. Superficial liver metastasis equals
              stage III.
              – tumour is limited to the true pelvis but with
              histologically proven malignant extension to
              small bowel or omentum.

Stage IV   – growth involving one or both ovaries with
              distant metastases. Pleural effusion with
              positive cytology is allotted to Stage IV.

Different subgroup criteria are used for allotting cases into a, b, and c in each stage. For details, refer to the *Annual Report of Gynecological Cancer FIGO*, Vol. 20 (1988).

Management of ovarian tumours

In the reproductive phase, women presenting with an ovarian tumour that is greater than 5 cm in size and persists for 2 months should have the tumour removed. Any ovarian tumour found in postmenopausal women should also have laparotomy to remove the tumour.

If the tumour appears to be clinically benign, it should be shelled out of the ovary (cystectomy) in reproductive women. In postmenopausal women, both ovaries should be removed.

If the tumour appears to be malignant then a frozen section examination should be carried out at the time of operation. If malignancy is confirmed then a bilateral salpingo-oophorectomy and hysterectomy should be performed as well as exploration of the upper abdomen. Any secondary deposits should be removed together with omentum and a peritoneal debulking operation. Surgery should be followed by a course of chemotherapy – presently a combination of cyclophosphamide and cis-platinum/or carboplatin for six cycles gives the best response. The overall survival rate for ovarian malignancy is only 30% – most patients die following bowel obstruction, ureteric involvement and cachexia. The only patients with a good prognosis in ovarian cancers are those with early Stage I disease and complete surgical excision.

17.8 UTERINE TUMOURS

Fibromyoma

Fibromyomas, as the name suggests, are tumours composed of muscle and fibrous connective tissue. They are the most common type of genital tract tumour, and in about 99% of cases are associated with the uterus.

They are usually hard, spherical masses that may range in size from a few millimetres up to 30 cm in diameter. They are surrounded by a pseudocapsule, consisting of compressed myometrial tissue, in which run the blood vessels that supply the tumour.

It is rare to find a fibromyoma in women aged under 30; and most are detected in women aged over 35 – about one-third of all women over this age will be found to have a fibromyoma.

However, in the majority of cases the tumours are relatively small and do not cause any symptoms, so no treatment is required.

The three common sites for uterine fibromyoma are (Fig. 17.1):

1. **Subserous.** The tumour has grown and extruded through the serous surface of the uterus, forming a sessile or a pedunculated tumour covered by peritoneum.

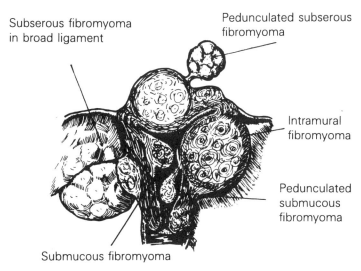

Figure 17.1 Fibromyoma of the uterus. (After Jeffcoate.)

2. **Intramural.** The tumour is found within the uterine musculature and apart from enlarging the uterus, produces only a localized thickening in the wall.
3. **Submucous.** The tumour has grown into the cavity of the uterus, the surface being covered by endometrium.

Symptoms and signs

The symptoms depend on the site and the size of the tumour:

1. Many fibromyoma are asymptomatic and are discovered at a routine examination.
2. These tumours may produce symptoms related to their size, pressure on surrounding organs or due to degeneration. Rarely they may reach the size of a football, producing a distended abdomen, bowel symptoms, heavy dragging ache and marked urinary frequency.
3. If the fibromyoma reaches a large size, the uterus itself will increase in size, and this will increase the length and surface area of the uterine cavity. This increased endometrial surface area leads to an increase in blood loss with each menstrual flow, often causing anaemia over a prolonged period of time. Fibromyomas that produce menstrual problems are mainly submucous and intramural tumours. They rarely cause intermenstrual or irregular bleeding, and the symptom complained of most commonly is heavy regular periods. Subserous fibromyomas never cause menorrhagia, but as fibromyomas are often multiple it is common to find an enlarged irregular uterus with tumours at all three sites (see Fig. 17.1).
4. Fibromyomas may undergo hyaline, cystic or fatty degeneration due to interference with the blood supply to the tumours. Red degeneration is a rare complication associated with pregnancy – the fibromyoma becomes necrotic and haemorrhagic, causing acute pain and discomfort.
5. Colicky uterine pain may occur with pedunculated submucous fibromyoma. The fibromyoma may act as a foreign body (like an IUCD), and the uterus actively tries to pass the tumour. The cervix will then dilate and the fibromyoma may present into the vagina as a red, bleeding or degenerating tumour. Pain may also occur in pregnancy if red

degeneration occurs or there is torsion of a subserous fibromyoma.
6. Other complications associated with pregnancy are:
   (a) Incarceration of a retroverted gravid uterus, causing
       urinary retention and abortion.
   (b) Obstruction to labour when a fibroid involves the
       cervix or lower uterine body.
   (c) Increased risk of postpartum haemorrhage.
7. Submucous fibroids may produce infertility, but intramural
   and subserous fibromyomas usually do not interfere with
   conception.
8. Fibromyomas are easily diagnosed by simple bimanual palpation when the normal uterine size was enlarged by one or
   more smooth, round and firm masses which moved when
   the uterus is moved up and down. The diagnosis may be
   confirmed by an ultrasound examination of the pelvis.

Management

Fibromyomas that are found during a routine examination and
have given no symptoms should not be treated unless they are
larger than a 12–14-week pregnancy.

Fibromyomas that cause symptoms should be removed by
myomectomy when the woman is aged under 35, and by hysterectomy when the woman is older. However, individual variations to this will arise due to the desire for further
pregnancies, size of family, request for symptomatic relief and
occasionally when sterilization is a concomitant request. Gonadotrophin-releasing hormone (GnRH) agonist has been shown
to be effective in producing regression of uterine fibromyomas;
however, the effect is short-termed and regrowth occurs after
completion of treatment.

Whatever method of management is used, prior hysteroscopy
and/or diagnostic curettage should be performed so that
submucous fibromyomas, polyps or endometrial neoplasia can
be excluded. Submucous fibromyamata, if not too big, may be
removed by hysteroscopic resection and the patient may be
cured of her symptoms. Myomectomy, if performed, should
be done with caution as morbidity such as haematoma formation, excessive uterine damage and infection can occur. Recurrence of residual small fibroids is always a possibility after

myomectomy. Therefore patients should be warned about these complications before the operation.

17.9 ADENOMYOSIS

Adenomyosis is a peculiar disease of the uterus, caused when the basal layer of endometrial cells grows into the myometrium, producing crypts and glandular invasion of the muscle. Each crypt or gland is connected to the uterine cavity from which it has arisen, and the endometrium that is shed eventually finds its way into the endometrial cavity of the uterus.

This condition produces a range of symptoms and signs, varying from none to extreme discomfort. About 10% of all women who have a hysterectomy are found to have evidence of adenomyosis on pathological examination, but only one-third of these women will have complained of symptoms referable to the disease.

Most women with symptoms of adenomyosis are aged over 35, have a history of normal fertility and pregnancies, and present with dysmenorrhoea. The dysmenorrhoea is heavy, dragging and congestive, beginning on the first day of each period, reaching a peak of discomfort on day 2 or 3, and gradually subsiding as the menses cease. Because there is a menstrual loss into each crypt and gland in the myometrium, these glands become distended during menses and produce tension on the surrounding myometrial cells. The blood within each crypt finds its way slowly to the endometrial cavity, so that patients with adenomyosis will have a prolonged menses that is only occasionally heavy.

The signs that may indicate adenomyosis are:

1. Slight enlargement of the uterus. (It is unusual for adenomyosis to cause uterine enlargement beyond the size of a 12-week pregnancy.)
2. Generally firm consistency and regular uterine shape rather than a nodular uterine enlargement. (Occasionally there may be a single focus of adenomyosis, which can resemble an intramural fibromyoma.)
3. Tenderness of the uterus when it is squeezed, particularly during a period. (The uterus is generally a non-tender organ.)

Pathologically, the uterus has a whorled, striated appearance with much fibromyomatous material surrounding blood-filled clefts. It can be distinguished from fibromyomas in that there is no 'capsule' of compressed myometrium. Most areas of adenomyosis can be found close to or connected to the uterine cavity, and very few areas are detected near the serosal surface.

Management

Symptomatic adenomyosis does not respond well to hormonal therapy, as the offending cells are derived from the basal layers of the endometrium. However, younger women may be treated with a course of progesterone (e.g. 5 mg norethisterone daily) for 3–6 months. If there is no improvement at the end of this course, then hysterectomy is indicated.

17.10 ENDOMETRIOSIS

Endometriosis is often confused with adenomyosis, but is similar only in that both originate from the same cellular layer.

There have been several hypotheses put forward to account for the development of endometriotic cysts. However, the most popular and plausible hypothesis is that put forward by Sampson. He suggests that endometrial cells spill out through the tubes onto the ovaries and peritoneum of the pouch of Douglas, and implant in these sites to form cysts containing endometrial fluid. The cause of spill of endometriotic cells is not confirmed, but probably involves an increase in uterine contractions against a tightly closed internal cervical opening. When the menstrual flow exceeds the capacity of the uterine cavity, and the excess flow may flow into the tubes and spill onto the peritoneal cavity.

Supportive evidence for this hypothesis is to be found in the following:

1. Most patients are of reproductive age between 25 and 35 when the signs are first detected.
2. Retrograde menstruation is observed in women with patent tubes and endometriosis during laparotomy.
3. There is a high incidence of endometriosis among women with cryptomenorrhoea or other outflow tract obstruction.

4. Early pregnancy, which leads to dilatation of the cervical sphincter, usually relieves the dysmenorrhoea and the subsequent development of endometriosis. Women who have their families early in their reproductive life have less evidence of endometriosis.
5. Women with a history of spasmodic dysmenorrhoea and subsequent infertility are often found to have endometriosis and extensive adhesions in the pelvis.
6. Intentional implantation of endometrium onto peritoneal surfaces in animals can initiate endometriosis.
7. The common sites for endometriosis are the ovary (70%), uterosacral ligaments (30%) and the pouch of Douglas (20%).

However, the Sampson's spill theory fails to explain the rare cases of endometriosis in the umbilicus, lung, brain or in women with congenitally absent uteri. Other theories, coelomic cell metaplasia and lymphatic or haematogenous embolism are worthy of consideration. It is likely that all may be involved in the development of endometriosis.

Symptoms

Endometriosis may produce a multitude of symptoms. There is, however, no relationship between the extent of the disease and the symptoms it produces. The most extensive of disease processes may be found at laparoscopy with virtually no symptoms.

1. Dysmenorrhoea is a common associated factor. Initially patients often give a history of spasmodic, first-day cramp or colic (due to the increased uterine muscle activity), but after 5–10 years (when the endometriotic cells implant and begin to grow into cysts) the pattern of period pain changes. The dysmenorrhoea begins several days before each period, is congestive in nature and reaches a peak towards the middle or end of each cycle, subsiding gradually over several postmenstrual days.
2. Dyspareunia is also a common symptom. This occurs due to the penis pressing on and moving the cysts and the associated adhesions or implants on the uterosacral ligaments.

3. Infertility occurs due to fibrosis and adhesions around the ovary. There is no tubal obstruction, but the tube and ovary may be so involved in adhesions that the ova cannot freely enter the fimbrial end of the tube.
4. Abdominal pain and discomfort, particularly on defaecation and micturition are common.

There is only occasionally a disturbance in menstrual function and flow, which is probably due to coincidental ovarian or uterine pathology.

Pathologically the tumours are blood-filled 'chocolate cysts' whose walls are composed of flattened endometriotic cells. The cyst itself is surrounded by dense, fibrotic material and adhesions, which may simulate infection, neoplasia, myoma, diverticulitis, hernia or any other abdominal tumour or obstruction.

Diagnosis

Endometriosis should be suspected whenever a patient presents with one or more of the above symptoms. The diagnosis is usually confirmed by pelvic findings of nodules or small tumours in the pouch of Douglas, the utero-sacral ligaments, the recto-vaginal septum or on the ovaries. Often the uterus is retroverted, fixed and very tender to move. Any history or physical findings suggestive of endometriosis should be followed up with a laparoscopy or laparotomy to confirm the diagnosis.

Management

Initially the management should be conservative. The aim of hormonal therapy is to create a 'pseudopregnancy' state by pills, progestogens, weak androgens or GnRH agonists, to 'burn out' the endometriotic deposits. Progestogens (medroxyprogesterone, 10 mg three times a day) prevent further growth of endometrium and produce hypoplasia of the glands. If continued for 6 months or more, any small lesions in the pelvis may regress and disappear. The use of progestogens is successful in 25% of cases where the lesions are very small. An alternate drug is the weak androgenic progestogen (Danazol/ Danacrine). It has marked anti-oestrogenic activity on endometrial cells and has been found to be most useful in the treatment of endometriosis. The dosage of danazol is 600–800 mg daily in three divided doses until the complete suppression of menstruation. However, the drug produces unwanted side effects like acne, deepening of voice, weight gain, increased hair growth and depression.

The administration of gonadotrophin-releasing hormone agonists has also shown to be effective. It causes marked hypoestrogenaemia that suppresses the growth of endometriosis. Because of its high cost and equal efficacy, GnRH treatment may be no better than other hormonal manipulation.

Larger endometriotic deposits, result in dense capsular fibrosis, will not regress in spite of prolonged progestogen therapy. The offending tissue should be removed surgically. Smaller deposits can be treated laparoscopically with diathermy or laser. Large deposits and larger cysts may need to be surgically removed at laparotomy. However, in spite of all measures taken, the endometriosis, fibrosis and accompanying symptoms often persist, and will remain a cause for discomfort until after the menopause.

17.11 CARCINOMA OF THE ENDOMETRIUM

Carcinoma of the endometrium commonly affects postmenopausal women, the average age of presentation being in the early 60s.

The endometrium may show all the features of neoplastic atypia, ranging from atypical hyperplasia, well-differentiated change to poorly-differentiated adenocarcinoma – and the gross features may vary from papillary overgrowth to necrotic ulceration. Squamous metaplasia may occur with well-differentiated adenocarcinomas, and this condition is termed adenoacanthoma.

Aetiology

Although the cause for carcinoma of the uterus is not known, a number of associated factors have been noted:

1. Late menopause. Women who menstruate beyond the age of 50 have a higher incidence of carcinoma of the endome-

trium than women who reach the menopause earlier. Prolonged exhibition of hormones, especially oestrogen, may play a part.

2. Relative infertility. Women who have a long history of infertility have a higher incidence of neoplasia. Again, anovulation and unopposed oestrogen are thought to be factors.

3. Dysfunctional uterine haemorrhage due to oestrogen influence or anovulation is also implicated. The action of unopposed oestrogen is to produce endometrial and cystic hyperplastic. Occasionally the cells and glands are associated with stromal hyperplasia and atypical hyperplasias, which are thought to be pre-malignant conditions.

4. Feminizing tumours of the ovary such as granulosa and theca-cell tumours are associated with a higher incidence of carcinoma of the endometrium.

5. Recent evidence suggests that exogenous unopposed oestrogen given for post-menopausal symptoms is also associated with an increased (2–3 times greater) incidence of neoplasia of the uterus.

Other factors such as race, parity, diabetes and pregnancy have been implicated in the past, but recent studies have suggested that these factors are not as important.

Clinically, carcinoma of the uterus presents with abnormal uterine bleeding. Any irregularity of menstrual function, intermenstrual or postmenopausal bleeding should be investigated by a hysteroscopy and/or dilatation and curettage. Some women ignore the slight haemoserous discharge, which may present for some months, and only attend when frank blood is visible. Any amount of bleeding should be regarded as potentially derived from a malignant site.

The uterus may enlarge or become softer, but only when the tumour is growing and is more extensive. Occasionally the endocervical canal may become occluded and haematometra (or even pyometra) may result. Extension to the bladder or to the peritoneal surface suggests a poor prognosis.

Metastases occur primarily to the pelvic lymph nodes, the para-aortic nodes and occasionally to the inguinal nodes, or there may be widespread haematogenous dissemination. Direct spread to other pelvic organs or trans-peritoneal migration to

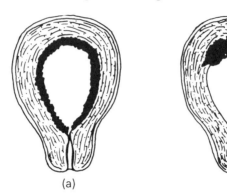

(a)   (b)

Figure 17.2 Carcinoma of endometrium. (a) Diffuse involvement of uterine cavity; (b) Localized tumour involving myometrium.

abdominal cavity sites is very common in the late stages of the disease.

Pain is a late symptom in the disease, as is bowel involvement.

Staging of carcinoma of the endometrium (Fig. 17.2)

FIGO staging

Stage   Ia (G123) Tumour limited to endometrium.
          Ib (G123) Invasion to <1/2 myometrium.
          Ic (G123) Invasion >1/2 myometrium.
Stage   IIa (G123) Endocervical glandular involvement only.
          IIb (G123) Cervical stromal invasion.
Stage   IIIa (G123) Tumor invades serosa and/or adnexa
            and/or positive peritoneal cytology.
          IIIb (G123) Vaginal metastases.
          IIIc (G123) Metastases to pelvic and/or para-aortic
            lymph nodes.
Stage   IVa (G123) Tumour invasion bladder and/or bowel
            mucosa.
          IVb (G123) Distant metastases including intra-
            abdominal and/or inguinal lymph node.

Diagnosis

The diagnosis is made by examining tissue obtained by endometrial biopsy or by curettage for evidence of histological neo-

plasia, and the staging of the disease is made by clinical examination and chest X-ray (cystoscopy and proctoscopy, if
advanced).

Management

The basic management depends on several factors:

1. Age. No bar to surgery if medically fit.
2. Stage of the disease. Early diagnosis and early staging
   allow more curative management to be undertaken.
3. Availability of appropriate therapy.

Stage 1. The ideal management of Stage I carcinoma of the
uterus is to perform a total abdominal hysterectomy with bilateral salpingo-oophorectomy. While performing this surgery,
gland biopsy and peritoneal cytology should be obtained to
determine if any extension has occurred. If the postoperative
histopathological examination demonstrates any evidence of
tumour in the lymph glands, the peritoneum, or there has been
myometrial invasion deeper than one-half, then postoperative
radiotherapy should be administered.

Stage 2. Stage 2 tumours require a radical hysterectomy with
removal of as much pelvic/parametrial tissue as possible. A
course of preoperative irradiation is sometimes given before
attempting a hysterectomy and bilateral salpingo-oophorectomy.

Stages 3 and 4. Stage 3 and 4 tumours are usually treated with
radiotherapy and palliative surgery only. If following a combined radiotherapeutic and surgical approach, there is evidence
of extension of the disease then the use of progesterone
(medroxyprogesterone – Provera 100–200 mg, t.i.d.) may cause
reversion of the neoplastic changes in some women.

Prognosis

Stage 1 tumours treated adequately have a 5-year cure rate of
80% while Stage 2 tumours have a 5-year cure rate of 65%.
Stage 3 and 4 tumours of the endometrium have a generally
poor prognosis with a cure rate of 15–25%.

17.12 TUMOURS OF THE CERVIX

The most common benign lesion of the cervix is ectopic columnar epithelium. Normally, the endocervix is lined by mucus-secreting columnar epithelium, which is under the influence of oestrogen. The ectocervix is covered by flat squamous epithelium, which normally is of a mid-pink colour, and is smooth and regular. Under the influence of oestrogen (during menarche, pregnancy, the taking of certain oral contraceptives, exogenous oestrogen, endogenous oestrogen-producing tumours), the endocervical glands proliferate and grow onto the ectocervix. This outgrowth of columnar epithelium (erythroplakia) produces a velvety red or orange, roughed epithelium which secretes a profuse clear mucous discharge. Occasionally the mucus epithelium may become infected with coliform bacilli, trichomonas or other pathogens and then a yellow or brownish mucus discharge is evident. Because columnar epithelium is usually only one to two cell layers thick, it is easily broken and eroded, leading to bleeding and a pus-like discharge.

The ectopic columnar epithelium is continually undergoing metaplastic change to squamous epithelium, and may be more susceptible to influences such as human papilloma virus. Regular Papanicolaou (PAP) smears should be performed on all women, especially those who have evidence of ectopic columnar epithelium. Ectopic columnar epithelium is in fact not an 'erosion' although it is often discussed in this context when

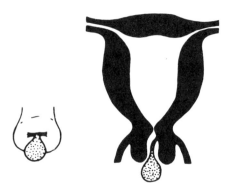

Figure 17.3 Demonstrating how an endocervical polyp presents at the cervical os.

describing cervical lesions. (A true erosion occurs when the whole of the epithelium is lost, leaving a 'raw' area of granulating or stromal tissue.)

Ectopic columnar epithelium, particularly following a pregnancy, may become involved in a chronic infective state and lead to chronic cervicitis. More commonly, however, the cervix is mildly inflamed or not even infected.

When metaplasia to squamous epithelium occurs naturally, a number of glands and crypts will be buried under the surface and so lead to occluded glands. These eventually become round, firm, discrete cysts known as Nabothian follicles. They are seen round the external os of a cervix that has undergone metaplastic change to squamous epithelium – they are benign and require no treatment.

POLYPS

Occasionally, under the influence of oestrogen, the endometrial or endocervical glands hypertrophy until the tissue is thick and polypoidal. These polyps usually develop stalks and protrude out through the cervical os (Fig. 17.3). The majority are less than 0.5 cm in size, but some may grow to 5 cm diameter. They usually cause abnormal bleeding (e.g. menorrhagia, intermenstrual bleeding or postcoital bleeding) or are occasionally associated with colicky abdominal pain (as the uterus attempts to expel the polyp).

The treatment is simply to twist the polyp or cauterize its base. The polyp must be examined histologically, as about 1–3% have evidence of neoplastic change in the base.

17.13 CARCINOMA OF THE CERVIX

This is the second most common cancer affecting females, accounting for almost 10% of neoplasia of women. It should be entirely preventable by encouraging all women from the time they become sexually active to have PAP smears every 1–2 years.

The most common age for detection of carcinoma of the cervix is 45–55, when most other abnormal bleeding symptoms are also commonly found. It is important to be aware of the symptoms and signs of carcinoma of the cervix so that the disease may be diagnosed early and appropriate management initiated.

Factors associated with carcinoma of the cervix

1. The most common factor associated with the development of carcinoma of the cervix appears to be the papillomavirus. There are more than 70 known strains of wart virus but four or five are known to have a malignant influence on cervical cells (strains 16, 18, 31 and 33 are particularly oncogenic).
2. Intercourse. Women who have intercourse with multiple partners have a higher incidence of neoplasia than women who have infrequent or no intercourse. It is believed that sperm, semen, bacterial or viral infection may all predispose to change within the metaplastic cells. It has also been shown that prostitutes have over 100 times greater risk of developing carcinoma of the cervix than do nuns.
3. Childbirth appears to increase the risk of carcinoma about 5–10-fold.
4. Other viral infections such as herpes genitalis may be associated with an increased incidence of abnormal change in the cervix.
5. Early age at first and subsequent intercourse increases the risk.

It was once thought that circumcision of the male partner reduces the incidence of carcinoma of the cervix. However, the evidence for this suggestion was the low incidence of carcinoma among orthodox Jewesses, who rarely have intercourse when 'unclean' (i.e. when menstruating, bleeding for 12–16 weeks postpartum, or having profuse vaginal discharge). But during these times ectopic columnar epithelium is undergoing metaplasia to squamous epithelium, so by avoiding intercourse during these periods, the incidence of carcinoma of the cervix is reduced. The incidence among liberal Jewesses, who do not necessarily refrain from intercourse at these times, is the same as that among Gentile women.

The actual causative agent for carcinoma of the cervix is still unknown. However, large population studies of women in various age groups suggests that there may be a latent phase of

5–10 years, during which cervical epithelium is undergoing a change to dysplasia, carcinoma-*in-situ*, and finally to invasive carcinoma. If a PAP smear is taken regularly from the squamo-columnar junction, then these changes can be identified by detecting abnormal cells with large irregular pyknotic nuclei, or even mitotic divisions, and unusual cell shape. If appropriate treatment and follow-up is instituted at the stage, cervical cancer may be preventable.

An abnormal smear result may be found in a slide prepared from the cells taken from a clinically normal cervix. This common finding occurs because the initial cellular changes are intraepithelial and therefore the early disturbance of the normal surface is macroscopically not visible. PAP smears do, however, have a false-negative rate and up to 10% of cases with cervical cancer may have a false-negative smear. This is because the cancer contains necrotic tissue and slough which may prevent the malignant cells from being sampled.

Clinical symptoms and signs

Pre-invasive lesions

(Cervical intraepithelial neoplasia – CIN 1, 2 or 3).
Because the abnormal lesion is still intraepithelial, it usually has no presenting symptomatology. All abnormal PAP smears including those that are only atypical or those which have human papilloma virus present should be sent for colposcopic examination by an appropriately trained person. The use of a colposcope allows magnification of the cervix and therefore easier visualization of any abnormal epithelium (Figs 17.4–17.8). When the site is painted with acetic acid, the abnormal epithelium will appear white (an aceto-white lesion) and alternatively Schiller's iodine will mark the abnormal epithelium as iodine negative area. (Glycogen-containing squamous epithelial cells normally take up iodine and stain a mahogany–brown colour, whereas neoplastic or mucus-secreting cells remain non-staining.) When an abnormal smear is reported in the absence of a visible cervical lesion, then a colposcopy, selective biopsy should be performed.

If the diagnosis of pre-invasive lesions (CIN 1, 2, 3) is con-

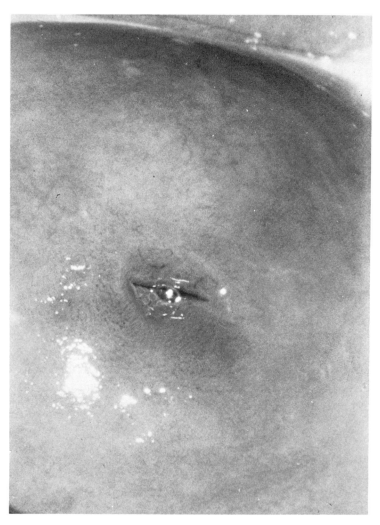

Figure 17.4 The ectocervix is covered by original squamous epithelium. The external os is in the centre of the colpophotograph. The white areas are due to light reflection. (Figures 17.4–17.8 are from Coppleson, Pixley and Redi (1978) *Colposcopy*, 2 edn, Charles C. Thomas, Springfield MA.)

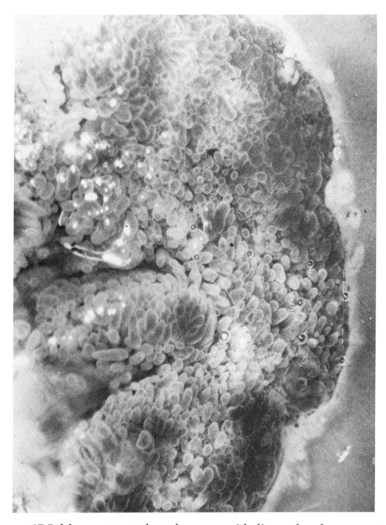

Figure 17.5 More commonly columnar epithelium also forms part of the cervical covering and here displays the characteristic grape-like or villous colposcopic appearance, which in pregnancy is even more conspicuous. The external os is seen in the centre on the left. Columnar epithelium is laid down on the ectocervix either during embryogenesis or by eversion in the first pregnancy. It appears red to the naked eye and is commonly referred to, incorrectly, as cervical erosion.

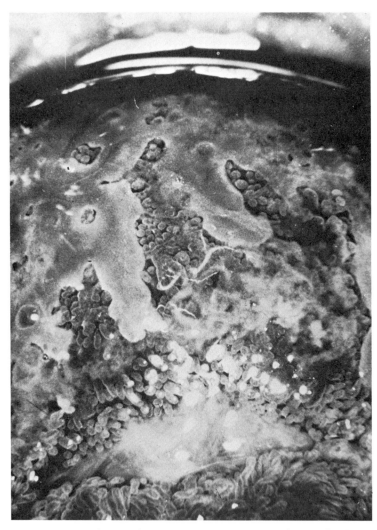

Figure 17.6 Typical transformation zone. Due to the acid pH in the vagina, the exposed columnar epithelium undergoes metaplasia. Mature normal metaplastic squamous epithelium is seen to form fingerlike processes replacing the columnar epithelium which is still visible as islands in the metaplastic epithelium and near the cervical os below. A plug of white mucus is present at the os.

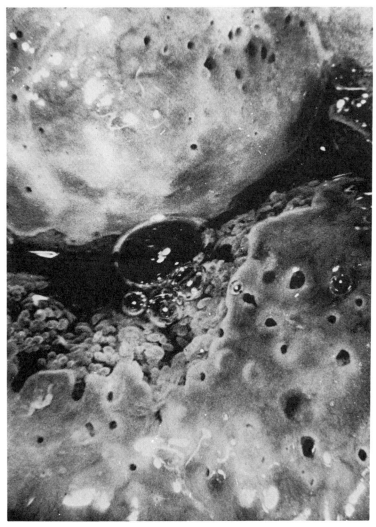

Figure 17.7 Typical transformation zone (fully developed). Mature normal metaplastic epithelium has completely replaced the columnar epithelium previously present on the ectocervix. Several gland openings, representing the remnants of the pre-existing glands in the columnar epithelium can be seen. Where these glands are occluded by the metaplastic epithelium, retention cysts (Nabothian follicles) result. This change is irreversible and this woman is now almost free of risk of developing squamous cancer of the cervix.

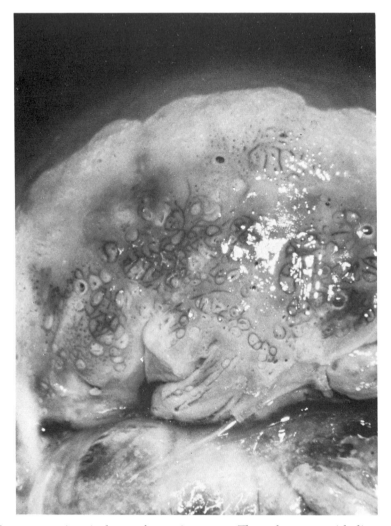

Figure 17.8 Atypical transformation zone. The columnar epithelium on the ectocervix has been completely replaced by the less common atypical metaplastic squamous epithelium. White epithelium and mosaic structure, the characteristic colposcopic attributes of dysplasia and CIN 3 are seen. The atypical transformation zone is 'the field of neoplastic potentials'.

firmed, cautery, laser or large-loop excision of transformation zone (LLETZ) should be performed. Cryosurgery can be used for less severe abnormalities such as CIN 1. A cone biopsy should be performed if there is no colposcopic evidence of abnormality of the ectocervix or the whole transformation zone of the cervix is not fully visualized.

Follow-up

Following any treatment for an abnormal PAP smear, all women should be seen for regular follow up visits. PAP smears should be taken at 6-monthly intervals for 2 years and then annually thereafter.

Invasive carcinoma

This may present with symptoms, such as intermenstrual bleeding, postcoital bleeding, postmenopausal bleeding, brown or haemoserous discharge or occasionally (in extensive cases) bladder or bowel symptoms. However, early invasive carcinoma or carcinoma of the endocervix may be detected only at a routine check-up, when a PAP smear suggests an abnormality and a subsequent cone biopsy proves early invasion to be present. The signs of the disease are a reflection of the stage of the tumour:

(a) Visually, there may be an exfoliating growth, an ulcer or an intra-epithelial spread of the cancer over the cervix and the vagina. Bleeding is common, and any trauma produces a steady ooze of frank haemorrhage.

(b) Digital vaginal examination usually discloses a firm, often friable mass or ulcer which may extend onto the vaginal epithelium, laterally into the paracervical tissue, to the side walls and pelvic nodes or to the bladder or the rectum.

(c) Occasionally there may be spread to pelvic glands, liver, scalene node or other sites.

(d) Rectal examination may disclose parametrial thickening and extension of the pelvic walls or the lymph nodes.

Pathology

Carcinoma of the cervix is usually of the squamous type, although 5–10% of tumours are derived from columnar epi-

thelium and have the usual characteristics of an adenocarcinoma.

The tumours may vary from well-differentiated squamous-
cell carcinomas to poorly differentiated anaplastic lesions, the
response to treatment and the survival rate depending not only
on the stage of the tumour but on the degree of cell differentiation.

They usually spread by direct invasion to surrounding tissue
– by lymphatic spread and occasionally by the haematogenous
route. Direct invasion of the paracervical tissues, parametrium,
uterus and vagina is the most common extension – spread to
the pelvic lymph nodes (obturator, internal, external, common
iliac and pre-sacral nodes) is frequent but the bladder and
rectum are rarely involved.

Staging of carcinoma of the cervix

FIGO staging of the cervix

Pre-invasive carcinoma

Stage 0: Carcinoma-*in-situ* (CIN 3). Carcinoma cells found
within the cervical epithelium, but no invasion of the
underlying tissue has taken place.

Invasive carcinoma

Stage 1: The carcinoma is strictly confined to the cervix.
  Ia   Preclinical carcinoma of the cervix – those
       diagnosed only by microscopy
       Ia1 – minimal stromal invasion
       Ia2 – lesion with invasion less than 5 mm (depth)
             × 7 mm horizontal spread)
  Ib   Clinical lesions of greater dimensions than Ia.
Stage 2: The carcinoma has extended beyond the cervix, but
       has not reached the pelvic walls. It may involve the
       vagina, but not the lower third.
  IIa No obvious parametrial involvement
  IIb Obvious parametrial involvement
Stage 3: The carcinoma has extended to the pelvic side-walls
       or has involved the lower third of the vagina.
  IIIa No extension to the pelvic wall

IIIb Extension to pelvic wall and/or hydronephrosis
or non-functioning kidney.

Stage 4: The carcinoma has involved the bladder, the rectum
or spread to tissue outside the pelvis.
IVa Spread to adjacent organs   bladder, a rectal mucosa
IVb Spread to distant organs   outside the pelvis.

All staging is performed clinically, and before the results of
investigations or treatment are available.

Diagnosis

When a history, physical examination or PAP smear suggest
that a carcinoma of the cervix may be present, the definitive
pathological diagnosis depends on the results of a biopsy taken
from the cervix.

An abnormal smear in the presence of a cervical lesion indicates that a punch biopsy should be taken from the edge of the
lesion. However, when the same smear results are obtained
from a relatively normal-looking cervix, then a colposcopy and
biopsy should be performed to make certain that all the
squamo-columnar junction is examined. If the squamo-columnar junction is not readily visualized or if no abnormal lesion is
seen, then a cone biopsy should be performed if the PAP smear
is persistently suspicious.

In both cases, curettage should also be performed to eliminate the possibility that the abnormal PAP smear is derived
from adenocarcinoma of the endocervix or uterus.

Management

For squamous-cell carcinoma of the cervix, the management
depends entirely on the stage of the tumour.

Stage 0

If colposcopy is available, the most obvious abnormal area is
easily identified and biopsied. The whole transformation zone of
the cervix can be treated by extensive radical diathermy or laser
ablation as the method of choice in management. Recently, a
large loop electrosurgical excision procedure (LLETZ) has
become popular, which can eradicate the abnormal lesion as
well as to provide tissue for pathological confirmation.

However, if the cervix appears to be clinically normal to inspection after an abnormal PAP smear, then a cone biopsy or LLETZ should be performed. If the histopathology suggests complete excision, then follow-up should be taken every 6 months for 2 years, with a yearly smear after that time.

An incomplete excision requires a repeat cervical smear to document persistent disease, then followed either a second LLETZ, cone biopsy, or even a hysterectomy. Following a hysterectomy, vaginal vault cytology should be performed regularly to check that recurrence has not taken place.

Stages 1 and 2a
These are treated by one of the following methods:

1. Radical hysterectomy with bilateral pelvic lymph nodes dissection and a generous cuff of the vagina.
2. Combined external irradiation or intracavity radium/cesium followed by extended surgery.
3. Using external and internal irradiation only to treat the cancer.

In the best of hands all techniques appear to give a 5-year survival rate of about 80–90%.

Stages 2b and 3
These are usually treated by external radiation followed by intracavity radium/cesium. The survival rate varies from 40–60% depending on the stage of the tumour.

Stage 4
These are also treated by intracavity and external irradiation. Survival rates are low and depend on whether only the bladder and rectal mucosa are involved.

17.14 VAGINA

There are very few pathological lesions that affect the vagina, because it is resistant to any epithelial change. However, benign cysts may be found:

1. A cystocoele or urethrocoele is relatively common in multiparous women. This lesion is invariably in the midline anteriorly and is easily diagnosed. This is discussed in Chapter 6 under the title 'prolapse'.

2. Inclusion cysts may occur near the vaginal introitus following episiotomies and surgery on the vagina. They cause no problems and do not require treatment.

3. Gartner's duct cysts may be seen in the antero-lateral area of the vagina and are the result of cystic dilatation of the vestigial mesonephric duct (Wolffian duct). They are generally asymptomatic and require no treatment unless very large and distorting the vagina or urethra. They are thin-walled, translucent, greyish, soft cystic swellings which should not be opened until after an IVP excludes any urinary tract connection.

4. Peri-urethral cysts may enlarge and protrude from the anterior wall of the vagina, simulating a urethrocoele. However, they are usually firm and cystic. They should not be incised as it may lead to a urinary fistula.

Carcinoma of the vagina

This is relatively rare and is usually of the squamous-cell type. The treatment is generally by radiotherapy. The only exception is the treatment of clear cell adenocarcinoma of the vagina which is usually found in diethylstilboestrol (DES)-exposed young women. Exploratory laparotomy, radical hysterectomy and upper vaginectomy are the preferred treatment for this special group.

Staging of carcinoma of the vagina

FIGO staging of carcinoma of the vagina

Stage 0   Intra-epithelial carcinoma.
Stage I   Carcinoma limited to the vaginal wall.
Stage II Carcinoma has involved the subvaginal tissue, but has not extended to the pelvic wall.
Stage III Carcinoma has extended to the lateral pelvic wall.
Stage IV Carcinoma has extended to involve adjacent organs or it has metastasized to distant organs.

17.15 VULVA

Infective lesions of the vulva may include:

1. Bartholin's abscess.
2. Vulval warts.
3. Herpes genitalis.
4. Lymphogranuloma inguinale.
5. Granuloma venereum.

Bartholin's disease

This usually starts as small cysts which become infected and presents with an acute, tender, painful swelling in the posterior third of the labia. The duct becomes obstructed following inflammatory invasion by bacteria (usually coliform or *Neisseria gonorrhoea*).

It is an acute condition requiring emergency admission and treatment. Although the abscess tends to 'point' outside the vagina, the surgical drainage of a Bartholin's abscess should be into the vagina itself.

The operation to drain a Bartholin's abscess is called 'marsupialization' (Fig. 17.9). The technique is to incise into the abscess and then sew the margins of the incision so that the abscess wall is allowed to unite to the vaginal epithelium, to form a pouch. In this manner the abscess continues to drain

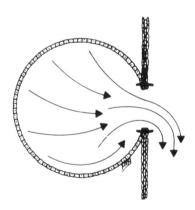

Figure 17.9 Bartholin's abscess – demonstrating drainage by incision and marsupialization.

into the vagina and when it resumes functioning, the Bartholin's gland secretions empty into the vagina. However, recurrence of Bartholin's cyst is common.

Vulval warts

These are usually due to viral infection and can be transmitted venereally. All warts in the vaginal/vulval area appear to increase rapidly in size and extent in moist conditions or during pregnancy so that when other vaginal discharges are present, the warts (condylomata accuminata) appear to flourish profusely. They are often painful irritating or itchy and are best treated by cautery, laser or painting with 25% podophyllin in tincture of benzoin. The use of podophyllin in pregnancy should be avoided because of its teratogenic effect. Vulval and vaginal warts in pregnancy can be eradicated with laser ablation, electrocautery or cryosurgery.

Urethral carbuncle

This is usually due to prolapse or overgrowth of the urethral mucosa. A small inflamed polypoid-like lesion is seen at the urethral introitus. It can be treated with cautery or excision if symptoms warrant its removal. Occasionally it may be due to a trichomonal infection.

Vulval dermatoses and vulval malignancy

A number of vulval lesions present with symptoms and some with signs. All of these conditions require careful investigation, as some are due to pre-malignant or malignant conditions and some are benign dermatoses.

A unifying classification of vulvar disease has been recommended as follows:

1. Vulval dystrophies
   Non-neoplastic epithelial disorders of skin and mucosa (hyperplastic dystrophy, lichen sclerosus, leucoplakia, kraurosis vulvae).
2. Neoplastic epithelial disorders
   (a) Squamous: vulvar intraepithelial neoplasia (VIN)

VIN1 (mild dysplasia)
VIN2 (moderate dysplasia)
VIN3 (severe dysplasia or carcinoma in situ)
  (b) Non-squamous
      Paget's disease
      Tumours of melanocytes

The most common presenting symptom of these lesions is an itch or an irritation, while bleeding, ulcerations, papules or warts may be manifestations of vulval lesions.

Diagnosis: All patients need to have colposcopy and a biopsy from the most suspicious areas to exclude invasive cancer. Often multiple 2–3-mm drill biopsies need to be taken under local anaesthesia.

Treatment: This is by laser ablation or wide local excision.

Hyperplastic dystrophy

This is a chronic inflammation of the subdermis, which leads to ischaemia, increase in keratinization and hypertrophic changes in the epithelium. There is a typical appearance of white plaques and patches in the epithelium, and often the intra-dermal cells may resemble cancer. It is thought that hyperplastic dystrophy may lead to squamous-cell carcinoma of the vulva.

If a malignant change does not occur, the hyperplastic dystrophy eventually leads to atrophy and fibrosis. This causes the vaginal introitus to shrink, leading to stenosis, 'hooding' of the clitoris and urethra, and eventually to almost complete closure of the vagina.

Hyperplastic dystrophy should be treated with oral oestrogen (in postmenopausal women), together with a local fluorinated corticosteroid ointment. If any areas appear suspicious, i.e. associated with a crack or fissure, a biopsy of the site should be performed to exclude a malignant change.

Hypoplastic dystrophy

Lichen sclerosis
The skin shows white papules which progress to atrophic skin lesions around the perineum and peri-anal skin.

Kraurosis vulvae (primary atrophy)

This is a condition often mistaken for hyperplastic dystrophy, as it also causes stenosis of the vulva with atrophic changes. However, although the epithelium is pale, there are no plaques. The condition is not pre-malignant.

Diagnosis

This can only be made for certain by biopsy.

Treatment

If marked atrophic vaginal changes are present, local oestogens will help. However, most atrophic dystrophies will respond best to regular application of testosterone ointment.

Mixed dystrophies

Leukoplakia

This accounts for about 20% of vulval dystrophies. The vulval skin has thick and hard white lesions which crack easily. It affects areas around the clitoris, the labia and the perineum. Histologically leukoplakic vulva may show hypertrophic or atrophic epithelial lesions with or without atypia.

Treatment

These respond best to the use of either fluorinated corticosteroids or testosterone ointment.

Other dermatoses

Women who suffer from chronic dermatological conditions such as psoriasis, intertrigo, fungal infections, vitiligo, etc., may manifest the disease in the vulval and pubic areas. Close inspection is required to diagnose a dermatological cause.

Malignant vulval lesions

The most common vulval malignancy is squamous-cell carcinoma. This condition is unusual before the age of 65, and usually presents itself as an ulcerated, bleeding lesion. It is slow growing and the disease tends to progress from carcinoma-*in-situ* to invasion.

Staging of vulval carcinoma

FIGO staging of vulval carcinoma

Pre-malignant

Stage 0   Carcinoma-*in-situ* (VIN 3)

Malignant

Stage I   Tumour confined to the vulva – 2 cm or less.
           Nodes are not palpable.
Stage II   Tumour confined to the vulva – >2 cm.
           Nodes are not palpable.
Stage III Tumour of any size.
           (1) Adjacent spread to lower urethra, and/or the
                vagina, or the anus, and/or
           (2) Unilateral regional lymph node metastasis.
Stage IV   Tumour invades any of the following:
           (a) Upper urethra, bladder mucosa, rectal mucosa,
                pelvic bone and/or bilateral regional node
                metastasis.
           (b) Any distant metastasis including pelvic lymph
                nodes.

Stages I to III should be treated with radical vulvectomy,
with the removal of extensive inguinal and pelvic nodes. Some
patients are, however, old and frail and unable to tolerate the
major surgical procedure necessary to remove the tumour and
the affected glands. Radiotherapy is an alternative treatment.
Most women (90–100%) with early carcinoma of the vulva will
be alive after 5 years. Radiotherapy and chemotherapy have a
palliative role to play in advanced lesions.

18

Human sexuality

18.1 GENERAL INSTRUCTIONAL OBJECTIVE

The students should understand the psychology and physiology of human sexuality and the principles of available therapy for patients with sexual problems so that they can initiate appropriate management.

18.2 SPECIFIC BEHAVIOURAL OBJECTIVES

1. Describe the physiological changes that occur in the human sexual response cycle.
2. Describe deviations from the normal anatomy that cause physical sexual problems.
3. Discuss factors that may modify the human sexual response cycle:
   (a) Physical.
   (b) Psychological.
   (c) Social.
   (d) Cultural.
4. Discuss factors that influence libido and sexual arousal in the individual and partners:
   (a) Physiological disturbances (illness, fatigue, depression, anxiety).
   (b) Personality differences.
   (c) Attitudinal differences.
   (d) Hormonal influences (both exogenous and endogenous).
   (e) Sexual techniques.
   (f) Effects of drugs and alcohol.
5. Discuss how a couple's general relationship influences their sexual behaviour.

6. Discuss factors affecting satisfactory intercourse, e.g. impotence, rapid ejaculation, loss of libido, vaginismus.
7. Discuss the physical and emotional factors affecting the achievement of orgasm.
8. Discuss the principles of psychosexual counselling.
9. Elicit, present and discuss the history of a patient with a psychosexual problem.

18.3 REASONS FOR LEARNING ABOUT HUMAN SEXUALITY

Every medical practitioner at some stage will be confronted by a patient who complains directly of a sexual problem, or who presents with a problem that on deeper inquiry will be found to be due to some psychosexual cause. These multiple presentations may be as varied as depression, pelvic pain, loss of libido or vaginismus. Women may complain of absence of orgasm or headaches due to marital conflict. Most often, the patient and her partner require a full investigation and counselling to allow them to understand their mutual problems, although occasionally therapy directed to one partner only, may help to resolve the issue. The medical practitioner must have the knowledge and skill to recognize the presentation, explore its cause and direct the couple to the correct mode of management. It is important to be sympathetic and appear to have the time to listen to any problems.

18.4 HUMAN SEXUALITY

Sexual drive or libido is generated in the brain and can occur without requiring any stimulus outside the body. However, sexual drive is capable of being affected by the emotional state, past experiences, environment and by many influences external to the body. Every person has a sexual urge or libido and the level of the response to this basic urge depends on many factors. These can be grouped into two separate but interrelated parts:

1. **Biological.** The brain contains centres that enhance or stimulate sexual drive. In this regard, sexual drive is regulated like other biological drives such as thirst and hunger. The centre located in the brain, stimulates or depresses the

physical reflex in the sacral portion of the spinal cord.
When erogenous zones are stimulated impulses are transmitted to the sacral portion of the spinal cord. Return
impulses then stimulate the blood vessels in the genital
region, so that engorgement occurs.
2. **Psychological.** This is a reflection of the need or motivation
to engage in sexual activity at a given time. Psychological
need for sex is a complex issue, as emotional state, environment and experiences, play an important role.

18.5 THE SEXUAL RESPONSE CYCLE

The response cycle consists of five phases. The duration of each
of the phases varies greatly with the individual and the circumstances. There are marked differences between the male and
female sexual response cycles with respect to timing. Men are
rapidly arousable while women are slower to arouse. While a
young man can become rapidly aroused (a full erection in 3
seconds), a young inexperienced woman may take up to half
an hour to become aroused. As women become more sexually
experienced their time to arouse shortens but they usually still
require 15 to 20 minutes to reach plateau phase. Men have a
refractory period after orgasm where they cannot re-erect or
have another orgasm. For this reason the male is usually
unable to have repeated orgasms over a short space of time.
This refractory period may well be due to inhibitory impulses
from the ejaculatory reflex centre in the lumbar portion of the
spinal cord. Women do not have a refractory period and may
enjoy continued stimulation. Between 15 and 30% of women
are capable of multiple orgasms.

Vasocongestion and myotonia

Vasocongestion and myotonia are the two underlying mechanisms in both sexes which lead to the various organ responses.
Vasocongestion is the engorgement of blood vessels in superficial and deep tissues, but especially in the genital organs. It
begins at the start of sexual excitement and precedes myotonia,
the second response. Myotonia is increased muscle tension.
Myotonia affects both smooth and skeletal muscles, and occurs
both voluntarily and involuntarily. With continual stimulation,

muscle tensions build up to a certain point and then a reflex stretch mechanism causes the muscles to contract vigorously. The result of these contractions is a release of muscular spasm and a decrease of vasocongestion. At the time these contractions are occurring, the individual experiences the peak of physical pleasure known as orgasm.

1.   The desire phase

Both men and women experience sexual drive but men's sexual drive is more urgent and undistractable than women's. Desire is affected by many factors: courtship, children, unemployment, illness, fatigue, depression, anxiety. Sex drive fluctuates throughout the lifespan according to the individual's circumstances. Women's sex drive tends to fluctuate more than men's does. For this reason it is unrealistic to expect that two people will have the same sexual drive just because they are in a relationship.

2.   The excitement phase

In all individuals there is a base level of sexual drive, which is variable. Starting from this, within 10–30 seconds of the beginning of any effective mechanical or psychological sexual stimulation, there is marked vasocongestion. This produces vaginal lubrication in the female and erection of the penis in the male. At the same time in the female there is lengthening and distention of the inner two-thirds of the vagina. As the plateau phase is approached the uterus is elevated as the pelvic floor contracts and rises and the inner two-thirds of the vagina balloons and expands. The spongy tissue in the labia minora and clitoral shaft also undergo vasocongestion and the nipples become erect. This phase is variable in duration and dependent on the form of stimulation.

3.   The plateau phase

The outer third of the vagina becomes markedly engorged, so that the vaginal opening decreases by at least one-third. The clitoris retracts under the clitoral hood, almost inaccessible to direct stimulation but still responding to pressure from traction of the clitoral hood. The engorged labia minora undergo a vivid colour change, from pink to bright red in nulliparous women and red to deep wine colour in parous women.

4. The orgasmic phase

This usually lasts 5–10 seconds, and begins with contractions in the outer third of the vagina. Uterine contractions may also begin at this time. At the same time, respiration, heart rate and blood pressure have all increased. During orgasm, there is a release of muscular spasm and engorgement of blood vessels, and a peak of physical pleasure.

5. The resolution phase

During this time, in the female the plateau and orgasmic phase may be reactivated by adequate stimuli. Following orgasm, the clitoris that has been retracted returns to its normal position within 5–10 seconds. The contraction in the outer third of the vagina ceases and slowly all the organs return to their previously unstimulated state. Unlike the female, who maintains higher levels of stimulative susceptibility during the immediate post-orgasmic period, the male has a unique refractory period where sexual tension is reduced to low excitement phase levels. Due to the post-orgasmic loss of stimulation response, the male viscera tend to lose superficial and deep vasocongestion more rapidly than the female.

18.6 FACTORS AFFECTING HUMAN SEXUALITY

Various factors affect basic sexual drive and the subsequent sexual response cycle. They are discussed here as two separate but inter-related parts – physical factors and the effect of psychological factors.

Physical factors

1. Physical touch
Touch is the only type of stimulation to which the body can respond reflexly and independently of higher psychic centres. If

a man is unconscious or has a spinal cord injury preventing impulses to and from the brain, an erection can still be obtained by stimulation of the genitals or inner parts of the thigh. This is a reflex from nerve endings to the cord, with resultant vasocongestion and myotonia. The reflex is centred in the sacral portion of the cord. The degree of response depends upon the intensity of the mechanical stimulus and the area of stimulation. Although touch receptors are the same in all areas of the body, they are much more concentrated in those parts that are commonly called the erogenous zones (e.g. breasts, inner parts of the thigh, genitals, etc.). Many women who are orgasmic are only able to respond to the point of orgasm by direct manipulation (manual or oral) of the clitoral region.

2. Organic factors

Aging is a good example. A man usually achieves peak sexual drive at about the age of 19–20 and this slowly decreases, but sexual drive is still present in old age.

In the female this drive tends to reach its maximum somewhat later and then slowly decreases.

3. Hormones

Hormones play a significant role in the development and maintenance of our sexuality. Oestrogen decreases sexual drive in the male, but testosterone has been reported to increase drive in a female by increasing the clitoral response mechanisms. Progesterone in high dosages tends to decrease libido in the female, as may oestrogen. This is probably related to increasing levels of sex hormone binding globulin.

4. Pathological

Pain, fatigue, chronic debilitating diseases and neurological diseases.

5. Drugs

Particular drugs include:

- Anticholinergics.
- Anorexiants.
- Anti-epileptics.
- Some cardiovascular drugs.
- Some CNS depressants.
- Psychotropic drugs (antidepressants, neuroleptics).

Psychological factors

Psychological factors are primarily related to our education and past experiences. There is no doubt that one of the stronger factors in sustaining sexual drive is satisfaction of previous relationships and experiences.

However, other important factors can lead to a depression of sexual response, such as fear. This may be fear of discovery, fear of pregnancy, fear of contracting a sexually transmitted disease, injury, heart attack, or fear of failure, guilt or shame.

Self-esteem and perceived body image are also important factors. If lack of self-esteem or poor body image is an issue, then there may be marked depression in the ability to respond sexually.

The way in which individuals regard themselves as sexual persons also has an important effect on the ability to abandon themselves and enjoy sexual activity. Development of sexual attitudes during childhood and adolescence can vary greatly depending on the cultural and individual environment and influence sexuality. General attitudes of the community are also of importance and can affect response.

Interpersonal problems: Some which might be encountered as a cause for sexual problems include:

1. Failure to communicate.
2. Failure to arouse emotionally.
3. Poor sexual technique or boredom with the technique.
4. Poor sex education and lack of sexual experience.
5. Aversion and dislike of partner.
6. Fear of interruption by children or relatives, etc.
7. Fear of pregnancy.
8. Financial pressures.
9. Cultural, social and religious differences.
10. Sexual aversions and perversions.

18.7 SEXUAL COUNSELLING

Sexual counselling involves both therapists and clients in a detailed exploration of the problems causing the sexual inadequacy and then the therapist using a reflective approach, allowing the client to understand the factors which have caused the problem.

Counselling requires skill and patience on the part of the therapist and motivation and involvement by the couple. Used in conjunction with behaviour modification, excellent results may be achieved in the majority of motivated couples. Both counselling and behaviour modification by themselves have high failure rates.

How to counsel

1. Counselling is best done by having both members of the client partnership attend for all visits, creating the understanding that all problems are shared problems.
2. Make sure that you have allowed sufficient time to listen to the problem and have both partners express their interpretation of the problem. It is difficult to conduct any counselling session in less than 1 hour.
3. Make the session a relaxed, non-threatening experience – the more relaxed you appear to be, the more productive the session will be.
4. Do not attempt to clarify, but allow both parties equal time to present their differing viewpoints.
5. Do not take sides or favour one point of view, even though you may feel strongly that one or the other person is incorrect or being imposed upon.
6. Provide a setting in which the couple learn by self-discovery and awareness, rather than by you being too directive in your approach.
7. Encourage the couple to take an active role in the solutions to their problems. Stress the need for their participation and motivation in problem solving. If they are not sufficiently motivated to work together, their problems will be difficult to solve.
8. Always give client couples a task to complete before they return for their next visit. These tasks may relate to communication activities (verbal, non-verbal and sexual) or to behavioural modification exercises.
9. Always begin each new session by asking about the homework which has been set at the previous counselling session.

A simple graded counselling model has been developed called the PLISSIT model. PLISSIT is a mnemonic standing for:

P = PERMISSION.
LI = LIMITED INFORMATION, e.g. sex education.
SS = SPECIFIC SUGGESTIONS, e.g. reading a relevant book, Squeeze technique or Sensate Focus.
IT = INTENSIVE THERAPY – these cases need referral to an experienced sex therapist.

All practitioners can counsel to the level of their expertise using the PLISSIT model.

18.8 HUMAN SEXUAL PROBLEMS

Sexual problems may be:

- Primary (always present).
- Secondary (arising after a period of normal sexual function).
- Total (occurring at all times and in all situations).
- Situational (occurring at specific times and in specific situations).

Common male problems

Rapid ejaculation
This is defined as a problem where a man does not have control over when he ejaculates. Rapid ejaculation is common in younger men with little ejaculatory control. Some men never get control or lose control due to a traumatic event.

Treatment: More frequent ejaculation helps the problem, making the man less 'trigger-happy'. Stop–start technique through masturbation or intercourse is helpful. This involves stimulation to high arousal with cessation just before the point of ejaculatory inevitability. Stimulation is restarted, with the aim being 15 minutes of stimulation with three stops. In more difficult cases the squeeze technique may be used. Results are generally very good.
   N.B. The average length of intercourse is 2 to 6 minutes. There are many harmful myths about how long a man should last. Reassurance may be all that is needed.

Erectile difficulties
Erectile difficulties have a 55% psychological and 45% organic basis. Psychological erectile difficulties may result from performance anxiety, depression, guilt or problems in the relationship. Organic problems may be due to *physical disease*: vascular (arterial inflow or venous outflow problems); neurogenic (diabetes, MS, spinal cord injury, radical prostatectomy or pelvic surgery or irradiation); hormonal (hyper or hypothyroidism, prolactin-secreting tumour, low testosterone, diabetes); or *chemical agents* such as alcohol, nicotine or prescribed drugs.

A full assessment should be made including a sexual history, physical examination and, if necessary, blood tests. Further investigations may be needed as specialist level.

Treatment: Options include counselling, chemically induced erections using injections into the penis, use of vacuum constrictor devices or surgical treatment with vascular surgery or implant surgery. Couples may choose not to recreate erection but to alter their sexual practices to enjoy 'outercourse' rather than intercourse.

Delayed and retrograde ejaculation
Delayed ejaculation occurs when the man has difficulty achieving an orgasm, usually with a partner. It may be due to unusual masturbatory techniques, e.g. gripping penis too hard or due to some underlying emotional, psychological or relationship problem. These men often suffer from inhibited sexual arousal. Retrograde ejaculation occurs when the bladder neck has been damaged usually through surgery. Emission occurs into the bladder rather than through the penis.

Low libido, inhibited sexual interest, disparate desires
Treatment of desire problems involves a thorough sex education with an emphasis on what is normal. Couples can be taught to negotiate differences in sex drive.

Common female problems

Low sexual interest, inhibited sexual desire, disparate desires
About 30% of women will rarely experience any driving urge for sex but they can still enjoy sexual activity and even orgasm if they are willing to participate sexually with an under-

standing partner. In some women desire may be quite strong but female libido is usually more sensitive to outside pressure than male desire. Female desire can be enhanced by eradicating negative influences, e.g. stress, resentment, unresolved conflict, fatigue and promoting positive influences such as communication, attention, time spent together, intimacy, non-demand affection and romance.

Orgasmic dysfunction
Orgasm in women results from clitoral stimulation, either directly or indirectly. Not all women are orgasmic through intercourse. Some 30% of women will never have an orgasm with a partner, 30% of women have an orgasm during intercourse and the remaining 40% can achieve orgasm through clitoral stimulation either before, during or after intercourse, manually, orally or with a vibrator. Treatment involves:

- A thorough sex education, with particular emphasis on female anatomy and how it responds sexually.
- Self-exploration by the woman of her genitals at home.
- Kegel's exercises – pelvic floor exercise to heighten orgasmic capacity and awareness.
- Masturbatory training with or without a vibrator.
- Sensate focus techniques to incorporate the partner.

Vaginismus
Vaginismus is the inability to achieve penetration of the penis into the vagina due to involuntary spasm of the muscles of the pelvic floor. Attempts at penetration are so painful that intercourse is impossible. Patients have often had little sexual education, restrictive upbringing, have a negative attitude to sex or less commonly may be the victim of sexual assault.

Treatment:

- Sex education.
- Self-exploration.
- Insertion of graded trainers or fingers with relaxation by doctor and/or patient.
- Sensate focus exercises.
- Insertion of fingers/trainers by partner.

Dyspareunia (painful intercourse)
Causes are either physical or emotional. Pain may be super-

ficial or deep. Exclude physical reasons for superficial tenderness such as vaginitis, Bartholin's cyst, tender episiotomy scar, etc. or cervicitis, salpingitis, endometriosis or ovarian cyst, etc. for deep discomfort.

The most common cause is inadequate arousal – during full arousal the vulva swells and the labia evert, making penetration by the erect penis comfortable and pleasurable. Lubrication forms inside the vagina so that a woman must ensure the introitus is well lubricated, otherwise the labia will get caught and pain will occur. Inadequate arousal is often due to anxiety – the more anxious a woman feels the less aroused she will become. Women need 15 to 20 minutes of sustained pleasuring to achieve good arousal – a good arousal is extremely important for comfortable intercourse – with good arousal there is elevation of the pelvic floor, lifting the uterus, tubes and ovaries up out of the pelvis and out of the way of a thrusting penis.

Treatment

- Education.
- Self-exploration.
- Kegel's exercises.
- Sensate focus to increase arousal.
- Use of water-based lubricant may be necessary in early stages.
- If appropriate, avoidance of positions with deep penetration.

Management

The aims of the initial consultation are:

1. Establishment of rapport with patient and partner preferably (the relationship must allow interchange between patient and doctor and be non-directive in approach).
2. Taking a sexual problem history, including:
   (a) Description of current problem.
   (b) Onset and course of problem.
   (c) Patient's perception of cause and maintenance of problem.
   (d) Past treatment and outcome (professional and self-treatment) and why the patient feels it did not work.

(e) Expectation and goals of treatment.
3. Relieve immediate anxiety by reassurance and limited relevant information.
4. Decide if referral to sex therapist is necessary. (Grounds for referral may be insufficient time or resources, poor relationship with patient, or the case being too complicated.)

In almost all cases, the basic problem is compounded by anxiety, either related to inadequate sexual knowledge or to fear of failure. Often all that is necessary is reassurance and limited related information, showing that myths regarding sex (e.g. penis size, coincidental orgasm, etc.) are incorrect, and explaining that any sexual behaviour which is perhaps producing guilt is also practised by others and may be continued without misgivings.

In conducting sex therapy the overall aims should encompass:

1. Comprehensive sex education.
2. Reducing anxiety.
3. Overcoming performance pressure.
4. Making expectations about sex more realistic.
5. Improving a couple's communication skills.
6. Providing an opportunity for couples to learn what kind of stimulation is pleasant and arousing.

The classic example of this approach is the sensate focus programme, which is a graded approach to intercourse involving all the above concepts. It usually consists of three separate stages. The first is each partner exploring and stimulating the other partner's non-genital regions, and communicating their feelings. Once complete relaxation and confidence is obtained by both partners they move to the second stage, genital stimulation, and finally the third stage, intercourse.

A cooperative partner is required for this or similar programmes. The patient must have some assertive skill, and both participants must feel comfortable with their own body. This type of graded massage programme is helpful to encourage sensuality and communication. It may also be used as an adjunct in the management of the other common problems listed.

Other simple programmes use desensitization in addition to

sensate focus. For example the stop–start and the squeeze technique are used in the treatment of premature ejaculation and the use of progressively larger trainers is used to help women with vaginismus to learn to accommodate penetration. The squeeze technique also requires cooperative partners, and is based on the fact that squeezing for 10–15 seconds just below the head of the penis before ejaculation removes the desire to ejaculate. Progressive desensitization to vaginal containment may be carried out using fingers or trainers made of glass or plastic of increasing sizes. This desensitization may be carried out by the woman alone at home or with the help of a doctor.

18.9 SEXUALITY IN PREGNANCY

Pregnancy produces a further set of problems which might cause conflict and increased interpersonal disruption. These can be listed under the following headings:

1.   Nausea, vomiting and tiredness.
2.   Change in mental attitude to sexual intercourse.
3.   Fear of hurting 'the baby'.
4.   Feeling cumbersome.
5.   Repugnance of the whole sexual act.
6.   Feeling fat and ugly.
7.   Difficulty in maintaining a suitable position for intercourse.
8.   Worry and anxiety about managing a new infant in the house – will they be able to cope?
9.   Is the baby normal?

It must of course be remembered that pregnancy may also enhance a close sexual relationship for the following reasons:

1.   Sharing the feelings of producing a new life.
2.   Enhancing a close interpersonal relationship.
3.   Enhancing the physical appearance of women.
4.   Increasing the sexual response mechanism.

Advice on sexual activity in pregnancy and the puerperium

Women often experience a drop in interest in sex during pregnancy. Interest may rekindle during the middle trimester and then drop down again in the last trimester. A small percentage of women feel more interested in sex during pregnancy than at any other time. By the final trimester of pregnancy 30% of couples are abstaining from sex.

It is quite normal for couples to have sexual intercourse during pregnancy and you should advise that there is no contraindication to intercourse throughout pregnancy except if any of the following problems have occurred:

1. Antepartum haemorrhage.
2. Premature rupture of membranes.
3. History of premature labour or of premature rupture of membranes.
4. Vaginal infections such as trichomonas, monilia or venereal disease.
5. If the obstetrician specifically advises against intercourse for a specific reason.

In the puerperium, intercourse may be resumed when:

1. Vaginal cuts or lacerations have healed – usually 3–4 weeks.
2. Blood-stained discharge has ceased – usually 2–3 weeks.

Index

Page numbers in **bold** refer to figures; page numbers in *italics* refer to tables.

normal placenta has an active Sulphatase System.
urinary estriol levels reflect the pattern of plasma estriol.
foetal adrenal is involved indirectly in estriol production.